STATISTICAL ANALYSIS OF MEDICAL DATA

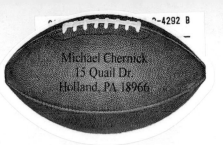

New Developments

Edited by

Brian S. Everitt
Department of Biostatistics and Computing,
Institute of Psychiatry,
London, UK

and

Graham Dunn
School of Epidemiology and Health Sciences,
University of Manchester,
Manchester, UK

A member of the Hodder Headline Group

LONDON • NEW YORK • SYDNEY • AUCKLAND

First published in Great Britain in 1998 by
Arnold a member of the Hodder Headline Group,
338 Euston Road, London NW1 3BH

http://www.arnoldpublishers.com

Copublished in the United States of America
Oxford University Press Inc.,
198 Madison Avenue,
New York, NY 10016

British Library Cataloguing in Publication Data
A catalogue record for this book is available from the British Library

Library of Congress Cataloging-in-Publication Data
A catalog record for this book is available from the Library of Congress

Publisher: Nicki Dennis
Production Editor: Wendy Rooke
Production Controller: Helen Whitehorn
Cover Designer: Terry Griffiths

ISBN 0 340 67775 9

Typeset in 10/12pt Times by AFS Image Setters Ltd, Glasgow
Printed and bound in Great Britain by J W Arrowsmith Ltd, Bristol

Contents

Preface   vii

List of contributors   ix

1. **Statistics in medical research**   *Brian S. Everitt and Graham Dunn*   **1**
    1.1   Introduction   1
    1.2   Four influential statisticians   3
    1.3   Recent advances in medical statistics   8
    References   11

2. **Regression models for survival data**   *Keith R. Abrams*   **13**
    2.1   Introduction   13
    2.2   Survival in end-stage renal disease (ESRD)   15
    2.3   Semi-parametric proportional hazards model   19
    2.4   Accelerated failure time models   29
    2.5   Bayesian models   34
    2.6   Discussion   54
    Acknowledgements   55
    References   55

3. **Frailty models**   *Odd O. Aalen*   **59**
    3.1   Introduction   59
    3.2   The proportional frailty model   61
    3.3   The effect of frailty on relative risk   63
    3.4   Multivariate survival data   67
    Appendix   71
    References   72

4. **Risk set sampling designs for proportional hazards models**   **75**
    Ørnulf Borgan and Bryan Langholz
    4.1   Introduction   75
    4.2   Model and inference for cohort data   77
    4.3   Sampling of controls   78
    4.4   Partial likelihood and estimation of the regression coefficients   83
    4.5   Estimation of cumulative hazard rates   84

4.6	Matching and pooling	86
4.7	Lung cancer deaths among uranium miners	87
4.8	Neighbourhood-stratified counter matching	91
4.9	Concluding comments	98
	Acknowledgements	98
	References	99

5. Tree-structured survival analysis in medical research 101
Mark R. Segal

5.1	Introduction	101
5.2	Motivation	101
5.3	Tree-structured regression methodology	103
5.4	Software	112
5.5	Examples	113
	References	123

6. Mixed and multi-level models for longitudinal data: growth curve models of language development 127
Alan Taylor, Kevin Pickering, Catherine Lord and Andrew Pickles

6.1	Introduction	127
6.2	Language ability in autism	128
6.3	Growth curve models	130
6.4	Growth curve model for parent report of expressive language	133
6.5	Ceilings and floors: mixed models for censored data	135
6.6	Ceiling effects in the parent report of receptive language	136
6.7	Ceiling and floor effects in the choice of measuring instrument	138
6.8	Multivariate growth curve models	139
6.9	Discussion	141
	Acknowledgements	142
	References	142

7. The analysis of longitudinal studies having non-normal responses 145
Charles S. Davis

7.1	Introduction	145
7.2	Layout and notation for longitudinal data	146
7.3	Examples	148
7.4	Distribution-free methods for the analysis of non-normal repeated measures	156
7.5	Applications to the examples	166
	References	169

8. Regression models for discrete longitudinal data 175
Garrett M. Fitzmaurice

8.1	Introduction	175
8.2	Notation	177

8.3	Marginal regression models	178
8.4	Conditional regression models	188
8.5	Conclusions	196
	Acknowledgements	197
	References	197

9. Dealing with missing values in longitudinal studies   **203**
Peter J. Diggle

9.1	Introduction	203
9.2	Simple solutions and their limitations	207
9.3	Modelling the missing value process	210
9.4	Case study	217
9.5	Discussion	226
	Acknowledgements	227
	References	227

10. Comparing institutional performance using Markov chain Monte Carlo methods   *E. Clare Marshall and David J. Spiegelhalter*   **229**

10.1	Introduction	229
10.2	Bayesian statistics and MCMC	231
10.3	Kidney transplant data	233
10.4	Basic cross-sectional analyses	233
10.5	Alternative forms of random effects distribution	237
10.6	Models using survival rates from previous epoch as a predictor	242
10.7	Computation	244
10.8	Discussion	246
	Acknowledgements	247
	References	247

11. Bayesian meta-analysis   *Larry V. Hedges*   **251**

11.1	Introduction	251
11.2	Models for effect sizes	253
11.3	All effect sizes exchangeable	254
11.4	The general case	265
11.5	Prior distributions	271
11.6	Conclusions	273
	References	273

12. Functional neuroimaging and statistics   **277**
Ian Ford and Andrew P. Holmes

12.1	Introduction	277
12.2	Statistical methods for ROI data in cross-sectional studies	280
12.3	Functional mapping – voxel-level approaches	285
12.4	Discussion	303
	References	304

13. Localizing brain activation in a single subject using functional magnetic resonance imaging   **309**
S. Rabe-Hesketh, M. J. Brammer and E. T. Bullmore
13.1   Introduction   309
13.2   Image quality and preprocessing   310
13.3   Experimental design   313
13.4   Modelling the experimental effect   314
13.5   Detecting activation   319
13.6   Localizing activation anatomically   322
13.7   Concluding remarks   324
Acknowledgements   325
References   325

Author index   **329**

Subject index   **335**

Preface

If for medical journals the 1960s and 1970s seem likely to be remembered as the era when the importance of ethics was emphasised, the last 10 years of this century promises to be that of statistics.

This prediction, made by Lock in the early 1980s (Lock, 1982 – see Chapter 1), has turned out to be surprisingly accurate. Editors of medical journals, stung perhaps by criticisms of the previously unacceptably poor level of the statistical analyses reported in many papers (see, for example, White, 1979, in Chapter 1), have implemented stricter statistical guidelines for potential authors and often taken a statistician onto their editorial boards. One of the consequences of this move has been a more ready acceptance of the use of increasingly sophisticated methods of analysis. This is fortunate since during the last decade statisticians have developed a large number of techniques which have particular importance for the analysis of data from medical investigations. In fact medical statistics has become such an active research area for statisticians that two specialist journals have arisen, namely *Statistics in Medicine* and *Statistical Methods in Medical Research*. The latter (which we co-edit with Professor Theodore Holford) publishes review papers dealing with particular topics (past examples include the EM algorithm, crossover designs, longitudinal data, and screening trials), and the original plan for this collection was a series of revised papers from past issues. But in the end this plan was abandoned in favour of commissioning a completely new set of chapters to cover a range of topics, some of which have not been covered in the journal. The emphasis in each chapter is on the practical aspects of the analysis of medical data and we are extremely grateful to the contributors for producing such high quality material including some fascinating examples. We hope the collection will be of interest both to medical statisticians and to medical researchers who are not primarily statisticians but who understand that advances in statistical methodology create the opportunities for more informative analyses of their data.

B.S.E. and G.D.
August 1997

List of contributors

O. O. Aalen
Section of Medical Statistics, University of Oslo, PO Box 1122 Blindern,
N-0317 Oslo, Norway (o.o.aalen@basalmed.uio.no)

K. R. Abrams
Department of Epidemiology and Public Health, University of Leicester,
22–28 Princes Road West, Leicester LE1 6TP, UK (kra1@le.ac.uk)

Ø. Borgan
Institute of Mathematics, University of Oslo, PO Box 1093 Blindern,
N-0316 Oslo, Norway (borgan@math.uio.no)

M. J. Brammer
Department of Biostatistics and Computing, Institute of Psychiatry, De
Crespigny Park, Denmark Hill, London SE5 8AF, UK
(spbcmjb@iop.bpmf.ac.uk)

E. T. Bullmore
Department of Biostatistics and Computing, Institute of Psychiatry, De
Crespigny Park, Denmark Hill, London SE5 8AF, UK
(spbcetb@iop.bpmf.ac.uk)

C. S. Davis
Division of Biostatistics, University of Iowa, 2800 Steindler Building,
Iowa City, IA 52242–1008, USA (charles-davis@uiowa.edu)

P. J. Diggle
Department of Mathematics & Statistics, Fylde College, Lancaster
University, Lancaster LA1 4YF, UK (p.diggle@lancaster.ac.uk)

G. Dunn
School of Epidemiology and Health Sciences, University of Manchester,
Oxford Road, Manchester M13 9PT, UK (g.dunn@man.ac.uk)

B. S. Everitt
Department of Biostatistics and Computing, Institute of Psychiatry, De Crespigny Park, Denmark Hill, London SE5 8AF, UK (b.everitt@iop.bpmf.ac.uk)

G. M. Fitzmaurice
Department of Biostatistics, Harvard School of Public Health, 677 Huntington Avenue, Boston, MA 02119, USA (fitzmaur@hsph.harvard.edu)

I. Ford
Robertson Centre for Biostatistics, University of Glasgow, Glasgow G12 8QQ, UK (ian@stats.gla.ac.uk)

L. V. Hedges
The University of Chicago, 5835 South Kimbark Avenue, Chicago, IL 60637, USA (hedge@cicero.spc.uchicago.edu)

A. P. Holmes
Wellcome Department of Cognitive Neurology, 12 Queen Street, London WC1N 3BG, UK (a.holmes@fil.ion.ucl.ac.uk)

B. Langholz
Department of Preventive Medicine, University of Southern California, School of Medicine, 1540 Alcazar Street, CHP-220, Los Angeles, CA 90033, USA (langholz@hsc.usc.edu)

C. Lord
Department of Psychiatry, University of Chicago, Chicago, IL 60637, USA (cathy@yoda.bsd.uchicago.edu)

E. C. Marshall
MRC Biostatistics Unit, Institute of Public Health, Robinson Way, Cambridge CB2 2SR, UK (clare.marshall@mrc-bsu.cam.ac.uk)

K. Pickering
MRC Child Psychiatry Unit, Institute of Psychiatry, De Crespigny Park, Denmark Hill, London SE5 8AF, UK (kevin.pickering@iop.bpmf.ac.uk)

A. Pickles
MRC Child Psychiatry Unit and Department of Biostatistics and Computing, Institute of Psychiatry, De Crespigny Park, Denmark Hill, London SE5 8AF, UK (a.pickles@iop.bpmf.ac.uk)

S. Rabe-Hesketh
Department of Biostatistics and Computing, Institute of Psychiatry, De Crespigny Park, Denmark Hill, London SE5 8AF, UK (s.rabe-hesketh@iop.bpmf.ac.uk)

M. R. Segal
Division of Biostatistics, University of California, MU 420 West, 500
Parnassus Avenue, San Francisco, CA 94143-0560, USA
(mark@biostat.ucsf.edu)

D. J. Spiegelhalter
MRC Biostatistics Unit, Institute of Public Health, Robinson Way,
Cambridge CB2 2SR, UK (david.spiegelhalter@mrc-bsu.cam.ac.uk)

A. Taylor
MRC Child Psychiatry Unit, Institute of Psychiatry, De Crespigny Park,
Denmark Hill, London SE5 8AF, UK (A.Taylor@iop.bpmf.ac.uk)

1 Statistics in medical research

Brian S. Everitt and Graham Dunn

1.1 Introduction

All who drink of this remedy recover in a short time, except those whom it does not help, who all die. Therefore, it is obvious that it fails only in incurable cases.

The aphorism above, ascribed to Galen (AD 138–201), indicates the kind of invulnerability claimed by physicians until well into the seventeenth century. Uncritical reliance on past experience, *post hoc ergo propter hoc* reasoning and veneration of dogma proclaimed by authoritative figures (particularly Galen) largely stifled any interest in experimentation or proper scientific exploration. Even the few who did attempt to increase their knowledge by close observation or simple experiment often interpreted their findings in the light of the currently accepted dogma. When, for example, Andreas Vesalius, a sixteenth century Belgian physician, first dissected a human heart and did not find 'pores', said by Galen to perforate the septum separating the ventricular chambers, the Belgian assumed the openings were invisible to the eye. It was only several years after his initial investigation that he had the confidence to declare that 'pores' did not exist.

Similarly the announcement of the discovery of the circulation of the blood by an English physician, William Harvey, in 1628, met with violent opposition, since it contradicted Galen's view that blood flowed to and fro in a tide-like movement within arteries and veins. Even when it was admitted rather grudgingly that Harvey was probably correct, a defender of the established view wrote that if the new findings did not agree with Galen, the discrepancy should be attributed to the fact that nature had changed; one should not admit that the master had been wrong!

But contrast the statement above with the following material taken from

David Hume's *An Enquiry Concerning Human Understanding* (quoted in Senn, 1997):

> when the usual symptoms of health or sickness disappoint our expectation; when medicines operate not with their wanted powers; when irregular events follow from any particular cause; the philosopher and physician are not surprised at the matter, nor are even tempted to deny, in general, the necessity and uniformity of those principles by which the animal economy is conducted. They know that a human body is a mighty complicated matter, that many secret powers lurk in it, which are to us altogether beyond our comprehension . . .

> . . . nor has rhubarb always proved a purge, or opium a soporific to everyone who has taken these medicines.

And medicine's progress from dogmatic, even mystical, certainty to scientific uncertainty which began with the challenge to Galenism in the seventeenth century has continued almost unabated to the present day. The key to this progress is the collection and valid interpretation of evidence and, particularly in the context of the present book, quantitative evidence as is nicely summarized in Lord Kelvin's well-known assertion that:

> When you can measure what you are speaking about, and express it in numbers, you know something about it; but when you cannot measure it, when you cannot express it in numbers, your knowledge is of a meagre and unsatisfactory kind.

But the use of statistics in medical research is not free from controversy. Even approaching the twenty-first century some clinicians might still claim that statistical information contributes little or nothing to the progress of medicine, because the physician is concerned at any one time with the treatment of a single patient and every patient is unique. Such an attitude is reflected in the following quotation from a letter by an eminent psychiatrist (we are too kind to give a name) to the *Lancet*:

> One must go on repeating the fact that if, in the past thirty years, one had ever paid very much attention to statistics, especially when they were not supported by clinical bedside findings, treatment progress in this country would not have got very far.

Fortunately, this type of 'facts speak louder than statistics' attitude is increasingly rare amongst clinicians since most are aware of the contribution that statistics and statisticians have made to medical research. But controversy remains. Not everyone is convinced by the claims of the modern evidence-based medicine (EBM) movement as articulated by, for example, Sackett *et al.* (1997), although to us they seem to be self-evidently worthwhile. Nor is everyone convinced by the need for experimental approaches (including randomization) to the evaluation of all forms of intervention whether they be surgical procedures, psychotherapies or healthcare reforms. And many are still happy to rely on the pronouncements of authority rather than critical appraisal of the evidence.

Before introducing the main part of this book, we thought we would highlight the development of medical statistics from its early beginnings to the middle of the present century, by describing briefly the contributions of four eminent statisticians. Two of them, Adolphe Quetelet and Florence Nightingale, epitomize the nineteenth century move to the collection of quantitative evidence in order to make sense of the world and to inform change. The other two, John Arbuthnot and Ronald Fisher, illustrate the (eventual) parallel move to the widespread use of probabilistic reasoning and statistical inference.

1.2 Four influential statisticians

1.2.1 John Arbuthnot and divine providence

Described by Karl Pearson as 'a wit in the age of wits', John Arbuthnot was born on 29 April 1667 in Arbuthnot, Kincardineshire, Scotland. A close friend of Jonathan Swift and all the literary celebrities of the day, he was also a distinguished doctor and writer of medical works, and a physician to Queen Anne. In 1712 he published five statistical pamphlets against the Duke of Marlborough, called *The History of John Bull*, which was the origin of the popular image of John Bull as the typical Englishman. He helped to found the Scriblerus Club and was the chief contributor to the *Memoirs of Martinus Scriblerus* (1741).

But in addition to his roles as clinician and writer, Arbuthnot had a capability in mathematics and an eagerness to apply mathematics to the real world, and his statistical claim to fame originates largely from the paper he presented to the Royal Society of London on 19 April 1711 entitled 'An Argument for Divine Providence, taken from the constant regularity observ'd in the births of both sexes'. In it, he maintained that the guiding hand of a divine being was to be discerned in the nearly constant ratio of male to female christenings recorded annually in London over the years 1629–1710. Part of his reasoning is recognizable as what would now be called a *sign test*.

The data presented by Arbuthnot showed that in each of the 82 years, 1629–1710, the annual number of male christenings had been consistently higher than the number of female christenings, but never very much higher. Arbuthnot argued that this remarkable regularity could not be attributed to chance, and must therefore be an indication of divine providence. His representation of chance in this context was the toss of a fair two-sided die so that the distribution of births would then be

$$\left(\tfrac{1}{2} + \tfrac{1}{2}\right)^{82}$$

so that the observed excess of male christenings on each of 82 occasions had an extremely small probability.

Shoesmith (1997) makes the point that some of the features of the modern hypothesis test can be seen in Arbuthnot's probabilistic reasoning. He defined a null hypothesis ('chance' determination of sex at birth) and an alternative (divine providence) and calculated, under the assumption that the null hypothesis was true, a probability defined by reference to the observed data. Finally, he argued that the extremely low probability he obtained cast doubt on the null hypothesis and offered support for his alternative. Arbuthnot offered an explanation for the greater supply of males as a wise economy of nature, as the males are more subject to accidents and diseases, having to seek their food with danger. Therefore provident nature to repair the loss brings forth more males. The near equality of the sexes is designed so that every male may have a female of the same country and of suitable age.

But Karl Pearson (see Pearson, 1978) is relatively dismissive of Arbuthnot's paper which he refers to as 'rather slim' and expresses doubt that it represents the first use of the binomial to express birth ratios. He also points out that Arbuthnot fails to consider an alternative binomial, namely $(p + q)^{82}$ with $p \neq q$. Nevertheless Arbuthnot's argument tends now to be regarded as the first, explicitly set out and recognizable statistical significance test, although it is doubtful whether his contribution, and the debate it presented, provided any immediate stimulus to ideas of statistical significance testing.

Arbuthnot died on 27 February 1735 in London. Shortly before his death he wrote to Swift, 'A recovery in my case and in my age is impossible; the kindest wish of my friends is euthanasia'. After his death Dr Johnson offered the following epitaph:

He was the most universal genius, being an excellent physician, a man of deep learning and a man of much humour.

Rightly or wrongly, statistical significance testing plays a dominant role in present-day medical statistics; Arbuthnot might be thought of as its father figure.

1.2.2   Adolphe Quetelet and the average man

Lambert Adlophe Jacques Quetelet was born in Ghent, Belgium, on 22 February 1796 and became one of the nineteenth century's most influential voices. He received a doctorate of science in 1819 from the University of Ghent, with a dissertation on conic sections. From 1819 on he taught mathematics in Brussels, founded and directed the Royal Observatory and dominated Belgian science for half a century from the mid 1820s to his death in 1874.

Although Quetelet's principal career within Belgium was as an astronomer and meteorologist at the Royal Observatory in Brussels, his international reputation was achieved as a statistician and a sociologist. According to Stigler (1986), Quetelet's first awakening to the variety of relationships latent in society many have come with his investigation of population data, but his interests soon spread. Stigler continues his account of this aspect of Quetelet's work thus:

From 1827 through 1835 he examined scores of potentially meaningful relationships through the compilation of tables and the preparation of graphical displays. With few exceptions he compared only two characteristics at a time, but within this constraint his curiosity was seemingly boundless. He examined birth and death rates by month and city, by temperature and by the time of day. He calculated the month of conception from the birth month and tried to relate it to marriage statistics. He investigated mortality by age, by profession, by locality, by season, in prisons and in hospitals. He considered other human attributes: height, weight, growth rate and strength. Quetelet's interests also extended to moral qualities: statistics on drunkenness, insanity, suicides and crime.

The result of such studies was Quetelet's *magnus opum, Sur l'homme et le développement de ses facultés, au essai de physique sociale.* This was translated into English in 1842 as *A Treatise on Man and the Development of His Faculties.* In his book Quetelet coined the term 'social physics' and his aim was clear, that is to conduct a rigorous, quantified investigation of the laws of society that might some day stand with astronomers' achievements of the previous century. But 150 years on the work is best known for the introduction of that now famous character the 'average man' (*l'homme moyen*). The average man began as a simple way of summarizing some characteristics of a population (usually a national population) but took on a life of its own and to this day still lives in headlines of our daily papers. In a more subtle form it underlies the rationale for reference ranges, and so on, where it is assumed that abnormality (deviation from the average) implies pathology – and quite often it does!

Quetelet was a prolific writer and editor and carried on an immense correspondence with scientists and others all over Europe. He was instrumental in founding the Statistical Society of London and was the first foreign member of the American Statistical Association. According to Sarton (1935), Quetelet was the 'patriarch of statistics'; certainly his place in history is ensured by his creation of the 'average man'.

1.2.3 Florence Nightingale, the Passionate Statistician

Florence Nightingale was born on 12 May 1820 in Florence, Italy. Raised in England, she trained as a nurse in Kaiserworth and Paris, and in the Crimean War, after the Battle of the Alma (1854), led a party of 38 nurses to organize a nursing department at Scutari. There she found grossly inadequate sanitation, but soon established better conditions and had 10 000 wounded under her care. She returned to England in 1856, where she formed an institution for the training of nurses at St Thomas' Hospital and spent several years on army sanitary reform, the improvement of nursing, and public health in India.

In her efforts to improve the squalid hospital conditions at Scutari during the Crimean War and in her subsequent campaigns to reform the health and living conditions of the British Army, the sanitary conditions and administration of hospitals, and the nursing profession, Florence Nightingale was not dissimilar from many other Victorian reformers. But in one important respect she was very different: she mustered massive amounts of data, carefully arranged and tabulated, to convince ministers, viceroys, secretaries, undersecretaries and parliamentary commissioners of the truths of her cause. No major national cause had previously been championed by the presentation of sound statistical data. One example, quoted by Read (1997), which clearly illustrates her approach, is her finding that 'those who fell before Sebastopol were about seven times the number who fell by the enemy'. The opposition lost because her statistics were unanswerable and their publication led to an outcry.

In 1850 no scientific system of tabulating or reporting mortality or morbidity statistics existed. Florence Nightingale introduced such a system in Scutari in 1854 and quickly became aware that mortality statistics should be age specific and that crude death rates are often highly misleading. The following is taken from Nightingale (1859):

> In comparing the deaths of one hospital with those of another, any statistics are justly considered absolutely valueless which do not give the ages, the sexes and the diseases of all the causes. There can be no comparison between old men with dropsies and young women with consumptions.

Florence Nightingale was instrumental in the founding of a statistical department in the army. Her pioneering use of statistical tables and charts to back her calls for reform establishes her right to be placed firmly in the forefront of the history of statistics. Although more widely known as the Lady of the Lamp, her less common accolade, the Passionate Statistician, is also well deserved.

1.2.4   Sir Ronald Aylmer Fisher and randomization

Born in East Finchley, London, on 17 February 1890, Ronald Aylmer Fisher became arguably the most influential statistician of the twentieth century. His general intelligence and mathematical precocity were apparent early and in 1909 he won a scholarship in mathematics to Cambridge. In 1912, he graduated as a Wrangler and began a study of the theory of errors, statistical mechanics and quantum theory. In the same year he published a paper in which the method of maximum likelihood was introduced, although not yet by that name. One of the results of this paper was the start of a correspondence with W. S. Gosset ('Student'), the mutual topic of which concerned Gosset's use of $n-1$ for the denominator of the standard deviation. At about the same time Fisher became interested in evolutionary theory, especially as it affected man, an interest which led to him forming the Cambridge University Eugenics Society. After work teaching mathematics and physics during the First World War, Fisher joined the staff of Rothamsted Experimental Station in 1919. There he developed his techniques for the design and analysis of experiments where it is not possible to control every element that could affect the outcome. His analysis of variance has become standard practice in medical, biological and agricultural research and the associated principle of randomization has had a massive impact on medical research involving treatment comparisons where it has led to what has been described by Sir David Cox as 'the most important contribution of 20th Century statistics', that is the randomized controlled clinical trial in which patients are randomly allocated to alternative therapies.

Prior to adopting Fisher's randomization principle, most of the early experiments to compare competing treatments for the same condition involved arbitrary non-systematic schemes for assigning patients to treatments. The first trial with a properly randomized control group was that for streptomycin in the treatment of pulmonary tuberculosis (see Fox *et al.*, 1954). Initially not all clinicians were convinced of the need for such trials, as is evidenced by the following quotation from a letter to the *British Medical Journal* commenting on a trial involving depressed patients.

There is no psychiatric illness in which bedside knowledge and long clinical experience pays better dividends; and we are never going to learn about how to treat depression properly from double blind sampling in an MRC statistician's office.

There are, of course, ethical problems associated with randomized trials (see, for example, Pocock, 1983), but most clinicians now accept that any other system of treatment allocation is likely to cause more problems than it solves. Randomization serves several purposes: it provides a method of allocating patients to treatments free from personal biases and it ensures a firm basis for the application of significance tests and most of the rest of the statistical methodology likely to be used in assessing the results of a trial. Most importantly randomization distributes the effects of concomitant variables, both measured and unobserved (and possibly unknown), in a chance, and therefore impartial, fashion amongst the groups to be compared. In this way, random allocation ensures a lack of bias, making the interpretation of an observed group difference largely unambiguous – its cause is very likely to be the different treatments received.

Fisher made massive contributions to the theory of statistics, to genetics and to the design of experiments. But it is in the introduction of his principle of randomization to medical research that his work has had its greatest impact on the twentieth century's equivalent of Adolphe Quetelet's average man.

1.3   Recent advances in medical statistics

In the last two decades the field of medical statistics has grown rapidly and the number of medical statisticians increased accordingly. At least two specialized journals, *Statistics in Medicine* and *Statistical Methods in Medical Research*, have arisen to publish accounts of the methodological advances being made. Adequate coverage of the whole range of medical statistics could only be achieved in a text containing many hundreds of articles. We have, therefore, chosen to be highly selective. The choice is, inevitably, largely personal, but we have attempted to select areas in which there is currently much active research and additionally that are of clear importance to the development of the subject.

1.3.1   Survival analysis

The duration of a patient's survival is one of the most important response variables in many medical investigations (certainly from the patient's viewpoint). The methodology for analysing survival times was radically altered with the publication in 1972 of Cox's landmark paper describing the proportional hazards model and the use of partial likelihood to estimate the model's parameters. Since then the literature on survival analysis has increased dramatically and the variety of techniques that have evolved represents one of the most important methodologies in medical research.

This book opens with four chapters discussing various aspects of survival analysis. The first, by Abrams, presents an overview of the use of regression models for survival-type data, including both semi- and fully parametric regression models. Both maximum likelihood and Bayesian methods of estimation are considered including Markov chain Monte Carlo. The methods are illustrated in a fascinating example involving survival of patients with end-stage renal failure who are receiving dialysis treatment.

In the second chapter concerned with survival analysis, Aalen considers the problems caused by heterogeneity between individuals when applying methods such as Cox's proportional hazards model. High risk individuals, for example, will tend to have a short survival, and the remaining ones will have lower risk, giving a selection over time. This selection causes the hazard rate to decline, or to rise less rapidly. Such a decreasing hazard rate is often interpreted as expressing a biological phenomenon within the individual yielding a declining risk. But the hazard rate is not a pure measure; it expresses a mixture of the individual development and the previously mentioned selection effects. The problem is addressed by introducing a random variable known as frailty into survival models. The duration of dental fillings is used as an example.

In large epidemiological cohort studies of a rare disease, use of proportional hazards models requires collection of covariate information on all individuals in the cohort even though only a small fraction of these actually get diseased. This may be expensive, or even logically impossible, and in the third chapter of this section Borgan and Langholz consider cohort sampling techniques, where covariate information is collected for all failing individuals (cases), but only for a sample of the non-failing individuals (controls). Such an approach may drastically reduce the resources that need to be allocated to a study. The work is illustrated on examples involving lung cancer deaths among uranium miners and the possible association between childhood leukaemia and the presence of very high current configuration power lines.

In the last chapter in this section Segal offers an alternative to Cox's proportional hazards model for the analysis of survival data, based on tree-structured or recursive partitioning methods. The central thrust of such techniques is the formation of subgroups within which covariates are homogeneous. This means that in clinical settings with survival outcomes, interpretation in terms of prognostic group identification is frequently possible After a discussion of the relevant methodology and structure Segal describes two illustrative examples, one involving breast cancer and one concerned with HIV disease progression.

1.3.2   The analysis of longitudinal data

Longitudinal studies, in which repeated measures of some response variable of interest are obtained over time from each patient in the study, are particularly important in medical research – many, probably most, clinical trials, for example, are such. One indication of the importance of such studies both in medicine and as a rich source of interesting statistical problems is the recent publication of a spate of books dealing with the topic; these include Jones (1993), Lindsey (1993), Diggle *et al.* (1994), Davidian and Giltinan (1995), Kshirsagar and Smith (1995), Crowder and Hand (1995), Voresh and Chinchilli (1997) and Kenward (1997).

The first of the four chapters discussing longitudinal studies by Taylor *et al.* concentrates on the use of mixed models and growth curve models illustrating their use with an example involving language ability in autism.

The second chapter in this section, by Davis, reviews the methods available for analysis when the response variable is non-normal. A lot of useful techniques, both univariate and multivariate, are described and illustrated in several examples including ones where some subjects have missing values.

In the third chapter in this section, Fitzmaurice considers the analysis of discrete longitudinal studies data. The focus is on regression models, that is models in which the primary interest lies in relating the distribution of responses to a set of covariates or explanatory variables. Both marginal and conditional regression models are discussed. In the former, the regression parameters for the marginal expectation of each response separately are of primary interest. In the latter interest switches to the regression parameters modelling the conditional expectation of each response, conditional either on the values of previous responses or on a set of random effects. Data taken from the Six Cities Study of Air Pollution and Health, a longitudinal study designed to characterize the adverse health effects of exposure to air pollutants, are used to illustrate both types of model. The response variable is binary: the child's wheeze status (wheeze, no wheeze).

The final chapter in this section, by Diggle, addresses the difficult problem of longitudinal studies in which subjects drop out. Some common methods for dealing with the problem, namely complete case analysis and last observation carried forward, are considered and largely rejected. Instead the missing value process is modelled in an attempt to identify the type of drop-outs involved. The example used to illustrate the suggested modelling procedure is a trial comparing different drug regimes in the treatment of chronic schizophrenia.

1.3.3   Bayesian methods

In Bayesian inference both observables (data) and model parameters (unknowns which may include latent variables, missing data and so on) are treated as random quantities so that both a probability model for the data and a prior distribution for the model parameters have to be specified. Inferences regarding the model parameters are then based on the derived posterior distributions determined by Bayes's theorem. Until recently the often high dimensional integration needed to evaluate relevant characteristics of the posterior distribution posed severe practical difficulties. But over the last five years or so use of Markov chain Monte Carlo methods has largely overcome the problem and Marshall and Spiegelhalter give a fascinating account of the application of such methods in comparing institutional performance.

The second chapter in which Bayesian methods are central is that by Hedges on meta-analysis. This procedure for combining information from different clinical trials or epidemiological studies has become widespread in the biomedical sciences. In his chapter Hedges gives a comprehensive account of the Bayesian approach to the random effects models usually considered most suitable for meta-analysis. One of the examples considered involves the controversial area of the effects of environmental tobacco smoke on lung cancer.

1.3.4   Statistics in imaging

One of the most exciting developments in clinical research in the last decade has been the introduction of non-invasive techniques that produce neuro- and other images. A medical image consists of a very large set of measurements taken of some part of the body and arranged in an array (two- or three-dimensional) so that the spatial relationship between the elements of the array (called pixels or voxels) reflects the spatial relationship between the corresponding surface or volume elements of the body. Such an image may be acquired by any of a large number of different imaging modalities including, for example, magnetic resonance imaging (MRI), computed X-ray tomography (CT) and emission tomography (PET and SPECT). Depending on the imaging modality and the precise imaging parameters used, the image may reflect different aspects of the body such as anatomy, physiology or chemistry.

The first chapter in this section, by Ford and Holmes, provides a description of the role of statistics in the construction and analysis of neuroimages. In some cases interest lies in clarifying regions in the image, for example into tumour and healthy tissue, which may be important for diagnosis and treatment planning. Other studies seek to investigate the structure–function relationship of the healthy brain. Ford and Holmes consider a number of possible models and several extremely interesting examples.

The second chapter, by Rabe-Heskith *et al.*, considers functional magnetic resonance imagery (fMRI), which is a non-invasive technique for measuring changes in cerebral blood oxygenation related to brain activity. In about 5 minutes a sequence of three-dimensional images is acquired from which the temporal and spatial characteristics of neuronal activity can be deduced. The most important objective is usually to determine which brain regions are associated with a given mental task. Rabe-Heskith *et al.* consider issues of data quality and preprocessing, experimental design, modelling and detecting activation, and localizing the activated regions anatomically. A variety of models are described and illustrative examples given.

References

Arbuthnot, J. 1710: An argument for Divine Providence, taken from the constant regularity observ'd in the births of both sexes. *Philosophical Transactions of the Royal Society of London* **27**, 186–90.

Cox, D. R. 1972: Regression models and life tables. *Journal of the Royal Statistical Society (B)* **34**, 187–220.

Crowder, M. J. and Hand, D. J. 1995: *Practical longitudinal data analysis.* London: Chapman & Hall.

Davidian, M. and Giltinan, D. M. 1995: *Nonlinear models for repeated measurement data.* London: Chapman & Hall.

Diggle, P. J., Liang, K. Y. and Zeger, S. L. 1994: *Analysis of longitudinal data.* Oxford: Oxford University Press.

Fox, W., Sutherland, I. and Daniels, M. 1954: A five year assessment of patients in a controlled trial of streptomycin in pulmonary tuberculosis. *Quarterly Journal of Medicine* **23**, 347.

Jones, R. H. 1993: *Longitudinal data with serial correlation: a state space approach.* London: Chapman & Hall.

Kenward, M. G. 1997: *Analysis of repeated measurements.* New York: Oxford University Press.

Kshirsagar, A. M. and Smith, W. B. 1995: *Growth curves.* New York: Marcel Dekker.

Lindsey, J. K. 1993: *Models for repeated measurements.* New York: Oxford University Press.

Lock, S. 1982: Preface. In *Statistics in practice*, Gore, S. M. and Altman, D. G. (eds), London: British Medical Journal.

Nightingale, F. 1859: *Notes on nursing: what it is and what it is not.* London: Harrison.

Pearson, E. S. 1978: *The history of statistics in the 17th and 18th centuries. Lectures by Karl Pearson given at University College, London.* London: Charles Griffin.

Pocock, S. J. 1983: *Clinical trials.* John Wiley: Chichester.

Quetelet, A. 1835: *Sur l'homme et le développement de se facultés au essai de physique sociale.* Paris: Barchelier.

Read, C. B. 1997: Florence Nightingale. In Johnson, N. L. and Kotz, S. (eds), *Leading personalities in statistical services.* New York: John Wiley.

Sackett, D. L., Richardson, W. S., Rosenberg, W. and Hayes, R. B. 1997: *Evidence-based medicine.* New York: Churchill Livingstone.

Sarton, G. 1935: *Isis* **23**, 6–24.

Senn, S. 1997: *Statistical issues in drug development.* New York: John Wiley.

Shoesmith, E. 1997: John Arbuthnot. In Johnson, N. L. and Kotz, S. (eds), *Leading personalities in statistical science.* New York: John Wiley.

Stigler, S. M. 1986: *The history of statistics: the measurement of uncertainty before 1900.* Cambridge, MA: Harvard University Press.

Voresh, E. F. and Chinchilli, V. M. 1997: *Linear and nonlinear models for the analysis of repeated measurements.* New York: Marcel Dekker.

White, S. J. 1979: Statistical errors in papers in the British Journal of Psychiatry. *British Journal of Psychiatry* **135**, 336–42.

2 Regression models for survival data

Keith R. Abrams

2.1 Introduction

In many areas of health care research the main outcome of interest is time to an event. For example, in cancer the event of interest is often death, though it could also be recurrence of disease. In a transplant setting the event could be failure of a graft or organ. In nursing-related studies the event is often discharge from hospital. In all of these settings, although the event of interest is the time from entry into a study/treatment/admission to the event in question, for some patients this event might not be observed, only that it would have occurred at some time point beyond the observed time. Such patients are termed *censored*. It is the presence of censoring that makes the analysis of survival data, as such data are often referred to, so different and complex.

Whilst graphical and descriptive methods are initially useful in exploring the data, there is often a primary hypothesis to be tested, for example whether two treatments differ in terms of survival in a trial or whether there are differences with respect to a covariate in epidemiological studies. One of the most widely used tests is the log-rank test (Mantel and Haenszel, 1959). Whilst such tests can be extended to the case when there are either multiple patient groups to be compared or possible confounding factors that may be treated as strata, they are limited in their ability to describe (and model) the data fully. Therefore, a number of regression models for survival data have been proposed.

Essentially there have been two groups of models considered to date. The first has worked with the hazard function and modelled the hazard functions in patient groups compared with a baseline population by means of a multiplicative model on the log hazard scale. The multiplicative factor is often assumed to be constant over time, and therefore the model induces the hazards in the different patient groups to be proportional, thus yielding a *proportional hazards regression model*. The second group of models have considered modelling the survival functions directly, with covariates assumed to act multiplicatively directly on the time scale, thus accelerating or decelerating time to failure, and are termed *accelerated failure time models*. Within each of these two broad groups of models, either the baseline hazard in the proportional hazards models, or the baseline survivor function in the accelerated failure time models, can be assumed to be either fully parametric or modelled non-parametrically, though traditionally proportional hazards regression models have been thought of as semi-parametric, with the baseline hazard assumed non-parametric, and accelerated failure time models have been fully parametric.

Until recently much of the practical analysis of survival data, using the methods and models outlined above, has been from a classical perspective, that is to say using maximum likelihood methods. However, as with many areas of health care research, the last few years have seen interest in the use of Bayesian methods increase (Breslow, 1990). The Bayesian approach to statistical inference uses the data in the form of the likelihood function, which, when combined with a joint prior distribution for all the model parameters using Bayes's theorem, yields a joint posterior distribution for the model parameters. The posterior distribution is then used to make inferences about either specific model parameters or combinations of parameters. There are a number of advantages to the Bayesian approach, the first, and probably the most crucial and controversial, being the use of a prior distribution. The prior distribution essentially conveys all the available evidence about parameters a priori to the study in question. This has the advantage of being able to incorporate information that, although relevant, could not be formally incorporated into the likelihood, for example information from other pertinent studies in the field. The question of which prior distribution to use is a complex one, and one that will be discussed later. A presentational advantage of the Bayesian approach is that the posterior distribution enables probability statements to be directly made regarding the treatment comparison in a trial, say, or associated risk in epidemiological studies. Such information is often crucial in answering questions in a clinically meaningful manner. Finally, the Bayesian approach leads naturally into prediction of future data, through calculation of the predictive distribution, though this latter point is not used directly here.

The methods considered in this chapter are illustrated using data from a cohort study of patients with end-stage renal disease (ESRD) entered into a renal replacement treatment (RRT) programme in Leicestershire, a county in England, with a population of approximately 1 million.

The rest of this chapter is organized with Section 2.2 giving a more detailed background to the Leicester ESRD study, including descriptive methods. Section 2.3 considers the use of classical semi-parametric proportional hazards regression models, whilst Section 2.4 considers the use of fully parametric accelerated failure time models. Section 2.5

considers both semi- and fully parametric models from a Bayesian perspective. Finally, Section 2.6 discusses the models considered, their limitations and possible extensions.

2.2   Survival in end-stage renal disease (ESRD)

2.2.1   Background

Normal renal function is required so waste material may be eliminated, and so that the volume and composition of body fluids may be regulated. The first stage of renal failure is a diminished renal reserve; there is a reduction in the glomerular filtration rate (GFR) caused by a progressive loss of nephrons, the functional unit of the kidney, and thus ability to eliminate waste material and regulate body fluid levels will decline. Early renal failure occurs at a GFR of approximately 30 ml/min, and end-stage renal failure occurs at 5 ml/min. It is estimated that about 72 patients per million population below age 70 reach end-stage renal failure in the UK each year, and will die if *renal replacement therapy* (RRT), in the form of either *haemodialysis* or *peritoneal dialysis*, is not provided. The aim of RRT is to mimic the excretory function of normal kidneys. For some types of renal disease there are marked ethnic and regional differences in incidence. For Leicester, where approximately 25% of the population is of Indo-Asian origin, ethnic differences, in terms of incidence of ESRD and outcome whilst receiving RRT, are therefore of crucial importance.

Obviously when patients are receiving dialysis treatment, monitoring of renal function is important. In particular, one protein of the blood, *serum albumin*, which is formed by the liver, has been suggested as a means of monitoring renal function. Albumin exerts an intravascular oncotic pressure that influences fluid exchange between the interstitial and intravascular compartments. It is also responsible for increasing the viscosity of the blood. Normal levels of serum albumin are between 40 and 50 g/l.

2.2.2   Prior information

Prior to the current study being undertaken there were two sources of information available: expert clinical opinion and evidence from other studies in which the role of ethnicity had been explored.

A priori to the current study, and indeed the rationale for it, was the fact that clinical opinion was that Indo-Asian patients in Leicestershire were seen more often on the renal dialysis unit with treatment-related complications. Given that patients are dependent upon RRT for their survival, it was feared that a higher complication rate could lead to a detrimental prognosis, in terms of survival, for Asian patients compared with non-Asian patients. Such beliefs were quantified, after discussion with renal specialists, into a prior distribution which was equivalent to a 10%

survival disadvantage over non-Asian patients, but which were also consistent with there being either a 20% reduction in survival or no difference. In turn this distribution can be used to construct a prior distribution for the log hazard ratio, for Asian patients compared with non-Asian patients, and making a further assumption of normality, with a mean of 0.1 and a variance of 0.0025. This prior distribution will be termed a *clinical prior* in subsequent sections.

In terms of a priori data-based evidence four previous studies considered the effect of ethnicity on overall mortality (Cowie, 1993, Lowrie, 1993, Agodoa and Eggers, 1995, Medina *et al.*, 1996). These studies suggest that, even after allowing for the effect of age, there appears to be a survival advantage to non-Caucasian patients over those of Caucasian patients. In terms of how this information might be used formally in an analysis, a prior distribution, in this case for the log hazard ratio, is required. Performing a random effects meta-analysis (Fleiss, 1993) of the four studies yields a pooled estimate of the log hazard ratio of -0.411 with an approximate 95% confidence interval of -0.56 to -0.26. Thus, assuming the log hazard ratio to be normally distributed, a data-based prior distribution would have a mean of -0.411 and a variance of 0.0061.

In the models considered below, two further prior distributions will be considered. The first, referred to as a *reference prior*, assumes that the log hazard ratio is centred on zero, but that a plausible range extends from -200 to $+200$. The final type of prior distribution considered is termed an *equivalence prior*, and as with the reference prior distribution is centred on zero, but this time has a plausible range which extends from -0.5 to $+0.5$ on the log hazard ratio scale, which corresponds to a range from 0.60 to 1.65 on the hazard ratio scale. The equivalence prior distribution reflects beliefs that would indicate it being unlikely for there to be a difference between the ethnic groups, but that if such a difference did exist then it would be plausibly between a 40% relative reduction in survival and a 65% relative increase in survival for Asian patients compared with non-Asian patients.

2.2.3   Study design

The ESRD study followed up 252 patients who entered the renal dialysis programme in Leicestershire between January 1982 and December 1991, with completed follow-up until December 1994. Table 2.1 shows some of the covariates that were collected as part of the study; these included co-morbidity at entry into the study, mode of first-choice dialysis, either peritoneal dialysis or haemodialysis, and albumin levels. Albumin levels were also recorded annually, as an indication of renal function.

On examining the baseline covariate information for the two ethnic groups separately, there appeared to be few differences with the exception of age (mean age for non-Asians 60.5 years (SD 10 years) and Asians 55.5 years (SD 13.6 years)), diabetes (11.4% for non-Asians and 23.5% for

Table 2.1 Covariates, and their meaning, collected in the ESRD study

Covariate	Meaning
Asian	1 = Indo-Asian origin, 0 = other
Age	Age in years at entry
Cardiac	1 = any cardiac complications at entry, 0 = none
Vascular	1 = any vascular complications at entry, 0 = none
Cancer	1 = any history of cancer at entry, 0 = none
Diabetes	1 = diabetic at entry, 0 = non-diabetic
Albumin	Albumin levels measured at entry and then annually
Mode	First-choice treatment; 1 = peritoneal dialysis, 0 = haemodialysis
Gender	1 = male, 0 = female

Asians), and cardiac complications (19.6% for non-Asians and 22.1% for Asians). Therefore, in any analysis of survival outcome it might be anticipated that such covariates would need to be taken into account.

2.2.4 Descriptive methods

One of the most common methods for displaying survival data is the Kaplan–Meier survival curves. For the ESRD study Fig. 2.1 displays the

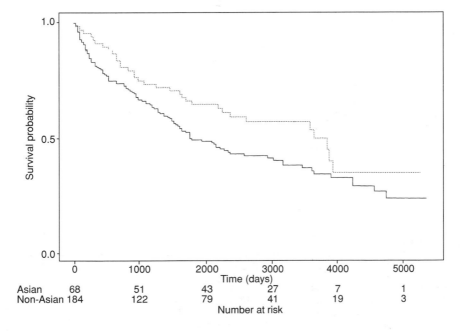

Fig. 2.1 Kaplan–Meier survival curves of all-cause mortality for ESRD study: ———, non-Asian; ······, Asian

estimated Kaplan–Meier survival curves for the two ethnic groups separately. It can be seen from the figure that such a plot would appear to indicate that the Asian patients did considerably better than the non-Asian patients in terms of survival. However, as we have seen there is a

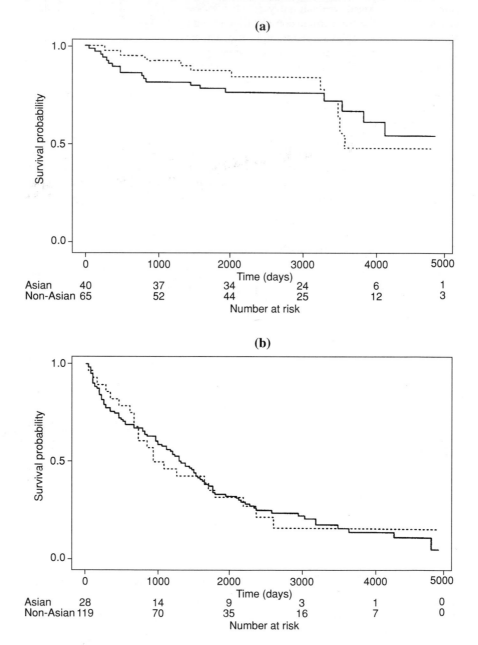

Fig. 2.2 Kaplan–Meier survival curves of all-cause mortality for ESRD study, stratified by age (a) ≤65 and (b) >65: ———, non-Asian; · · · · ·, Asian

considerable imbalance in terms of the average ages of the two patient groups, which could possibly bias the comparison of the survival times. Figure 2.2 shows the Kaplan–Meier estimated survival curves again for the two ethnic groups but this time stratified according to age, that is ≤65 and >65, and we can see that within each of the two age groups there appears to be less of a difference between the ethnic groups than in Fig. 2.1.

2.2.5 log-rank test

Although the graphical methods outlined above are useful initial methods for visually comparing the survival experiences of the two patient groups, we also wish to test formally the hypothesis that there is a difference in survival between the groups. A common non-parametric test that is used in survival analysis is the *log-rank test* for comparing two or more groups (Collett, 1994). Applying the log-rank test to the ESRD study data yields a test statistic of 4.8, and an associated P value of 0.028, suggesting that there is a statistically significant difference in the survival experiences between the two groups.

As we saw from Figs 2.1 and 2.2, however, an important potential confounding factor is age at entry into the study, which the log-rank test above has so far ignored. One way of accommodating age is to perform a *stratified log-rank test*, stratifying patients into ≤65 and >65 age groups. Performing a stratified log-rank test in the ESRD study, stratifying for age, yields a test statistic of almost zero, with an associated P value of 0.99, suggesting that, after allowing for the effects of differing ages at entry, there appears to be little evidence of a difference between the two ethnic groupings.

Whilst the log-rank and stratified log-rank test are relatively easy to implement and interpret, they do not give an estimate of the differences in survival between groups, neither do they extend to the case when there are numerous potential confounders that we wish to allow for, as is often the case in epidemiology. In order to address both of these issues some form of regression model needs to be considered, and the most widely used to date is the Cox proportional hazards regression model described in the next section.

2.3 Semi-parametric proportional hazards model

In this section we consider the construction of a regression model based on the idea of the hazard function. The particular model considered is a proportional hazards model, first advocated by Cox (1972), which has been widely used in survival analysis and medical applications in particular (Altman *et al.*, 1995). One of the main reasons why this particular model has been so widely adopted is that although it does make quite a stringent assumption about the hazard rates being proportional, it makes no assumption about the underlying distribution of the survival times, and thus is often referred to as a semi-parametric model. However, the particular formulation of the model here makes use of *counting process notation* (Anderson and Gill, 1982, Anderson and Borgan, 1985, Anderson *et al.*, 1992) which enables the model to be more easily extended to more complex situations.

2.3.1   Model and likelihood

In counting process notation each patient, for each type of event under consideration (in the ESRD study this is just death), has a counting process $N_i(t)$ which counts the number of events at time t. Similarly each patient also has an at-risk process, $Y_i(t)$, which is one if the ith patient is at risk at time t and zero otherwise. As can be seen this representation of each patient's event history can provide a flexible and comprehensive way of accommodating both repeated events within the same patient and different types of events. Governing the rate of change of the counting process, $N_i(t)$, is the *intensity process*, $\alpha_i(t)$, and it is the intensity process that is modelled in a similar manner to the hazard rate in traditional survival analysis. Whilst a variety of models for the intensity are possible, a frequently used model is what is termed a *multiplicative intensity model* which has algebraic form

$$\alpha_i(t) = Y_i(t)\,\alpha_0(t)\exp(\boldsymbol{\beta}^\top \mathbf{x}_i) \tag{2.1}$$

where $\alpha_0(t)$ is the baseline intensity process and $\boldsymbol{\beta}$ is a vector of regression parameters. For example, in the case of wishing to compare the Asian and non-Asian patients in the ESRD study, we might include a covariate, $x_{\text{ASIAN}i}$, which takes the value one if the ith patient is Asian and zero otherwise. Thus, model (2.1) becomes

$$\alpha(t|x_{\text{ASIAN}i}) = Y_i(t)\,\alpha_0(t)\exp(\beta x_{\text{ASIAN}i}) \tag{2.2}$$

and we can see that in this particular case $\alpha_0(t)$ refers to the intensity process for the non-Asian patients. Similarly, e^β represents the ratio of intensities for death of Asian patients relative to non-Asian patients. If e^β is greater than one, this indicates a survival advantage which favours non-Asians, whilst a ratio of intensities less than one favours Asians. The corresponding likelihood for (2.1), analogous to the *partial likelihood* originally advocated by Cox (1975), is of the form

$$\prod_{i=1}^{n}\left(\prod_{t\geq 0}\alpha_i(t)^{\mathrm{d}N_i(t)}\right)\exp\left(-\int_{t\geq 0}\alpha_i(t)\mathrm{d}t\right) \tag{2.3}$$

where as above $Y_i(t)$ is the at-risk process and $\mathrm{d}N_i(t)$ is the change in the counting process $N_i(t)$ for individual i in the interval $[t, t+\mathrm{d}t)$. If we are only interested in a single non-recurrent event then $\mathrm{d}N_i(t)$ is one if the ith individual experiences the event in the interval $[t, t + dt)$ and zero otherwise. Such a model formulation may be re-expressed as $dN_i(t)$ having a Poisson distribution with mean $\alpha_i(t)dt$, which is defined by

$$\alpha_i(t)dt = Y_i(t)\exp(\boldsymbol{\beta}^{\mathsf{T}}\mathbf{x}_i)d\Lambda_0(t)$$

where $d\Lambda_0(t) = \lambda_0(t)dt$ is the increment in the baseline integrated hazard function in the interval.

Under the assumption of non-informative censoring the intensity process, $\alpha_i(t)$, can be considered as a hazard function, and (2.1) can be thought of in terms of a semi-parametric proportional hazards model. Therefore, in the sections that follow, making the assumption of non-informative censoring, $\lambda(t)$ represents the intensity process $\alpha(t)$, and multiplicative intensity models of the form (2.1) are termed semi-parametric proportional hazards models.

Whilst models such as (2.2) enable us to replicate an analysis that we may have performed using the log-rank test discussed above, they also enable us to estimate the actual difference in terms of survival, on a hazard scale, between groups. In addition, they also enable us to consider a larger number of covariates than would be possible using hypothesis tests such as the log-rank test.

2.3.2 Comparing models

As with other regression techniques, although models such as (2.1) allow us to consider a variety of covariates, they also raise the question of how to obtain an appropriate model. As with regression generally, there are a variety of techniques available, including forward, backward and stepwise procedures. However, as in many other situations, the blind application of any automatic model building technique has to be treated with caution. A number of points need to be made, not least of which is that how a model is developed often depends upon the use to which the 'final' model is to be put. For example, if the objective of the modelling exercise is to produce a relatively simple model to be used to predict patient prognosis in clinic or whether further treatment or tests are necessary, then although a particular modelling strategy might identify a large number of covariates, some of which themselves require laboratory tests to be performed, it will be of limited clinical value. Similarly, in randomized trials it might be considered inappropriate to include covariates which should be balanced between treatment groups by randomization (Pocock, 1983). The main point is that a balance has to be struck between over-complicated modelling of the data and the study objectives. A final comment is that often when modelling strategies are adopted a large number of covariates are considered and a 'final' model identified, the results of which are then interpreted as if this model is 'correct'. This issue of conditioning on models being 'correct' will be discussed later from a

Bayesian perspective, but should not be forgotten when adopting a classical framework.

Regardless of which modelling strategy we adopt, at some point we will need to compare alternative models. A number of methods exist for such model comparisons but we mention only one here.

One of the most frequently used methods for the comparison of nested models is to compare the change in deviances between the two models. The deviance for a particular model is given by minus twice the log likelihood evaluated at the maximum likelihood estimates. Thus, for (2.1) the deviance is computed by evaluating (2.3) at $\hat{\beta}$, and taking minus twice its value.

Although measures of deviance cannot be used for comparing the absolute fit of a model they can be used in a comparative manner for two competing models. Assuming that we have two models, one with p covariates and an alternative with $p + q$ covariates, then the models may be compared by testing whether the additional q parameter values are significantly different from zero. Therefore, under the null hypothesis that they are not, the following hypothesis test may be used:

$$-2\log_e\left(\frac{L_p(\hat{\beta})}{L_{p+q}(\hat{\beta})}\right) \sim \chi_q^2$$

2.3.3   Application

Applying the Cox proportional hazards regression model to the ESRD study data using the covariates in Table 2.1 gives the results displayed in Table 2.2. The first comment to make is that there would appear to be a few covariates that are very important in helping to explain survival differences. Age can be seen to the single most important covariate, as one might expect in such a patient population. Thus, the second set of models considered all contain Age and examine whether the addition of other covariates significantly improves the model's ability to explain the data. We can see that both the presence of diabetes and cardiac complications appear to improve the model. Finally, the addition of ethnicity, Asian, to a 'final' model containing Age, Diabetes and Cardiac produces a clearly non-significant improvement, thus suggesting that ethnicity has little influence on survival for this patient population.

Table 2.3 shows the parameter estimates for three of the models considered in Table 2.2, namely that which only included Asian, that which included just Asian and Age, and finally the 'final' model which included Age, Diabetes and Cardiac, plus Asian. As with the results of applying the log-rank tests in the above section, including just Asian on its own would suggest that there is a statistically significant difference in terms of overall survival between the two ethnic groups. However, as soon as Age is also entered into the model, this effect disappears; indeed, if

Table 2.2 Model fitting results for all-cause mortality using a semi-parametric proportional hazards regression model

Model	−2LL	Change	P value
Null	1480.9	–	–
Age	1380.0	100.9	<0.000 001
Diabetes	1468.9	12.0	0.0 005
Cardiac	1458.4	22.5	0.000 002
Cancer	1473.7	7.2	0.007
Vascular	1479.3	1.6	0.21
Gender	1479.6	1.3	0.25
Albumin	1400.9	2.8	0.09
Mode	1470.8	10.1	0.001
Age + Diabetes	1370.9	9.1	0.003
Age + Cardiac	1372.5	7.5	0.006
Age + Cancer	1377.2	2.8	0.09
Age + Mode	1375.1	4.9	0.03
Age + Diabetes + Cardiac	1364.6	6.3	0.01
Age + Diabetes + Cancer	1370.4	0.5	0.48
Age + Diabetes + Mode	1368.4	2.5	0.11
Age + Diabetes + Cardiac + Asian	1364.5	0.1	0.75

Table 2.3 Parameter estimates for semi-parametric proportional hazards regression models for all-cause mortality in the ESRD study

Model	Parameter	MLE	SD	95% CI	P value
Asian	Asian	−0.432	0.198	(−0.828, −0.036)	0.03
Asian + Age	Asian	+0.146	0.213	(−0.271, +0.563)	0.49
	Age	+0.065	0.008	(+0.049, +0.081)	<0.0001
Asian + Age +	Asian	+0.027	0.216	(−0.396, +0.450)	0.9
Cardiac + Diabetes	Age	+0.062	0.008	(+0.046, +0.078)	<0.00001
	Cardiac	+0.563	0.183	(+0.204, +0.922)	0.003
	Diabetes	+0.551	0.212	(+0.135, +0.966)	0.01

anything, such a model suggests that Asian patients do slightly worse than non-Asian patients, though the difference is small and not statistically significant. Finally, including all the covariates identified in the model building process summarized in Table 2.2, namely Diabetes, Age and Cardiac, and then estimating the effect of Asian, still suggests that the effect of ethnicity on overall survival in this study population is small in comparison with the effect of age, diabetes and cardiac complications.

2.3.4   Time-dependent covariates

In many medical studies information, such as the results of biochemical tests, is collected over a period of time on patients, as with albumin levels in the ESRD study. Such *time-dependent covariates* can be incorporated into the standard proportional hazards model (2.1)

$$\lambda(t|\mathbf{x}_i(t)) = Y_i(t)\,\lambda_0(t)\exp(\boldsymbol{\beta}^\top \mathbf{x}_i(t)) \qquad (2.4)$$

The likelihood for models such as (2.4) is analogous to (2.3), but the added complexity of including time-dependent covariates makes them computationally more difficult.

Referring back to the ESRD data set, one of the covariates considered in the previous analysis was albumin measured at entry into the study. As part of the study annual albumin levels were also recorded, because previous research had suggested that albumin levels can be used as a means of monitoring renal function. Therefore, entering albumin into the proportional hazards model as a time-dependent covariate which changes annually is of considerable interest.

Table 2.4 shows the parameter estimates obtained from including Albumin in a Cox regression model which contains Asian, Age, Diabetes and Cardiac, both at baseline and also as an annually time-varying covariate. In terms of the addition of Albumin, for the non-time-dependent model the corresponding log likelihood for the model without Albumin was −606.61 (note that this is different to that in Table 2.3 because for some patients no albumin level was recorded), and that for the model including Albumin at baseline was −606.22, clearly a non-significant improvement. For the models which did include Albumin as a time-dependent covariate the log likelihood value for the reference model was −632.87, and for the model with Albumin as a time-dependent

Table 2.4 Parameter estimates for semi-parametric proportional hazards regression models for all-cause mortality in the ESRD study including albumin as both a time-independent and time-dependent covariate

Model	Parameter	MLE	SD	95% CI	P value
Albumin at baseline	Asian	−0.073	0.234	(−0.532, +0.386)	0.75
	Age	+0.039	0.008	(+0.023, +0.055)	<0.00001
	Diabetes	+0.106	0.200	(−0.286, +0.498)	0.6
	Cardiac	+0.468	0.241	(−0.004, +0.940)	0.02
	Albumin	−0.016	0.018	(−0.051, +0.019)	0.4
Albumin as time-dependent covariate	Asian	−0.046	0.226	(−0.489, +0.397)	0.84
	Age	+0.033	0.008	(+0.017, +0.049)	<0.00001
	Diabetes	+0.172	0.237	(−0.293, +0.637)	0.4
	Cardiac	+0.513	0.198	(+0.125, +0.901)	0.01
	Albumin	−0.047	0.015	(−0.076, −0.018)	0.002

covariate it was −628.40, the resulting change in minus twice the log likelihood being 8.94 which yields a *P* value of 0.003. Thus, it would appear that whilst the effect of measuring albumin levels at baseline are of little prognostic value, the annual measurement of serum albumin does help in explaining some variation in survival times. The interpretation of the time-dependent modelling results are that a change of 1 gram per litre in serum albumin level at any time during the study leads to a 4.6% reduction in the subsequent risk of death. Inference in terms of a rate, for example the change in risk due to a change of 1 gram per litre in serum albumin level over the course of a month, say, could be obtained by including further time-dependent covariates in the model.

2.3.5 Stratified models

One assumption of the models considered so far, such as (2.1), is that the baseline hazard function has been assumed to be the same for all patients. Clearly in some situations this may not be so, and we wish to allow for the baseline hazard to be the same within *strata*. The functional form of such models is

$$\lambda_s(t|\mathbf{x}_i) = Y_{ts}(t)\,\lambda_{s0}(t)\exp(\boldsymbol{\beta}^\top\mathbf{x}_i) \tag{2.5}$$

where $\lambda_{s0}(t)$ refers to the baseline hazard function in stratum s. Note that the effect of the covariates, $\boldsymbol{\beta}$, remains the same across strata.

Use of stratified proportional hazards regression models relates mainly to the situation in which the assumption of proportional hazards does not hold for certain patient groupings, and these can then be used to define strata, satisfying the assumption of proportional hazards within strata. Extension of the definition of the strata to include time-dependent events enables the consideration of multi-state models to be accommodated within a proportional hazards framework. For computational reasons such an approach to the fitting of multi-state models requires software that can accommodate time-dependent strata to be used, for example BMDP 2L (Dixon, 1990).

2.3.6 Model checking and residuals

As with any modelling process, certain assumptions have been made in the adoption of a semi-parametric proportional hazards regression model. The two key assumptions are firstly that the hazards in the patient groups are proportional and secondly that the effect of covariates is additive on a log hazard scale. There are a number of methods available for checking these assumptions, and two will be considered here: simple plots and the use of residuals.

Obviously when there is only one covariate of interest in the model, the use of such graphical methods poses few problems. However, frequently in assessing assumptions, models will contain several covariates.

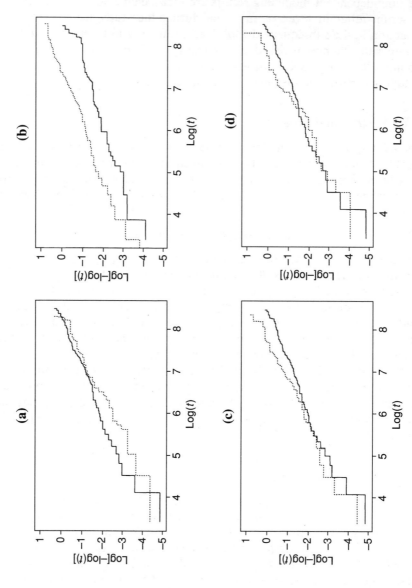

Fig. 2.3 Plot of log–log $S(t)$ versus log(t) for overall survival in ESRD study, stratifying by (a) Asian, (b) Age, (c) Cardiac and (d) Diabetes

In such circumstances, the model is required to be fitted several times, each time stratifying by the covariate to be checked, and including all other covariates as terms in the linear predictor. If the assumption of proportional hazards fails for any of the covariates then the 'final' analysis should be based on a model in which that covariate is treated as a stratum. Obviously when models contain continuous covariates decisions have to be made regarding formation of a factor with a number of levels.

As an illustration of such graphical methods consider the 'final' model in Table 2.3 which contained Asian, Age, Cardiac and Diabetes. On dichotomizing Age into either ≤ 65 or >65, Fig. 2.3 shows plots of log–log $S(t)$ versus $\log(t)$ for each of the four covariates in the model in turn, stratifying for each covariate and treating the three remaining terms as terms in the linear predictor. We can see that certainly for Age the plot produces two parallel lines, whilst for the other three covariates it is questionable as to whether the lines are parallel. Indeed for Diabetes the lines cross, and really Diabetes should be included in the model as a stratification variable.

As with other types of regression models we can consider the use of residuals for checking the adequacy of a particular model and verifying that the model assumptions are satisfied. A number of different types of residuals have been proposed for the Cox model (2.1). We consider essentially two: *martingale residuals* and *deviance residuals*.

Initially we have to define Cox–Snell residuals, r_{Ci}, which for the ith patient can be defined as

$$r_{Ci} = \exp(\hat{\boldsymbol{\beta}}^{\top} \mathbf{x}_i)\hat{\Lambda}_0(t_i) \tag{2.6}$$

where $\hat{\Lambda}_0(t_i)$ is an estimate of the cumulative baseline hazard function for a patient whose failure time was t_i. If the model is correct then r_{Ci} should follow a unit exponential distribution, regardless of the actual distributional form of $S(t_i)$. *Martingale residuals*, r_{Mi}, are then formed by taking the difference between the death/event indicator, d_i, and the Cox–Snell residuals. Thus

$$r_{Mi} = d_i - r_{Ci} \tag{2.7}$$

Martingale residuals can be used to assess whether any particular patients are poorly predicted by the model, with large negative or positive residuals indicating a lack of fit. They can also be used together with continuous covariates for assessing the functional form required for the covariate, with a random scatter about zero indicating that the variable does not need transforming. Calculating the martingale residuals for the ESRD study and plotting them against Age in Fig. 2.4(a) shows that Age appears to be quite adequate without transforming it.

Deviance residuals, r_{Di}, may be calculated from the martingale residuals (2.7) as follows:

$$r_{Di} = \text{sign}(r_{Mi})\sqrt{-2[r_{Mi} + d_i \log_e(d_i - r_{Mi})]} \tag{2.8}$$

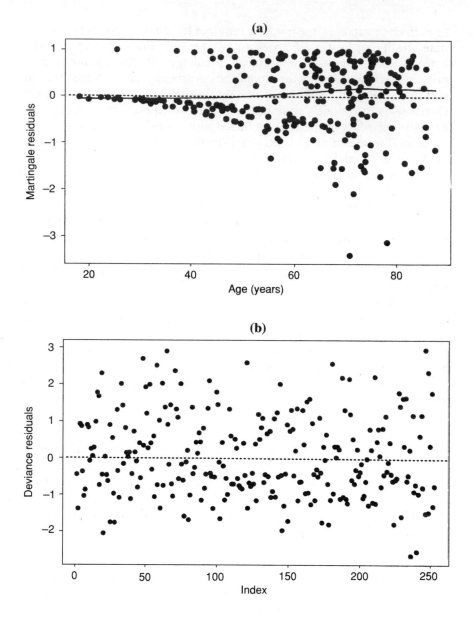

Fig. 2.4 Plots of (a) martingale and (b) deviance residuals for overall survival in ESRD study

They are also particularly useful in identifying patients who are poorly predicted by the model, with large negative or positive values of r_{Di} indicating individuals who can be deemed 'poorly' modelled. Figure 2.4(b) shows the deviance residuals plotted against patient number for the ESRD study. We can see that there is approximate random variation of the residuals about zero, and in particular there do not appear to be any patients who have unduly large negative or positive residuals.

As with any regression modelling process the identification of observations which may have an undue influence on the model results is of considerable importance; these observations are termed *influential observations*. For the semi-parametric proportional hazards regression model what are called *delta-betas* may be calculated, which are the scaled changes in each regression parameter in the model when one individual is removed from the analysis. Figure 2.5 shows the scaled changes in the coefficients for the four variables in the semi-parametric proportional hazards regression models for the ESRD study plotted against the patient number. We can see that although the removal of some patients does have a large effect on the coefficients, there does not appear to be any systematic influence of individual patients upon all of the coefficient estimates.

2.4   Accelerated failure time models

Although one of the more attractive reasons for using the semi-parametric proportional hazards regression models of Section 2.3 is the lack of parametric assumptions regarding the baseline hazard function, this also represents a lack of efficiency if the failure times do indeed follow a specific distribution. Even allowing for the possibility that we adopt a parametric proportional hazards model, with $\alpha_0(t)$ in (2.1) being replaced with a known functional form, it is quite conceivable that the assumption of proportional hazards might not be justified. Thus, an alternative model in which the effect of covariates is assumed to act multiplicatively directly on the survivor function might be considered. Such models are termed *accelerated failure time models*. The general likelihood for a parametric survival model can be formulated in terms of the survivor and density functions thus:

$$L(\beta, \theta) = \prod_{i=1}^{n} f(t_i|\beta, \theta)^{\delta_i} \, S(t_i|\beta, \theta)^{1-\delta_i} \tag{2.9}$$

where $f(t_i|\beta, \theta)$ and $S(t_i|\beta, \theta)$ are the density and survivor functions for the model respectively, and δ_i is an indicator function taking the value one if the ith patient was observed to fail and zero otherwise. Alternatively, the likelihood can be formulated in terms of the hazard and cumulative hazard functions

$$L(\beta, \theta) = \prod_{i=1}^{n} \lambda(t_i|\beta, \theta)^{\delta_i} \exp\left(-\int_0^t \lambda(u|\beta, \theta) \mathrm{d}u\right) \tag{2.10}$$

where $\int_0^t \lambda(u|\beta, \theta)\mathrm{d}u$ is the integrated hazard function.

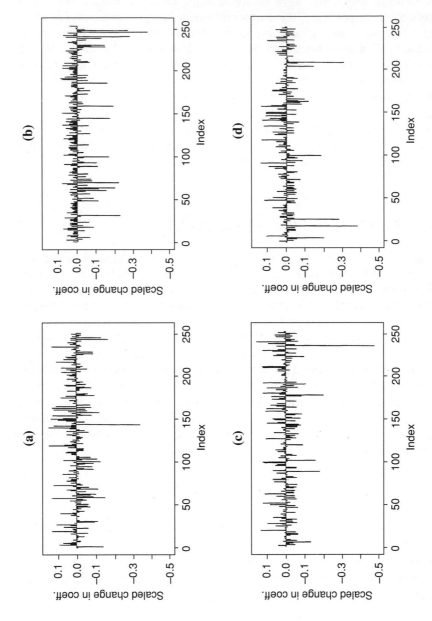

Fig. 2.5 Scaled changes in model coefficients on deleting individual patients for (a) Asian, (b) Age, (c) Cardiac and (d) Diabetes

2.4.1   Models

As we have seen in Section 2.3, often the assumption of proportional hazards is untenable, and alternative models, such as accelerated failure time models, have to be considered. Algebraically such models are of the form

$$S_i(t) = S_0(\phi_i t) \qquad (2.11)$$

where $\phi_i = \exp(\boldsymbol{\beta}^\mathsf{T} \mathbf{x}_i)$ is the *acceleration factor* of the ith patient compared with the baseline patient group. Model (2.11) can also be expressed in terms of the hazard functions

$$\lambda_i(t) = \exp(\boldsymbol{\beta}^\mathsf{T} \mathbf{x}_i)\, \lambda_0(\exp(\boldsymbol{\beta}^\mathsf{T} \mathbf{x}_i)t) \qquad (2.12)$$

For the exponential and Weibull distributions the respective parametric proportional hazards and accelerated failure time models coincide. The hazard for the Weibull distribution is given by

$$\lambda(t) = \theta \kappa t^{\kappa-1} \qquad (2.13)$$

where θ is termed the *scale parameter* and κ the *shape parameter*. We can see that if $\kappa = 1$ then the hazard function is constant over time, and the survival times are assumed to follow an exponential distribution. Similarly, the Weibull hazard function can accommodate both a hazard function that is increasing over time ($\kappa > 1$) or decreasing over time ($\kappa < 1$). The Weibull distribution can be a suitable distribution when the survival distribution can be assumed to have a heavy left tail, that is when events occur early on in the follow-up period. In this respect the Weibull distribution often leads to similar results as the gamma distribution.

Another distribution that is frequently used as a survival distribution is the log-normal distribution. The probability density function for the log-normal distribution, $f(t|\mu, \sigma^2)$, is given by

$$f(t) = \frac{1}{\sigma\sqrt{2\pi}}\, t^{-1} \exp\{-[\log(t) - \mu]^2 / 2\sigma^2\} \qquad (2.14)$$

where μ is the mean of the log-normal distribution and σ^2 is the variance. We can see that the hazard function will involve the evaluation of the integral of the normal cumulative function, making the estimation of the hazard function directly more problematical. The behaviour of the log-normal distribution is different to the Weibull distribution in that it tends to have a heavy right tail, a feature that it shares with the log-logistic distribution, and one that makes it particularly suitable for situations in which events occur later in the follow-up period.

Often the accelerated failure time model (2.11) is expressed in a log-linear form which makes computational implementation easier, and is the most frequent method with which software packages accommodate such models. Thus, letting the random variable T_i be the survival time for the ith patient

$$\log_e(T_i) = \mu + \alpha^\mathsf{T}\mathbf{x}_i + \sigma\epsilon_i \qquad (2.15)$$

where ϵ_i is assumed to have an appropriate distribution according to which distribution we wish to assume for T_i. In this way a variety of distributions can be accommodated including the exponential, Weibull, log-logistic, gamma and log-normal. Though this reformulation (2.12) is computationally easier, interest often focuses upon the parameters in the original model formulation. These, however, can be obtained by the following relationships: $\theta = -\mu/\sigma$, $\kappa = 1/\sigma$ and $\beta = -\alpha$. This method of fitting parametric survival models is used in both SAS (SAS Institute Inc., 1993) and Splus (Statistical Sciences Inc., 1990).

2.4.2   Comparing models

As with the proportional hazards models considered above, we often wish to compare a number of competing models. The first scenario is when we have a number of different covariates, as in the ESRD study, and we wish to select the most appropriate set of covariates. In this situation comparing deviances of the various models enables us to adopt a model building strategy, and the same methods as above are available: forwards, backwards, stepwise. The second scenario concerns the choice of survival distribution. A number of possibilities exist. There may be theoretical arguments for adopting certain distributions over others. For example, in diseases in which events are assumed to occur early in the follow-up period a distribution with a heavy left-hand tail would seem more appropriate than a symmetric distribution. Analogously, in diseases in which events are assumed to occur late in the follow-up period, for example breast cancer, a distribution with a heavy right-hand tail would seem appropriate. Choice of a distribution within each of these broad categories, say heavy left-hand tail, symmetric, heavy right-hand tail, might indeed be somewhat arbitrary, since each of these broad categories contains a number of distributions which might for practical purposes lead to similar results.

In terms of model checking, variants of the residuals outlined above may be calculated for the accelerated failure time models considered here, as they may all be derived from the estimated survivor function. However, in practice the use of residuals in a parametric framework is seen in the literature even less frequently than the Cox semi-parametric models.

Another issue that is rarely examined in practice is the inclusion of time-dependent covariates within a parametric regression model, and indeed little work has been done in this area with the exception of Petersen (1996).

2.4.3   Application to example

We now consider applying the two accelerated failure time models briefly described above, the Weibull and log-normal, to the ESRD study data.

Table 2.5 Model fitting results for all-cause mortality for Weibull and log-normal accelerated failure time models (* denotes comparisons based on a different number of patients owing to missing values)

Model	Weibull			Log-normal		
	−2LL	Change	*P* value	−2LL	Change	*P* value
Null	747.7	–	–	744.5	–	–
Asian	742.1	5.6	0.017	738.4	6.1	0.01
Age	642.2	105.5	<0.00001	660.8	83.7	<0.00001
Diabetes	735.6	12.1	0.0005	737.9	6.6	0.01
Cardiac	724.4	23.3	<0.0001	729.6	14.9	0.0001
Cancer	740.2	7.5	0.006	739.0	5.5	0.02
Vascular	746.8	0.9	0.34	742.6	1.9	0.17
Gender	746.3	1.4	0.24	743.4	1.1	0.29
Albumin	709.4	2.9	0.09*	704.3	5.3	0.02*
Mode	739.4	8.3	0.004	742.0	2.5	0.11
Age + Diabetes	635.5	6.7	0.01	657.8	3.0	0.08
Age + Cardiac	633.0	9.2	0.002	654.9	5.9	0.02
Age + Cancer	639.5	2.7	0.1	659.3	1.5	0.22
Age + Mode	640.6	1.6	0.21	–		
Age + Cardiac + Diabetes	627.5	5.5	0.02	652.6	2.3	0.13
Age + Cardiac + Cancer	631.5	1.5	0.22	653.8	1.1	0.29
Age + Cardiac + Asian	632.8	0.2	0.65	654.2	0.7	0.40
Age + Cardiac + Diabetes + Cancer	626.5	1.0	0.32			
Age + Cardiac + Diabetes + Asian	627.5	0.0	0.99			

The models were fitted using PROC LIFEREG in SAS (SAS Institute Inc., 1993). Table 2.5 shows minus twice the log likelihood for the various covariate models and adopts a forward selection procedure with the most highly significant covariate being entered into the model at each stage.

We can see from Table 2.5 that for both the Weibull and log-normal models Age is clearly the single most important covariate. Further models indicate that both Cardiac and possibly Diabetes also have a role to play. However, regardless of whether both Cardiac and Diabetes or just Cardiac are included in the model, in addition to Age, we can see that Asian, the effect of ethnicity, appears not to be helpful in explaining any variation in survival times.

Table 2.6 displays parameter estimates for both the Weibull and log-normal accelerated failure time models, which include Asian, Asian + Age and Asian + Age + Cardiac + Diabetes. We can see that the results are qualitatively similar, though there are slight differences between using the two distributions. In particular, we can see that regardless of which covariates, in addition to Age, are included in the models, the effect of ethnicity appears to be small, though whilst for the Weibull model Asian patients would appear to do less well compared with non-Asian patients,

Table 2.6 Parameter estimates for accelerated failure time regression models for all-cause mortality in the ESRD study

Model	Parameter	MLE	SD	95% CI	P value
Weibull					
Asian	Asian	−0.550	0.243	(−1.026, −0.074)	0.02
Asian + Age	Asian	+0.149	0.225	(−0.292, +0.590)	0.51
	Age	+0.069	0.008	(+0.053, +0.085)	0.001
Asian + Age + Diabetes	Asian	+0.027	0.221	(−0.406, +0.460)	0.90
+ Cardiac	Age	+0.063	0.008	(+0.047, +0.079)	0.0001
	Diabetes	+0.518	0.213	(+0.101, +0.935)	0.015
	Cardiac	+0.541	0.186	(+0.176, +0.906)	0.004
Log-normal					
Asian	Asian	−0.671	0.272	(−1.204, −0.138)	0.01
Asian + Age	Asian	−0.150	0.255	(−0.650, +0.350)	0.55
	Age	+0.068	0.008	(+0.052, +0.084)	0.0001
Asian + Age + Diabetes	Asian	−0.305	0.260	(−0.815, +0.205)	0.24
+ Cardiac	Age	+0.063	0.008	(+0.047, +0.079)	0.0001
	Diabetes	+0.503	0.291	(−0.067, +1.073)	0.08
	Cardiac	+0.597	0.252	(+0.103, +1.091)	0.018

for the log-normal model this is reversed with Asian patients doing slightly better than non-Asian patients.

2.5   Bayesian models

Whilst the classical models that have been considered in Sections 2.3 and 2.4 have provided a rich framework within which to explore the relationships between covariates and survival, we have not been able to include any of the background information described in Section 2.2. We now consider Bayesian models, in which we can formally include this information in terms of prior distributions for model parameters. Initially we consider a relatively simple Bayesian model, in which we model the log hazard ratio directly using a normal–normal conjugate model (O'Hagan, 1994a). We then consider Bayesian alternatives to the semi-parametric proportional hazards models of Section 2.3 and the fully parametric accelerated failure time models of Section 2.4.

2.5.1   Non-temporal models

Though the emphasis in this chapter is on developing regression models some simpler models should also be noted, especially in randomized

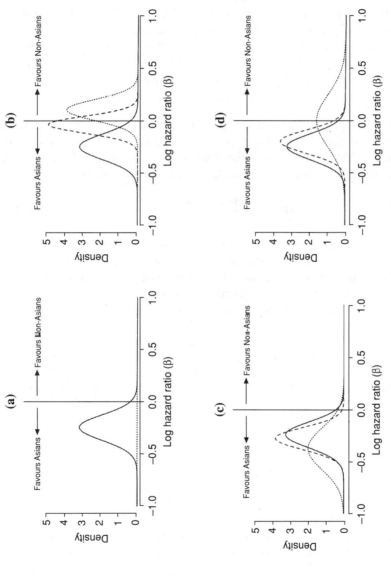

Fig. 2.6 Prior, standardized likelihood and posterior densities for log hazard ratio of Asians relative to non-Asians for all-cause mortality in ESRD study using (a) reference, (b) clinical, (c) data-based and (d) equivalence prior distributions in a normal–normal conjugate model: ——, standardized likelihood; ......, prior density; - - -, posterior density

controlled trials, as these can form the basis for an initial analysis (Spiegelhalter *et al.*, 1993, Abrams *et al.*, 1994). Consider that the survival experiences may be summarized by the statistic x_m, and that this statistic may be assumed to be normally distributed such that

$$x_m \sim N(\delta, \sigma^2/m)$$

Under the assumptions of proportional hazards x_m is the difference in observed and expected number of deaths in the treatment group, δ is the log hazard ratio, m is the total number of events and $\sigma^2 = 4$ (Tsiatis, 1981). Assume that prior beliefs regarding the log hazard ratio can also be expressed in terms of a normal distribution such that

$$\delta \sim N(\delta_0, \sigma^2/n_0)$$

where δ_0 is the prior mean and n_0 represents the size of a hypothetical trial such that it reflects the prior certainty surrounding δ_0. Using the fact that both the likelihood and prior distribution are normal distributions the posterior distribution for δ is also a normal distribution of the form

$$\delta|\text{data} \sim N\left(\frac{n_0\delta_0 + mx_m}{n_0 + m}, \frac{\sigma^2}{n_0 + m}\right) \tag{2.16}$$

Such a model has the advantage that the normal prior distribution is *conjugate* to the normal likelihood, thus enabling posterior summary statistics to be easily calculated. However, extension of the model to accommodate covariates is not straightforward.

Consider the prior distributions described in Section 2.2. Applying the conjugate model (2.16) above we obtain the posterior distributions in Fig. 2.6 and Table 2.7. We can see that first of all the model does not allow for Age and therefore we see that the reference posterior density, that is the standardized likelihood, indicates that Asian patients do better than non-Asian patients. However, we can see that both the vague, equivalence

Table 2.7 Prior to posterior analysis for normal–normal conjugate models for all-cause mortality in the ESRD study

Distribution		Mean	SD	95% CI
Vague:	prior	0.000	100.000	(−100.00, +100.00)
	posterior	−0.250	0.123	(−0.491, −0.009)
Equivalence:	prior	0.000	0.250	(−0.490, +0.490)
	posterior	−0.202	0.110	(−0.418, +0.014)
Clinical:	prior	+0.100	0.100	(−0.096, +0.296)
	posterior	−0.040	0.080	(−0.197, +0.117)
Data-based:	prior	−0.382	0.200	(−0.774, +0.010)
	posterior	−0.286	0.104	(−0.490, −0.082)

and clinical posterior distributions are shifted towards the likelihood, whilst the data-based posterior distribution changes little compared with the prior. Viewing all four posterior distributions we can see that there is a range of posterior beliefs regarding the likely effect of ethnicity on survival whilst on RRT. However, we must also appreciate that this model does not take account of the different age structures of the two ethnic groups that we know exist, and therefore ideally we wish to consider a formal regression model.

2.5.2 Semi-parametric models

Whilst models such as (2.16) can in theory accommodate more complicated models than considered above, by suitable specification of a likelihood, they do not readily provide an efficient means of considering regression models similar to the Cox proportional hazards or accelerated failure time models considered from a classical perspective in Section 2.3. For example, x_m in (2.16) above could be derived from a suitable regression model in which specific covariates could have been included. In this case, assuming that the effect of ethnicity was of primary interest, δ would represent the adjusted effect of ethnicity (adjusted for the covariates included in the model). However, such an approach raises a number of issues. The first is that any prior distributions specified for δ are prior distributions adjusted for the covariates, which in any elicitation exercise might not be a suitable way of obtaining a priori beliefs. The second issue is that such models would also make a strong, and sometimes untenable, assumption of the likelihood being approximately quadratic, corresponding to a normal distribution. The third, and final, issue is that whilst such an approach might indeed provide a suitable method for enabling inferences regarding δ to be made, it obviously cannot provide posterior summaries for other parameters, and perhaps more importantly it cannot provide information regarding the interaction between the different covariates considered.

Therefore, what is required is a unified modelling approach similar to the regression models considered above. However, as we saw in the comparison between the Cox models and the accelerated failure time models, one appealing advantage of the former model is its semi-parametric nature, which focuses attention on the regression nature of the model, rather than on modelling the underlying survival distribution.

Following the formulation of the semi-parametric proportional hazards regression model as a multiplicative intensity model (2.1) two approaches to Bayesian inference are possible. The first was advocated by Kalbfleisch (1978) who suggested assuming a gamma prior distribution for $d\Lambda_0(t)$, because given a Poisson likelihood, such a prior distribution would be conjugate (Bernardo and Smith, 1993). In particular, Kalbfleisch suggested defining $d\Lambda_0(t)$ as

$$d\Lambda_0(t) \sim \text{Gamma}[c \, d\Lambda_0^*(t), c]$$

where $d\Lambda_0^*(t)$ is an initial estimate of the underlying baseline hazard, whilst c represents the credibility of such an estimate, with small values c corresponding to weak prior beliefs.

An alternative approach is to assume that $d\Lambda_0(t)$ follows an independent-increments process, with $d\Lambda_0(t)$ in each defined interval having an independent prior distribution. In such a model formulation, specification of the cut-points to be used to define the time grid is required. In the simplest case, $d\Lambda_0(t)$ would be assumed to be constant within each interval, though such an assumption could be relaxed. A key issue with such an approach is the definition of the grid over which the baseline hazard is defined, that is the size of dt. If the grid is defined by the observed distinct failure times then a likelihood corresponding to the likelihood (2.3) is obtained. However, from an efficiency perspective, such a formulation may require considerable computational resources, and a more coarsely defined grid might be more appropriate from a practical point of view. The penalty for adopting such a grid is that if the baseline hazard is changing rapidly then such a model will only provide an approximation to it. However, as we have mentioned, interest primarily focuses upon the regression parameters, and therefore providing that we use a reasonably adequate grid, then our ability to make inferences about these parameters should not be unduly compromised.

2.5.3   Estimation

In estimating the parameters of Bayesian survival models, for which a conjugate analysis is not possible, there are essentially three classes of techniques available: asymptotic approximations, numerical integration (quadrature) methods and simulation methods (Thisted, 1988).

In terms of the first method, asymptotic approximation methods, Tierney and colleagues (Tierney and Kadane, 1986, Tierney *et al.*, 1989) have advocated the use of asymptotic approximations based on the work of Laplace (Stigler, 1986) and expanded by de Bruijn (1958). Specific implementations of the above Laplace approximations are `sbayes()` in Splus (Statistical Sciences Inc., 1990) and a suite of functions in XLISP-STAT (Tierney, 1990), both available as shareware (http://lib.stat.cmu.edu).

The second method is numerical integration methods or quadrature. Of particular prominence has been the use of Gauss–Hermite quadrature (Naylor and Smith, 1982, Naylor and Shaw, 1985) which assumes that joint posterior distributions can be approximated by the product of a suitable well-behaved polynomial and a Gaussian distribution.

Recently, Markov chain Monte Carlo (MCMC) methods of simulation have been proposed and Gibbs sampling in particular has become widespread (Gelfand and Smith, 1990, Gelfand *et al.*, 1990, Clayton, 1991, Gilks *et al.*, 1993, 1996). Gibbs sampling proceeds by sampling from the posterior conditional distributions, which under erodic theory should converge to the posterior marginal distributions.

In some situations random samples have to be generated from distributions for which only the functional form is known. Ripley (1987) suggests an *acceptance–rejection* criterion based on sampling from a ratio of uniform distributions, whilst Gilks and Wild (1992) have proposed a more efficient method for the case when the log likelihood or the log posterior is log concave.

Assessment of convergence criteria for the sampler has been proposed by a number of authors (Cowles and Carlin, 1996, Gelman, 1996). However, behaviour of the joint posterior density can have a profound effect upon convergence, especially when it is multi-modal, and parameterization is as important an issue as with the other parameter estimation methods (Hills and Smith, 1992). However, other issues need to be considered carefully, including how many 'burn-in' values to use, what initial starting values to use, and avoidance of serial autocorrelation.

In survival analysis problems Gibbs sampling proved to be computationally inefficient owing to the nature of the posterior conditional densities, caused by the presence of censoring. However, a method for overcoming these difficulties has been proposed by Kuo and Smith (1992) and Smith and Roberts (1993). Using these methods the censored observations are treated as additional unknown parameters, and a new set of conditional distributions are derived. Sampling from this new set of conditional distributions is then usually straightforward and does not require sophisticated sampling algorithms (Clayton, 1991).

In using Gibbs sampling, it is sometimes easier to think of models such as (2.1) graphically in what are termed *directed acyclical graphs* (DAGs) (Whittaker, 1990). Figure 2.7 shows the graphical model for (2.1) assuming a Poisson likelihood, and with β_{0j} representing the baseline intensity in the jth time interval.

The key message that should be borne in mind over and above all the specific points raised above is that the more that is known about the behaviour of the joint posterior distribution the better; for example, is it multi-modal, is it very flat?

Implementation of Gibbs sampling can be accomplished in any programming environment that allows random sampling from known distributions. However, recently development of the BUGS software (Thomas *et al.*, 1992) has provided a relatively user-friendly and unified method for implementing Gibbs sampling. In addition there is also an Splus (Statistical Sciences Inc., 1990) suite of functions CODA (Cowles *et al.*, 1994) which implements many of the diagnostic methods discussed above and which works directly with the output from BUGS.

2.5.4 Application

We now consider applying models such as (2.1) to the ESRD study. As

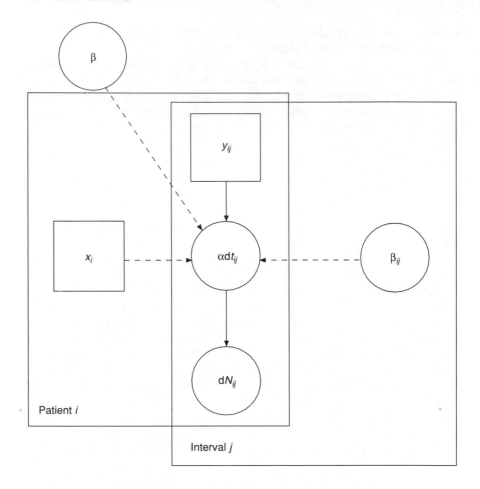

Fig. 2.7 Directed acyclical graph (DAG) for Bayesian semi-parametric proportional hazards model

in the classical analysis there are a number of potential confounding factors that we may wish to take into account, but for illustration we consider three models here, which include Asian, Asian + Age and Asian + Age + Cardiac + Diabetes. Tables 2.8 and 2.9 show the parameter estimates for the three models, in terms of the posterior means, standard deviations and 95% credible intervals using each of the four prior distributions outlined in Section 2.2.

We can see from Table 2.8 that even when we do not allow for any other covariates apart from Asian the 95% credible intervals for all the prior distributions except the data-based one include zero, the point of no difference. This analysis mirrors that of the normal–normal conjugate model above. This feature remains even when we allow for other covariates including Age, Cardiac and Diabetes, indicating the strength of

Table 2.8 Posterior estimates for the semi-parametric regression model, using a 'burn-in' of 500 and a sample of 2000

Model	Prior	Parameter	Mean	SD	95% CI	Geweke Z value
Asian	Reference	Asian	−0.282	0.228	(−0.737, +0.171)	−1.570
	Clinical	Asian	0.039	0.090	(−0.138, +0.209)	−0.562
	Data-based	Asian	−0.394	0.075	(−0.540, −0.252)	−0.585
	Equivalence	Asian	−0.143	0.165	(−0.481, +0.166)	−1.050
Asian + Age	Reference	Asian	0.393	0.247	(−0.109, +0.869)	0.893
		Age	0.072	0.009	(+0.054, +0.090)	0.497
	Clinical	Asian	0.143	0.093	(−0.043, +0.327)	−0.282
		Age	0.067	0.008	(+0.051, +0.084)	−0.845
	Data-based	Asian	−0.342	0.075	(−0.494, −0.194)	0.651
		Age	0.063	0.008	(+0.047, +0.079)	−0.611
	Equivalence	Asian	0.201	0.176	(−0.145, +0.551)	−0.208
		Age	0.069	0.009	(+0.052, +0.087)	−0.799

Table 2.9 Posterior estimates for the semi-parametric regression model including Asian, Age, Cardiac, Diabetes, and using a 'burn-in' of 500 and a sample of 2000

Prior	Parameter	Mean	SD	95% CI	Geweke Z value
Reference	Asian	0.282	0.246	(−0.224, +0.737)	−0.101
	Age	0.069	0.010	(+0.050, +0.089)	−0.082
	Cardiac	0.579	0.215	(+0.151, +0.997)	0.532
	Diabetes	0.767	0.239	(+0.302, +1.236)	−0.253
Clinical	Asian	0.125	0.091	(−0.061, +0.312)	−0.236
	Age	0.067	0.009	(+0.049, +0.085)	−0.765
	Cardiac	0.610	0.215	(+0.180, +1.030)	0.769
	Diabetes	0.789	0.246	(+0.285, +1.261)	0.215
Data-based	Asian	−0.356	0.075	(−0.509, −0.214)	0.496
	Age	0.060	0.009	(+0.043, +0.078)	−0.624
	Cardiac	0.625	0.222	(+0.201, +1.055)	0.237
	Diabetes	0.849	0.239	(+0.383, +1.300)	−1.080
Equivalence	Asian	0.142	0.177	(−0.203, +0.490)	−0.051
	Age	0.067	0.010	(+0.049, +0.086)	0.793
	Cardiac	0.597	0.222	(+0.160, +1.013)	−1.110
	Diabetes	0.783	0.241	(+0.305, +1.258)	0.916

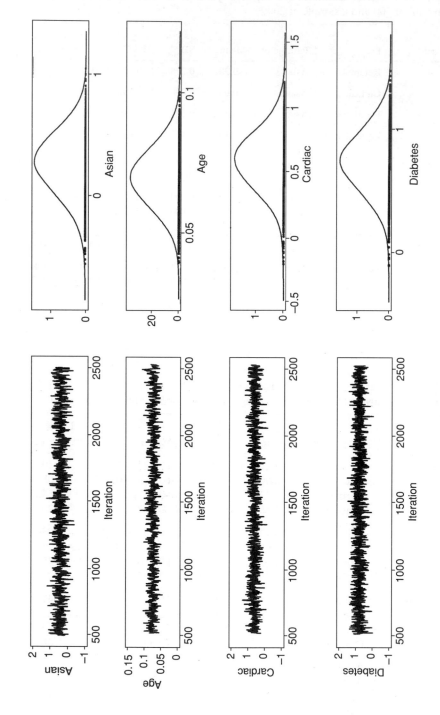

Fig. 2.8 Trace of samples from Markov chain and posterior kernel densities for semi-parametric model, including Asian, Age, Cardiac and Diabetes

evidence of the data-based prior distribution, so that the current study data, in the form of the likelihood, cannot substantially modify it.

In terms of the model properties, each of the models used a 'burn-in' of 500 iterations, and with the next 2000 samples being collected. A number of different starting values were tried, together with varying run lengths, but the results, in terms of the parameter estimates, were not qualitatively different. In terms of convergence, Fig. 2.8 shows the estimated posterior densities for the model which just included Asian, together with a trace of the samples for each of the model parameters. Whilst it can be difficult to interpret such traces there does not appear to be any evidence of systematic behaviour. Figure 2.9 shows auto-correlation plots for the same model, and we can see that there does not appear to be any serious autocorrelation between successive samples. Tables 2.8 and 2.9 also show the Geweke Z statistic (Geweke, 1992) as a means of assessing convergence. This statistic is simply based on dividing the sequence of samples into two halves and comparing them. Values of Z either below -2 or above 2 indicate evidence of a difference between the two halves. We can see from the tables that all the parameters would appear to have converged using that criterion.

As with the classical analysis of Section 2.3 we would like to extend the Bayesian semi-parametric model above to accommodate time-dependent covariates, which in the case of the ESRD study would enable us to consider the effect of albumin measured annually. In order to do this we have discretized the time scale into annual epochs, and assumed the baseline intensity to be constant within each epoch. For illustrative purposes we only consider an analysis here using a vague prior distribution for Asian, and Table 2.10 shows the results of including Albumin as both a non-time-dependent covariate and a time-dependent covariate.

We can see from Table 2.10 that the effect of Asian has changed slightly from that obtained using a much finer time scale (Table 2.8), but that qualitatively the results appear in agreement, certainly suggesting little evidence of an effect of ethnicity on all-cause mortality. In terms of the effect of albumin either at baseline or measured annually, there appears little evidence from these models that there is an effect on overall survival, though in comparing them with the classical models of Section 2.3 neither the effect of Cardiac nor Diabetes has been taken into account, and they use a different factorization of the time scale.

In terms of the model performance, again different starting values were used, together with differing lengths of 'burn-in' periods, but the model parameters appeared to be reasonably stable regardless. More specifically, the Geweke Z statistics for all the parameters in the two models are within acceptable bounds for convergence. Figure 2.10 shows the empirical and estimated hazards in each for the epochs for the first eight years of the cohort study.

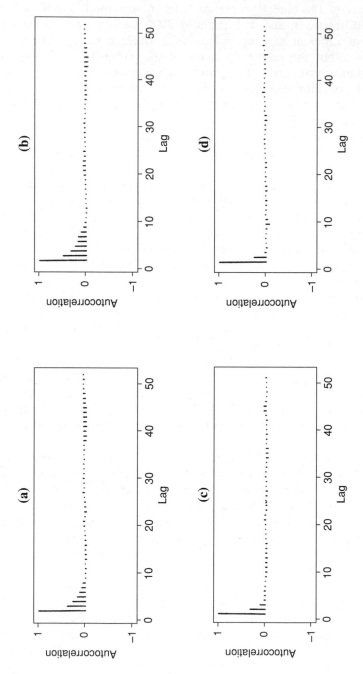

Fig. 2.9 Autocorrelations of samples from Markov chain for (a) Asian, (b) Age, (c) Cardiac and (d) Diabetes

Table 2.10 Bayesian estimates for semi-parametric regression models for all-cause mortality in the ESRD study including Albumin as both a time-dependent and independent covariate, using a 'burn-in' of 500 and a sample of 2000

Model	Parameter	Mean	SD	95% CI	Geweke Z value
Albumin at baseline	Asian	+0.430	0.258	(−0.087, +0.932)	−0.067
	Age	+0.073	0.010	(+0.054, +0.093)	−0.122
	Albumin	+0.019	0.017	(−0.015, +0.054)	0.255
Albumin as time-dependent covariate	Asian	+0.403	0.254	(−0.743, +0.894)	0.027
	Age	+0.073	0.010	(+0.055, +0.092)	0.681
	Albumin	+0.016	0.021	(−0.028, +0.059)	−0.007

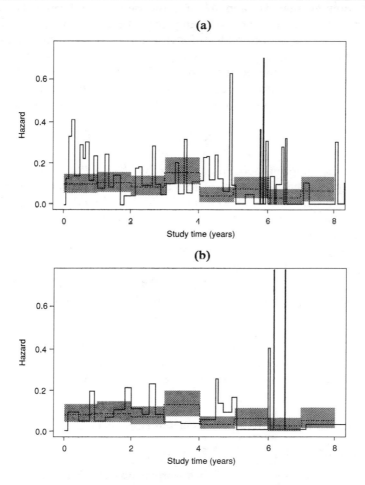

(a)

(b)

Fig. 2.10 Empirical and model-based hazard estimates for all-cause mortality in ESRD study, with follow-up restricted to eight years, (a) non-Asians and (b) Asians: ——, empirical; ······, model based)

2.5.5   Model comparison

As with the classical semi-parametric proportional hazards regression models of Section 2.3, we often wish to compare the various regression models that we have considered. One method of comparing models from a Bayesian perspective is to use what are termed *Bayes factors* (BFs) (Kass and Raftery, 1995). Consider the case when there are two models M_1 and M_2, each of which might contain different covariates (note that they are not necessarily assumed to be nested), and that we have collected data D. Then

$$\frac{P(M_1|D)}{P(M_2|D)} = \frac{P(D|M_1)}{P(D|M_2)} \times \frac{P(M_1)}{P(M_2)}$$

which, assuming that M_1 and M_2 are the only possible models under consideration, is equivalent to saying that the posterior odds of M_1 are equal to the prior odds of M_1 multiplied by the quantity $P(D|M_1)/P(D|M_2)$, which is termed the *Bayes factor*. Thus, the Bayes factor is the ratio of the posterior odds of M_1 to the prior odds of M_1 regardless of what the prior odds are. Though the role of the Bayes factor is similar to the likelihood ratio the actual calculation is different, as

$$P(D|M_1) = \int_{\Theta_1} P(D|M_1, \boldsymbol{\theta}_1)P(\boldsymbol{\theta}_1|M_1)d\boldsymbol{\theta}_1 \tag{2.17}$$

where $\boldsymbol{\theta}_1$ is the vector of model parameters for M_1 and $P(\boldsymbol{\theta}_1|M_1)$ is the joint prior density for the parameters of M_1. So in the calculation of the Bayes factor prior beliefs enter both in terms of the actual model parameters, as in the analysis, and in terms of prior beliefs regarding the plausibility of the various models.

There have been a variety of scales proposed on which to interpret Bayes factors, though one that appears to be a consensus is given in Table 2.11. Note, though, that the clear distinction between competing models in terms of hypothesis testing is not so evident in the interpretation of Bayes factors, but rather they convey the continuum between the plausibility of the various models.

Not only can Bayes factors be used in comparing and ultimately choosing a specific model from which to make inferences, but also they may be used in *averaging* over models, since assuming that the prior

Table 2.11 Interpretation of Bayes factors (Kass and Raftery, 1995)

$2\log_e(B_{10})$	B_{10}	Evidence against M_0
0 to 2	1 to 3	Not worth more than a bare mention
2 to 5	3 to 12	Positive
5 to 10	12 to 150	Strong
>10	>150	Decisive

probabilities of each of the models under consideration have been defined, and the Bayes factor calculated, then the posterior model probabilities will also be defined. Thus, if we wished to consider $k+1$ models $M_0, M_1, \ldots, M_k$, and had calculated Bayes factors $B_{10}, \ldots, B_{k0}$, then the posterior probability of the kth model is given by

$$P(M_k|D) = \frac{\alpha_k B_{k0}}{\sum_{j=0}^{k} \alpha_j B_{j0}}$$

where $\alpha_j = P(M_j)/P(M_0)$. If a priori we considered all models equally plausible, then $\alpha_0, \ldots, \alpha_k = 1$. Thus, if we obtain an estimate of a quantity of interest, say γ, from each model, then we can obtain an averaged estimate of this quantity, averaged over all the models under consideration. For example, the posterior mean of γ is given by

$$E[\gamma|D] = \sum_{j=0}^{k} E[\gamma|D, M_j]\, P(M_j|D)$$

and the variance of γ is given by

$$V[\gamma|D] = \sum_{j=0}^{k} \{V[\gamma|D, M_j] + (E[\gamma|D, M_j])^2\} P(M_j|D) - E[\gamma|D]^2$$

All of the above methods using Bayes factors for either comparing and choosing between competing models or averaging over models have assumed that we can calculate the Bayes factor. This is not always straightforward for a variety of reasons. The first, and most important, is that the integral in (2.17) requires evaluating. Obviously, as has been outlined above, there are a variety of estimation techniques that could be used, including the use of MCMC techniques. The second problem concerns the role of prior distributions for the model parameters. Whilst the Bayes factors are defined for the case when *proper* prior distributions are used for all parameters, when the prior distributions are *improper* the Bayes factor is not uniquely defined. This obviously raises problems, for example when we wish to perform a reference analysis using vague improper prior distributions. A number of possible solutions to the problem of Bayes factors when improper prior distributions are used have been proposed, including fractional Bayes factors (FBFs) (O'Hagan, 1994b) and intrinsic Bayes factors (IBFs) (Berger and Pericchi, 1995). However, a variety of approximations for the estimation of Bayes factors have also been proposed, and one of the most convenient is based on the Schwarz criterion/Bayes information criterion (BIC) (Kass and Raftery, 1995), which takes the form

$$\log(BF_{12}) \approx \log[P(D|\hat{\boldsymbol{\theta}}_1, M_1)] - \log[P(D|\hat{\boldsymbol{\theta}}_2, M_2)] - 0.5(d_1 - d_2)\log(n)$$

$$(2.18)$$

where $\hat{\boldsymbol{\theta}}_j$ is the MLE under M_j, d_j is the dimension of $\boldsymbol{\theta}_j$ and n is the sample

Table 2.12 Model comparison and averaging using Bayes factors for the ESRD study (γ – effect of ethnicity on all-cause mortality, model estimates obtained using vague proper prior distributions on all model parameters, all models a priori equally plausible)

Model		$\log(B_{j1})$	$P(M_j|D)$	$E[\gamma|D, M_j]$	$V[\gamma|D, M_j]$
M_1	Asian	0.0	0.00	−0.432	0.039
M_2	Asian + Age	45.8	0.06	+0.146	0.045
M_3	Asian + Age + Cardiac	47.6	0.34	+0.102	0.046
M_4	Asian + Age + Diabetes	46.6	0.12	+0.063	0.046
M_5	Asian + Age + Cardiac + Diabetes	47.9	0.48	+0.027	0.047
Model averaged		–	1.00	+0.064	0.048

size, or in a survival content the number of events. Whilst such an approximation ignores any prior distributions regarding model parameters, it is nevertheless easy to calculate and is often used as an initial analysis.

As an illustration consider the application of Bayes factors to the five models which include the covariates considered above in Table 2.8, using the approximation (2.18). Table 2.12 shows the results, including the log Bayes factor, model probabilities and the model averaged results. We can see that M_5 is the most favoured model, but with M_3 having 0.34 posterior probability, any averaged results should take account of this. The model averaged results indicate that the effect of ethnicity, as expected, is consistent with no effect, but that the level of uncertainty associated with this effect is slightly larger than if we had simply adopted a single model to make inferences from, even if this model had been M_5.

2.5.6   Parametric models

Analogous to the classical models of Section 2.4 we may wish to consider that the baseline hazard function, $\lambda_0(t)$, has a specific parametric form. Such an assumption may be made for a variety of reasons, but depending upon the aim of the analysis we may be interested in the prediction of the survival times of future patients, to which such a parametric approach leads more conveniently. Alternatively, assuming a semi-parametric model with the baseline hazard, or some function of it, modelled non-parametrically, when indeed a specific parametric model would have been more appropriate, will lead to a loss of efficiency.

Two particular approaches are possible. The semi-parametric proportional hazards model (2.1) could be extended so that $\lambda_0(t)$ is conditional upon a vector of baseline parameters, θ say, and then with suitable specification of prior distributions a posterior distribution for both θ and β could be derived. Such an approach has been considered by a number of authors (Greenhouse, 1992, Abrams *et al.*, 1996). Parameter estimation in such models can prove problematical, though for simple models in which a relatively well-behaved baseline hazard function is assumed (e.g. Weibull) and only a small number of covariates are included, model parameters may be estimated using a variety of techniques, including Laplace approximations, numerical integration techniques and MCMC outlined above. All three methods have been shown to provide consistent results in a number of applications (Abrams and Ashby, 1994).

An alternative model formulation would be to adopt the accelerated failure time models of Section 2.4. Representing the accelerated failure time model in the log-linear representation of (2.15), we can see that the model may be accommodated within a Bayesian framework by sampling from the assumed distribution of survival times either for those patients who were observed to die, or for those who are censored sampling from a left-truncated distribution, truncated at the time of censoring. In the case when we assume the survival distribution to be Weibull, such a model is of the form,

$$T_i \sim \text{Weib}[\mu_i, r]\, I[t_i, d_i]$$
$$\mu_i = \exp(\boldsymbol{\beta}^{\mathrm{T}} \mathbf{x}_i)$$
$$r \sim \text{Gamma}[a, b]$$
$$\boldsymbol{\beta} \sim N(\mathbf{c}, \Sigma)$$

where the hyperparameters a, b, $\mathbf{c}$ and Σ are specified so as to reflect a priori beliefs. In the case of the models presented $a = b = 0.001$, $\mathbf{c} = (0, \ldots, 0)^{\mathrm{T}}$, and $\Sigma_{ii} = 1000$, $\Sigma_{ij} = 0$ were used to reflect vague a priori beliefs. $I[-,-]$ is used to indicate truncation; that is, if patient i is censored then T_i is sampled from a left-truncated distribution, truncated at t_i. The four specific prior distributions outlined in Section 2.2 were used to define the elements of $\mathbf{c}$ and Σ corresponding to the effect of ethnicity. A similar model is obtained if instead the survival times are assumed to be log-normally distributed.

2.5.7   Application to example

Consider now the application of the Bayesian parametric models outlined above to the ESRD study using both a Weibull distribution and a log-normal distribution, and using the four prior distributions described in Section 2.2.

Tables 2.13–2.16 show the parameter estimates for models which include Asian, Age, Cardiac and Diabetes in the model, whilst Fig. 2.11 shows traces and kernel density estimates for the models' parameters when all covariates are included in a Weibull accelerated failure time model. We can see that the results are quite similar for the two different distribution models, certainly after taking into account the potential confounders. In

Table 2.13 Posterior estimates for the parametric regression model with Weibull baseline intensity, using a 'burn-in' of 500 and a sample of 2000

Model	Prior	Parameter	Mean	SD	95% CI	Geweke Z value
Asian	Reference	Asian	−0.467	0.198	(−0.866, −0.089)	−0.199
		Shape	0.823	0.073	(+0.707, +0.990)	−0.011
	Clinical	Asian	0.062	0.047	(−0.031, +0.158)	−0.239
		Shape	0.829	0.060	(+0.707, +0.945)	−0.507
	Data-based	Asian	−0.417	0.071	(−0.558, −0.269)	0.475
		Shape	0.819	0.055	(+0.707, +0.921)	0.543
	Equivalence	Asian	−0.134	0.101	(−0.330, +0.070)	−1.178
		Shape	0.831	0.051	(+0.721, +0.920)	3.308
Asian + Age	Reference	Asian	0.128	0.197	(−0.250, +0.525)	−0.269
		Age	0.065	0.007	(+0.051, +0.079)	−0.283
		Shape	0.923	0.074	(+0.785, +1.078)	−0.613
	Clinical	Asian	0.101	0.048	(+0.010, +0.197)	1.138
		Age	0.065	0.007	(+0.051, +0.079)	2.357
		Shape	0.951	0.071	(+0.815, +1.090)	4.692
	Data-based	Asian	−0.352	0.076	(−0.501, −0.207)	−1.676
		Age	0.060	0.007	(+0.047, +0.074)	−1.284
		Shape	0.929	0.061	(+0.791, +1.042)	−1.455
	Equivalence	Asian	0.037	0.109	(−0.172, +0.254)	0.821
		Age	0.065	0.007	(+0.051, +0.079)	1.809
		Shape	0.953	0.062	(+0.835, +1.089)	4.718

terms of the four different prior distributions we can see that for the reference, clinical and equivalence the posterior distributions are broadly in agreement, and certainly with respect to ethnicity there appears to be little evidence of an effect. However, for the data-based prior we can see that for all the six models considered, the posterior distribution for Asian is to the left of zero, indicating evidence of a beneficial effect towards Asian patients in terms of overall survival. We can see from Section 2.2 that although the standard deviation for the data-based prior is slightly larger than for the clinical prior, because of its location this has not influenced the posterior distribution sufficiently, so as to suggest the plausibility of there being no difference in survival between the two ethnic groups.

Table 2.14 Posterior estimates for the parametric regression model including Asian, Age, Cardiac and Diabetes with Weibull baseline intensity, including potential confounders using a 'burn-in' of 2000 and a sample of 8000

Prior	Parameter	Mean	SD	95% CI	Geweke Z value
Reference	Asian	−0.045	0.226	(−0.492, +0.390)	−0.756
	Age	0.061	0.008	(+0.046, +0.077)	−0.993
	Cardiac	0.523	0.182	(+0.156, +0.875)	0.168
	Diabetes	0.468	0.211	(+0.046, +0.870)	−0.158
	Shape	0.983	0.064	(+0.868, +1.132)	−0.558
Clinical	Asian	0.076	0.091	(−0.106, +0.257)	0.097
	Age	0.063	0.007	(+0.048, +0.078)	−1.730
	Cardiac	0.523	0.183	(+0.158, +0.875)	−1.050
	Diabetes	0.463	0.209	(+0.033, +0.857)	−0.866
	Shape	0.999	0.071	(+0.869, +1.142)	−1.590
Data-based	Asian	−0.374	0.074	(−0.518, −0.232)	0.106
	Age	0.056	0.007	(+0.042, +0.071)	−0.981
	Cardiac	0.555	0.185	(+0.188, +0.912)	−0.471
	Diabetes	0.513	0.214	(+0.082, +0.913)	−0.027
	Shape	0.994	0.072	(+0.862, +1.139)	−0.088
Equivalence	Asian	−0.026	0.171	(−0.364, +0.304)	−0.673
	Age	0.061	0.008	(+0.046, +0.077)	−0.385
	Cardiac	0.525	0.183	(+0.166, +0.875)	0.691
	Diabetes	0.458	0.211	(+0.031, +0.855)	0.152
	Shape	0.987	0.069	(+0.854, +1.126)	−0.238

Table 2.15 Posterior estimates for the parametric regression model with log-normal baseline intensity, using a 'burn-in' of 500 and a sample of 2000

Model	Prior	Parameter	Mean	SD	95% CI	Geweke Z value
Asian	Reference	Asian	0.671	0.278	(+0.115, +1.238)	−0.969
	Clinical	Asian	0.165	0.093	(−0.009, +0.345)	−0.715
	Data-based	Asian	−0.331	0.074	(−0.486, −0.189)	−0.080
	Equivalence	Asian	0.302	0.181	(−0.060, +0.636)	−0.089
Asian + Age	Reference	Asian	0.150	0.262	(−0.347, −0.687)	−0.943
		Age	−0.069	0.009	(−0.087, −0.053)	−1.010
	Clinical	Asian	0.105	0.095	(−0.072, +0.293)	−0.536
		Age	−0.069	0.008	(−0.086, −0.054)	−0.017
	Data-based	Asian	−0.364	0.076	(−0.516, −0.217)	0.170
		Age	−0.074	0.009	(−0.091, −0.058)	−0.416
	Equivalence	Asian	0.074	0.179	(−0.273, +0.419)	0.016
		Age	−0.069	0.008	(−0.087, −0.054)	−0.236

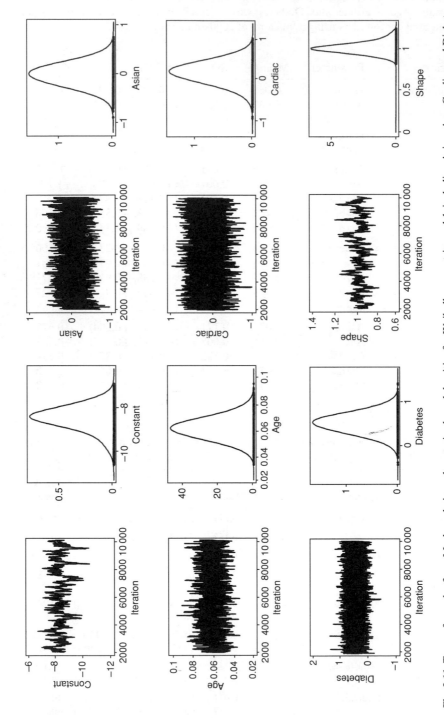

Fig. 2.11 Trace of samples from Markov chain and posterior kernel densities for Weibull parametric model, including Asian, Age, Cardiac and Diabetes

Table 2.16 Posterior estimates for the parametric regression model including Asian, Age, Cardiac and Diabetes with log-normal baseline intensity, allowing for potential confounders using a 'burn-in' of 2000 and a sample of 8000

Prior	Parameter	Mean	SD	95% CI	Geweke Z value
Reference	Asian	0.289	0.278	(−0.247, +0.839)	−0.684
	Age	−0.064	0.009	(−0.082, −0.047)	−0.391
	Cardiac	−0.616	0.257	(−1.125, −0.124)	0.436
	Diabetes	−0.482	0.304	(−1.082, +0.101)	−0.161
Clinical	Asian	0.122	0.094	(−0.064, +0.306)	0.325
	Age	−0.065	0.008	(−0.083, −0.049)	−0.276
	Cardiac	−0.609	0.256	(−1.115, −0.111)	−0.392
	Diabetes	−0.461	0.291	(−1.038, +0.111)	−0.177
Data-based	Asian	−0.360	0.076	(−0.508, −0.210)	−0.623
	Age	−0.071	0.009	(−0.089, −0.055)	−0.592
	Cardiac	−0.591	0.265	(−1.110, −0.063)	0.427
	Diabetes	−0.366	0.305	(−0.980, +0.234)	−0.462
Equivalence	Asian	0.128	0.183	(−0.237, +0.487)	−1.200
	Age	−0.065	0.009	(−0.083, −0.049)	0.603
	Cardiac	−0.610	0.257	(−1.105, −0.108)	−0.164
	Diabetes	−0.465	0.302	(−1.056, +0.124)	0.024

2.5.8 Model comparison

As with the Bayesian semi-parametric models, we are often interested in assessing the relative importance of the various covariates in the fully parametric models. However, another feature of the parametric models is that we would also like to assess the relative importance of the various survival distributions that have been assumed. In the example considered above these were a Weibull distribution and a log-normal distribution, though in many situations we may wish to consider a larger number of potential distributions. We could use the approximation techniques outlined above using BIC or we could use the fact that MCMC methods have been used to estimate the model parameters, and therefore we have a sample from the posterior distribution to estimate the Bayes factors and posterior model probabilities (Abrams and Sansó, 1997).

Suppose we have a sample θ_j, $j = 1, \ldots, m$, obtained using MCMC from the posterior distribution. Gelfand (1996) suggests that an approximation to the marginal density of the data, $P(D|\theta_k, M_k)$, for a particular model is given by

$$\hat{P}(D|M_k) = \frac{1}{(1/m) \sum_{j=1}^{m} h(\theta_j)/P(D|\theta_j)P(\theta_j)} \qquad (2.19)$$

where $h(\theta_j)$ is called an *importance density*. It turns out that $h(.)$ can be any proper density, but the better $h(.)$ approximates the posterior density the better will be the approximation to the marginal density of the data. Obviously in (2.19) if $h(\theta_j)$ and the prior density $P(\theta_j)$ are the same then they cancel and the approximation only utilizes the likelihood function. However, in such circumstances estimates of the marginal density can be unstable.

Consider the application of the methods above to the Weibull and log-normal models with just Asian and Age in them, denoting the Weibull model by M_1 and the log-normal model by M_2. Assuming that $h(\theta) = N[\hat{\mu}, \hat{\Sigma}]IG[\hat{\alpha}, \hat{\beta}]$ where $\hat{\mu}$, $\hat{\Sigma}$, $\hat{\alpha}$ and $\hat{\beta}$ are obtained from the classical analysis using maximum likelihood, an estimate for the log Bayes factor for M_1 compared with M_2 of 9.8 is obtained indicating strong evidence in favour of a Weibull model.

2.6   Discussion

This chapter has described the use of what are, currently, widely available classical regression models for the analysis of epidemiological data. The use of Bayesian regression models that allow for the formal incorporation of a priori information has also been demonstrated. Recent advances in parameter estimation techniques, in particular MCMC, now mean that these methods are becoming rapidly available in user-friendly packages such as BUGS (Thomas *et al.*, 1992). Though the use of MCMC methods allow otherwise intractable models to be applied in practice, potential users should be aware of some of the assumptions that must be verified. In particular, the issue of monitoring convergence of the Markov chain should be a mandatory requirement of any formal analysis.

The models discussed in Sections 2.2 and 2.3 have only considered one aspect of modelling survival or event data, namely the situation in which there is a single, non-recurrent, event of interest. In many situations in the ESRD study and other settings there are numerous events that are of interest, and we may be interested in estimating both the specific risks of events and the interrelationship between the various types of events. The situation in which we are interested in estimating the risk of specific events, in the presence of other (competing) risks, has an extensive literature (Collett, 1994). The situation in which we are interested in not only estimating the risks of specific events but also how the occurrence of such events affects the risk of other subsequent events, perhaps of the same type, has been less well developed (Clayton, 1988). Both of these scenarios may be included within a multi-state modelling framework, and the counting process framework outlined in Section 2.3 is ideally suited to such extensions, though, to date, such models have not been widely applied (Andersen, 1988, Abrams, 1992).

An alternative approach to the choice of survival distribution is to consider a very broad class of distributions characterized by an overall distribution, and to choose the most appropriate distribution based on the parameter estimates for that distribution. For example, the generalized *F* distribution (Stacy, 1962, Kalbfleisch and Prentice, 1980) encompasses all of the distributions mentioned above as special cases, and therefore could be initially considered to indicate which would appear to be the most appropriate. Though this approach can seem attractive, it is rarely used in practice, since the estimation of the parameters of the generalized *F* distribution can be computationally intensive, even when there is a relatively large number of events.

Another area of extension of both the Bayesian and classical models considered in this chapter is to allow for the often hierarchical nature of the data. We can think of either patients perhaps nested within centres, say in a multi-centre study, or observations nested within patients, in the case of repeated observations, such as the albumin levels recorded in the ESRD study. Such hierarchical models, which explicitly allow for the presence of within-patient/within-centre correlation, have been considered both from a classical (DeStavola, 1996) and Bayesian perspective (Stangl, 1994). One particularly important development within a Bayesian setting for such models has been in the monitoring of patients using laboratory tests by use of Bayesian hierarchical models that not only accommodate the hierarchical nature of the data (observations nested within patients), but also take advantage of the Bayesian approach in predicting future survival via the *predictive distribution* (Berzuini, 1996).

Acknowledgements

The author would like to thank Drs J. Feehally and C. B. Leung for permission to use the ESRD data and their clinical insights. He would also like to thank Peter Brecknock, David Clayton, Paul Lambert and Bruno Sansó for various discussions regarding the use of residuals and Bayesian methods in survival analysis.

References

Abrams, K. R. 1992: In discussion of Cox *et al.*: 'Quality-of-life: can we keep it simple?'. *Journal of the Royal Statistical Society (A)* **155**, 353–93.

Abrams, K. R. and Ashby, D. 1994: Parameter estimation in parametric survival models. *Technical Report*, University of Leicester.

Abrams, K. R., Ashby, D. and Errington, R. D. 1994: Simple Bayesian analysis in clinical trials – a tutorial. *Controlled Clinical Trials* **15**, 349–59.

Abrams, K. R., Ashby, D. and Errington, R. D. 1996: A Bayesian approach to Weibull survival models – application to a cancer clinical trial. *Lifetime Data Analysis* **2**, 159–74.

Abrams, K. R. and Sansó, B. 1997: Discrimination between competing parametric survival models – a Bayesian perspective. *Technical Report 97-03*, Department of Epidemiology and Public Health, University of Leicester.

Agodoa, L. Y. and Eggers, P. W. 1995: Renal replacement therapy in the United States: data from the United States renal data system. *American Journal of Kidney Diseases* **25**, 119–33.

Altman, D. G., DeStavola, B. L., Love, S. B. and Stepniewska, K. A. 1995: Review of survival analyses in cancer journals. *British Journal of Cancer* **72**, 511–18.

Andersen, P. K. 1988: Multi-state models in survival analysis: a study of nephropathy and mortality in diabetes. *Statistics in Medicine* **7**, 661–70.

Anderson, P. K. and Borgan, O. 1985: Counting process models for life history data – a review (with discussion). *Scandinavian Journal of Statistics* **12**, 97–158.

Andersen, P. K., Borgan, O., Gill, R. D. and Keiding, N. 1992: *Statistical models based on counting processes*. New York: Springer.

Anderson, P. K. and Gill, R. D. 1982: Cox's regression model for counting processes – a large sample study. *Annals of Statistics* **10**, 1100–20.

Berger, J. O. and Pericchi, L. R. 1995: The intrinsic Bayes factor for linear models. In Bernardo, J., Berger, J., Dawid, A. and Smith, A. (eds), *Bayesian statistics 5*. Oxford: Oxford University Press.

Bernardo, J. M. and Smith, A. F. M. 1993: *Bayesian theory*. Chichester: John Wiley.

Berzuini, C. 1996: Medical monitoring. In Gilks, W. R., Richardson, S. and Spiegelhalter, D. J. (eds), *Markov chain Monte Carlo methods in practice*. London: Chapman & Hall.

Breslow, N. E. 1990: Biostatisticians and Bayes (with discussion). *Statistical Science* **5**, 269–98.

Clayton, D. G. 1988: The analysis of event history data: a review of progress and outstanding problems. *Statistics in Medicine* **7**, 819–41.

Clayton, D. G. 1991: A Monte Carlo method for Bayesian inference in frailty models. *Biometrics* **47**, 467–85.

Collett, D. 1994: *Modelling survival data in medical research*. London: Chapman & Hall.

Cowie, C. C. 1993: Diabetic renal disease: racial and ethnic differences from an epidemiologic perspective. *Transplantation Proceedings* **25**, 2426–30.

Cowles, M. K., Best, N. G. and Vines, K. 1994: CODA – convergence diagnostics and output analysis software for Gibbs samples produced by the BUGS language version 0.30. *Technical Report*, MRC Biostatistics Unit, Cambridge.

Cowles, M. K. and Carlin, B. P. 1996: Markov chain Monte Carlo convergence diagnostics: a comparative review. *Journal of the American Statistical Association* **91**, 883–904.

Cox, D. R. 1972: Regression models and life-tables. *Journal of the Royal Statistical Society (B)* **39**, 187–220.

Cox, D. R. 1975: Partial likelihood. *Biometrika* **62**, 269–76.

de Bruijn, N. G. 1958: *Asymptotic methods in analysis*. New York: Dover.

DeStavola, B. L. 1996: Multilevel modelling for longitudinal variables prognostic for survival. *Lifetime Data Analysis* **2**, 329–47.

Dixon, W. J. E. 1990: *BMDP statistical software manual*, vol. 2. Berkeley, CA: University of California Press.

Fleiss, J. L. 1993: The statistical basis of meta-analysis. *Statistical Methods in Medical Research* **2**, 121–45.

Gelfand, A. E. 1996: Model determination using sampling-based methods. In Gilks, W. R., Richardson, S. and Spiegelhalter, D. J. (eds), *Markov chain Monte Carlo methods in practice*. London: Chapman & Hall.

Gelfand, A. E., Hills, S. E., Racine-Poon, A. and Smith, A. F. M. 1990: Illustration of Bayesian inference in normal data models using Gibbs sampling. *Journal of the American Statistical Association* **85**, 972–85.

Gelfand, A. E. and Smith, A. F. M. 1990: Sampling based approaches to calculating marginal densities. *Journal of the American Statistical Association* **85**, 398–409.

Gelman, A. 1996: Inference and monitoring convergence. In Gilks, W. R., Richardson, S. and Spiegelhalter, D. J. (eds), *Markov chain Monte Carlo methods in practice*. London: Chapman & Hall.

Geweke, J. 1992: Evaluating the accuracy of sampling-based approaches to calculating the posterior moments. In Berger, J. O., Bernardo, J. M., Dawid, A. P. and Smith, A. F. (eds), *Bayesian statistics 4*. Oxford: Oxford University Press, 169–94.

Gilks, W. R., Clayton, D. G., Spiegelhalter, D. J., Best, N. G., McNeil, A. J., Sharples, L. D. and Kirby, A. J. 1993: Modelling complexity: applications of Gibbs sampling in medicine. *Journal of the Royal Statistical Society (B)* **55**, 39–52.

Gilks, W. R., Richardson, S. and Spiegelhalter, D. J. 1996: *Markov chain Monte Carlo methods in practice*. London: Chapman & Hall.

Gilks, W. R. and Wild, P. 1992: Adaptive rejection sampling for Gibbs sampling. *Applied Statistics* **41**, 337–48.

Greenhouse, J. 1992: On some applications of Bayesian methods in cancer clinical trials. *Statistics in Medicine* **11**, 37–53.

Hills, S. E. and Smith, A. F. M. 1992: Parameterization issues in Bayesian inference. In Berger, J. O., Bernardo, J. M., Dawid, A. P. and Smith, A. F. M. (eds), *Bayesian statistics 4*. Oxford: Oxford University Press.

Kalbfleisch, J. D. 1978: Non-parametric Bayesian analysis of survival time data. *Journal of the Royal Statistical Society (B)* **40**, 214–21.

Kalbfleisch, J. D. and Prentice, R. L. 1980: *The statistical analysis of failure time data*. New York: John Wiley.

Kass, R. E. and Raftery, A. E. 1995: Bayes factors. *Journal of the American Statistical Association* **90**, 773–95.

Kuo, L. and Smith, A. F. M. 1992: Bayesian computations in survival models via the Gibbs sampler. In Klein, J. P. and Goel, P. K. (eds), *Survival analysis: state of the art*. Dordrecht: Kluwer Academic, 11–24.

Lowrie, E. G. 1993: Renal replacement therapy: practice, case-mix and outcome. *The Lancet* **341**, 412–13.

Mantel, N. and Haenszel, W. 1959: Statistical aspects of the analysis of data from retrospective studies of disease. *Journal of the National Cancer Institute* **22**, 719–48.

Medina, R. A., Pugh, J. A., Monterrosa, A. and Cornell, J. 1996: Minority advantage in diabetic end-stage renal disease survival on haemodialysis: due to different proportions of diabetic type? *American Journal of Kidney Diseases* **28**, 226–34.

Naylor, J. C. and Shaw, J. E. H. 1985: *Bayes four – user guide*. Department of Mathematics, University of Nottingham.

Naylor, J. C. and Smith, A. F. M. 1982: Applications of a method for the efficient computation of posterior distributions. *Applied Statistics* **31**, 214–25.

O'Hagan, A. 1994a: *Bayesian inference*, vol. 2b of *Kendall's advanced theory of statistics*. London: Edward Arnold.

O'Hagan, A. 1994b: Fractional Bayes factors for model comparison (with discussion). *Journal of the Royal Statistical Society* **56**, 99–138.

Petersen, T. 1996: Fitting parametric survival models with time-dependent covariates. *Applied Statistics* **35**, 281–88.

Pocock, S. J. 1983: *Clinical trials – a practical approach*. Chichester: John Wiley.

Ripley, B. D. 1987: *Stochastic simulation*. Chichester: John Wiley.

SAS Institute Inc. 1993: *Statistical analysis software*. Cary, NC: SAS Institute Inc.

Smith, A. F. M. and Roberts, G. O. 1993: Bayesian computation via the Gibbs sampler and related Markov chain Monte Carlo methods. *Journal of the Royal Statistical Society (B)* **55**, 3–23.

Spiegelhalter, D. J., Freedman, L. S. and Parmar, M. K. B. 1993: Applying Bayesian thinking in drug development and clinical trials. *Statistics in Medicine* **12**, 1501–11.

Stacy, E. W. 1962: A generalization of the Gamma distribution. *Annals of Mathematical Statistics* **33**, 1187–92.

Stangl, D. K. 1994: Hierarchical analysis of continuous time survival models. In Berry, D. A. and Stangl, D. K. (eds), *Bayesian biostatistics*. New York: Marcel Dekker.

Statistical Sciences Inc. 1990: *Splus for Sun workstations*. Oxford, UK, Version 2.3.

Stigler, S. M. 1986: Laplace's 1774 memoir on inverse probability. *Statistical Science* **1**, 359–62.

Thisted, R. A. 1988: *Elements of statistical computing – numerical computation*. New York: Chapman & Hall.

Thomas, A., Spiegelhalter, D. J. and Gilks, W. R. 1992: BUGS: a program to perform Bayesian inference using Gibbs sampling. In Bernardo, J., Berger, J., Dawid, A. and Smith, A. (eds), *Bayesian statistics 4*, Oxford: Oxford University Press.

Tierney, L. 1990: *XLISP-STAT – an object-oriented environment for statistical computing and dynamic graphics*. New York: John Wiley.

Tierney, L. and Kadane, J. B. 1986: Accurate approximations for posterior moments and marginal densities. *Journal of the American Statistical Association* **81**, 82–6.

Tierney, L., Kass, R. E. and Kadane, J. B. 1989: Fully exponential Laplace approximations of expectations and variances of non-positive functions. *Journal of the American Statistical Association* **84**, 710–16.

Tsiatis, A. A. 1981: The asymptotic joint distribution of the efficient scores test for the proportional hazards model calculated over time. *Biometrika* **68**, 311–15.

Whittaker, J. 1990: *Graphical models in applied multivariate analysis*. Chichester: John Wiley.

3 Frailty models

Odd O. Aalen

3.1 Introduction

Survival analysis has become one of the major fields of modern biostatistics. One might ask what justifies the image of this field as something separate from other parts of statistics. After all, survival times are measured variables just like body height, blood pressure and other quantities commonly present in medical studies.

The answer, of course, is that measuring the time of an event is actually very different from measuring some other quantity, like blood pressure. Blood pressure can be measured there and then. In order to make the time measurement, on the other hand, one has to wait for the event to occur. And one may discover that it never occurs owing to some intercepting event, or the study may end. This is the well-known problem of censoring. A host of methods have been developed to tackle this aspect, and their success is apparent when one considers how, nowadays, Kaplan–Meier plots and Cox analyses figure prominently in medical journals.

In fact there are deeper reasons for the usefulness of these special approaches. Measuring time is conceptually different from measuring other quantities. Survival curves are obviously useful descriptions of time to event data, but would not be so of blood pressure data. Cox analysis is based on the concept of hazard rate, which is a representation of the distribution function that is (almost) only of use for time to event data. The hazard rate specifies the likelihood of an event given the past, and this is meaningful precisely because past, present and future are essential aspects of time.

This brings us to the theme of this chapter. The passage of time means that features of the data that are usually ignored cannot be so anymore. One such feature is unmeasured heterogeneity between individuals. It is well known in statistical studies that even though one may have a number of explanatory variables, there is always an 'unexplained' remaining variation. In most parts of statistics this does not pose any problem, but in survival studies it does. The reason is precisely the flow of time. High risk individuals will tend to have a short survival, and the remaining ones will have lower risk, giving a selection over time. This selection causes the hazard rate to decline, or to rise less rapidly. High risk individuals may be termed 'frail'; hence the reason for the popular term 'frailty'.

One may ask why this simple and rather obvious phenomenon is seen as a problem, and a subject worth particular study. One reason is that it is very tempting to interpret the hazard rate as saying something about the development of risk within the individual. A decreasing hazard rate is often interpreted as expressing a biological phenomenon within the individual yielding a declining risk. The simple fact is that the hazard rate is not a pure measure; it expresses a mixture of the individual development and the above-mentioned selection effects. Mathematical studies have been undertaken to understand this phenomenon better; we will discuss this below.

The difficulty with the hazard rate has implications for other measures as well. In epidemiology one is interested in the ratio between hazard rates, and this is often termed relative risk (which is a term used in other senses as well). This relative risk is also vulnerable to selection. The fact that high risk individuals are selected out early may yield a decreasing relative risk between groups, even though at the individual level the importance of the risk factor does not decrease. Hence, one would usually not expect the proportional hazards assumption to hold, contrary to the general view. Even crossover phenomena may be observed where the high risk group appears, artificially, as a low risk group from a certain time on. Closely related to this is the 'false protectivity' phenomenon, where an adverse risk factor may appear, artificially, as protective. The term 'false protectivity' was introduced by Di Serio (1997).

The comparison of groups is a basic element in epidemiology. It is for instance common to compare the mortality in different countries. One may look at, say, those who are 70 years old in two countries and compare their present-day mortality. An obvious, although often ignored, complication is that in one country the people of age 70 may be a much smaller proportion of their original birth cohort than in the other country. The chances of survival may have been very different and the groups that remain may not be comparable owing to selection. This is just the phenomenon one tries to understand in frailty theory.

Hence the frailty phenomenon has fundamental implications for common statistical measures and methods in medicine and epidemiology.

We will end this introduction by returning to the difficulty of censoring. We will often have multivariate censored data (e.g. the survival of several dental fillings within an individual). This poses a problem for ordinary multivariate methods, which will have difficulty in handling censored data. If there is a large number of dependent survival times, with many of them being censored, for each of several individuals, then the normality-based variance component analysis will have a very hard time tackling this, if it is at all possible. However, the dependence may be modelled through a frailty variable, such that all survival times coming from a given individual have the same level of frailty attached to them. Such an approach to modelling dependence accommodates very well censored data and yields quite simple analysis. While for univariate data one will typically have an identifiability problem when attempting to estimate frailty models, no such problem exists in the multivariate case.

The effect of heterogeneity, or frailty, has been recognized for a long time, see, for example, Strehler and Mildvan (1960). Also the social science literature has discussions of this problem, for example Ginsberg (1971, 251–5). In fact, a very early frailty model was the 'mover–stayer' model of Blumen *et al.* (1955). The term 'frailty' was introduced by Vaupel *et al.* (1979). Other early contributors are Heckman and Singer (1982), Vaupel and Yashin (1985) and Hougaard (1984). The subject has even hit the general scientific literature (Barinaga, 1992, Carey *et al.*, 1992).

It should also be mentioned that frailty theory is closely related to the random effects models of statistics. In fact, frailty is just a random effect, or variance component. What makes it special is the role played by time and the ensuing selection effects that arise.

3.2 The proportional frailty model

The term 'frailty theory' has been primarily associated with one particular mathematical formulation of frailty: we study the time to the occurrence of a specific event, and assume that the hazard rate of an individual is given as the product of an individual specific quantity Z and a basic rate $\lambda(t)$:

$$\text{individual hazard rate} = Z \cdot \lambda(t) \tag{3.1}$$

Here Z is considered as a random variable over the population of individuals specifying the level of frailty. We will follow a common convention and assume that $E[Z] = 1$. What may be observed in a population is not the individual hazard rate, but the net result for a number of individuals with differing frailties The population survival function is

$$S(t) = E[e^{-Z\Lambda(t)}] = L(\Lambda(t))$$

where $\Lambda(t) = \int_0^t \lambda(u)\mathrm{d}u$, and $L(a)$ is the Laplace transform of Z. Of course, the population hazard rate may be derived by differentiating $-\log(S(t))$.

It was recognized by Hougaard (1984) that results in frailty theory are often elegantly formulated in terms of Laplace transforms. Hence, when applying the results one would naturally seek to use frailty distributions with a tractable Laplace transform. The most common choice is the gamma distribution with expectation 1 and variance δ, say, for which the Laplace transform, $L(a) = E[e^{-aZ}]$, is given as

$$L(a) = [1 + \delta a]^{-1/\delta} \tag{3.2}$$

The population survival and hazard rates corresponding to this Laplace transform are given as

$$S(t) = [1 + \delta \Lambda(t)]^{-1/\delta}, \quad \mu(t) = \frac{\lambda(t)}{1 + \delta \Lambda(t)} \tag{3.3}$$

respectively. It is clear from the formulae how the population hazard rate is a 'bent-down' version of the basic hazard rate. In fact, one often observes a decreasing population hazard rate when the individual hazard rate may well be increasing.

There exist many other suitable frailty distributions with explicit Laplace transforms. Hougaard (1986a) has demonstrated nice properties for the stable distributions, the inverse Gaussian distributions and also more general families. Frailty distributions of compound Poisson type were studied by Aalen (1992); these have the advantage of giving a group with zero frailty, corresponding to a non-susceptible subgroup.

What sort of shapes might one expect for actual frailty distributions? Corresponding to known risk factors, like high blood pressure and cholesterol, a log-normal or gamma frailty distribution may give a reasonable fit. It was suggested by Aalen (1988) that such a shape might be expected for the unknown risk factors too. However, this view may be too limited. With the present increasing knowledge of the importance of genetics in incidence of disease, one may possibly expect much more skewed distributions. For some diseases it has been found that a few individuals with single dominant genes might be at a much larger risk than the majority.

Unless specific assumptions are made the frailty distribution is not identifiable from univariate data. In fact, there will generally be at least two competing explanations for, say, a declining hazard rate: it could be a frailty phenomenon, and the underlying individual hazard rate could actually be increasing. The decline, however, could also reflect a real phenomenon on the individual level. For instance, the declining mortality rate for cancer patients when time from diagnosis exceeds a certain limit has been explained as reflecting a 'regenerative process operating in cancer' (Zajicek, 1983). Similarly, it has been suggested that the peak in the incidence of retinoblastoma and leukaemia in early childhood is due to the number of susceptible stem cells being at a maximum at this age (Little *et al.*, 1996, Moolgavkar and Knudson, 1981). Here, frailty would be an alternative explanation for the declining incidence from a certain age (Aalen, 1988). The dilemma is related to an old discussion on 'spurious contagion' (Feller, 1971, 57–8).

An interesting extension of the proportional frailty model with two frailty variables has been studied by Zahl (1997). Entirely different models may also be relevant (see, for example, Aalen, 1994).

3.3   The effect of frailty on relative risk

3.3.1   Declining population relative risk

The assumption of proportional hazards is very common in survival analysis. We will assume that this holds at the individual level; that is, conditioned on the frailty variables. It will be seen that the proportionality disappears at the population level. (Hougaard (1986a) has observed one exception to this, namely for stable frailty distributions.) This well-known phenomenon has implications for the Cox model: it means that if one covariate is unobservable, or excluded from the model, then proportionality is destroyed. Hence proportional hazards is a vulnerable assumption.

Assume that the basic rates in two risk groups are $\lambda(t)$ and $r \cdot \lambda(t)$, respectively, where r is a number greater than one; hence the latter group is the high risk group. With frailty variables Z_1 in group 1 and Z_2 in group 2 the simple proportional frailty model in equation (3.1) yields individual hazard rates equal to $Z_1\lambda(t)$ and $Z_2 r\lambda(t)$ respectively.

Assuming that the frailty variables have the same gamma distribution in both groups with variance δ, the population hazard rates $\mu_1(t)$ and $\mu_2(t)$ may be derived from equation (3.3) to give the following proportion:

$$\frac{\mu_2(t)}{\mu_1(t)} = r\frac{1 + \delta\Lambda(t)}{1 + r\delta\Lambda(t)} \tag{3.4}$$

This is a decreasing function in t, and hence a declining population relative risk will be observed. This observation is an old one; within the frailty framework an early paper is Vaupel *et al.* (1979).

3.3.2   Crossover phenomena

In the above case the population relative risk will always remain above one. However, with a slightly more complex situation, one may observe a *crossover*, that is the population relative risk may, after a while, fall below one, even though, at the individual level, the relative risk is always above one. This has been much discussed; see for instance the important paper by Manton and Stallard (1981). A review will be given here.

Crossover may happen in at least the following situations:

1. There is a non-susceptible subgroup (i.e. with frailty zero).

2. The relative risk at the individual level is declining.

3. The frailty variation in the two risk groups is different.

Case 1 will not be discussed here, but see for instance Aalen (1994).

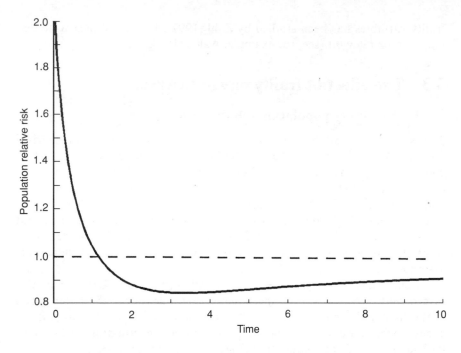

Fig. 3.1 Plot of the population relative risk for a decreasing value of the individual relative risk; see equation (3.5) with $\delta = 1$

Case 2, with a declining relative risk at the individual level, could arise for biological reasons. Maybe the damage that a risk factor could cause was most pronounced at the young ages and less pronounced at a more advanced age. To give an example, we shall assume the same situation as described in Section 3.3.1, but with r substituted by a function $r(t)$ which decreases but is always above one; that is, an individual in group 2 has all the time a higher risk than a comparable individual in group 1. To make things simple, let $\lambda(t) = 1$ and $r(t) = 1 + e^{-t}$, that is $r(t)$ declines from 2 towards 1. In this case one may derive

$$\frac{\mu_2(t)}{\mu_1(t)} = \frac{(1 + e^{-t})(1 + \delta t)}{1 + \delta t + \delta(1 - e^{-t})} \tag{3.5}$$

This function is plotted in Fig. 3.1 and is seen to fall below 1.

An interesting question, connected to the previous example, might be for which $r(t)$ might proportional hazards be observed on the population level. In fact, if the individual relative risk *increases* according to $r(t) = 2(1 + \delta t)$, then the population relative risk is exactly equal to two for all t.

We shall also give an example of case 3 above. Again, we assume the same situation as in Section 3.3.1, but with the change that Z_1 and Z_2 have different variances, denoted δ_1 and δ_2, respectively. Otherwise, they are

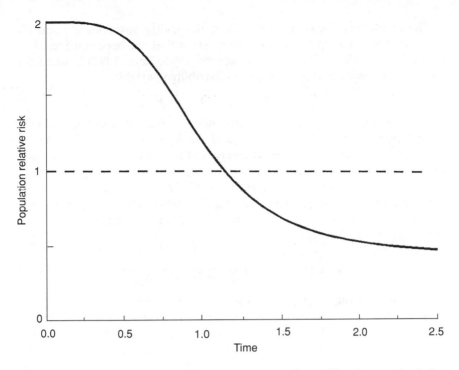

Fig. 3.2 Plot of the population relative risk when the variance differs between the frailty distributions; see equation (3.6) (parameters: $\lambda(t) = t^3, \delta_1 = 1.0, \delta_2 = 2.2, r = 2$)

gamma distributed, both with expectation 1. The population relative risk is given by a slight modification of equation (3.4), as follows:

$$\frac{\mu_2(t)}{\mu_1(t)} = r \frac{1 + \delta_1 \Lambda(t)}{1 + r\delta_2 \Lambda(t)} \qquad (3.6)$$

For an illustration we assume $\lambda(t) = t^3$, $\delta_1 = 1.0$, $\delta_2 = 2.2$ and $r = 2$. The result is shown in Fig. 3.2, which clearly demonstrates the crossover effect.

3.3.3   Competing risks and false protectivity

So far we have considered only one event that may occur to the individual. We will now consider briefly the possibility of several events, so that observation stops when the first event occurs. This is what is usually termed competing risks. An interesting discussion of competing risks in relation to frailty is given by Di Serio (1997), who also coined the term 'false protectivity' for certain paradoxical effects that may arise. A mathematical demonstration of this phenomenon is given below.

For simplicity, we will consider only two competing risks, corresponding to the two events A and B, with hazard rates at the individual level equal to $Z_A \lambda_A(t)$ and $Z_B \lambda_B(t)$.

The interesting situation arises when the frailty variables Z_A and Z_B are correlated. A simple model for correlation that has been considered by a number of authors (Yashin and Iachine, 1995, Zahl, 1997) is when the variables are sums of suitable gamma-distributed variables:

$$Z_A = Y_1 + Y_3, \qquad Z_B = Y_2 + Y_3$$

We assume that Y_1, Y_2 and Y_3 are independent and gamma distributed with expectation each equal to $1/2$, and with variances δ_1, δ_2 and δ_3 respectively. (This ensures that the expected frailty is one as elsewhere in the chapter.)

We will now concentrate on event A. Clearly, individuals at risk for experiencing this event at time t are only those for whom neither event A nor B has happened before t. The population hazard rate for event A at time t may be derived as

$$\lambda_A(t)\left(\frac{1}{2 + \delta_1\Lambda_A(t)} + \frac{1}{2 + \delta_3[\Lambda_A(t) + \Lambda_B(t)]}\right) \qquad (3.7)$$

Assume now that there is a covariate which has a causal influence on event B, but not on A. More precisely, say that $\lambda_B(t)$ increases positively with the covariate, but that $\lambda_A(t)$ is not influenced by it. From (3.7) it is apparent that the population hazard rate of A is then negatively dependent on the covariate. Hence, there is a false impression of a protective effect of the covariate on event A. This is similar to what Di Serio (1997) calls false protectivity.

A numerical example can be given as follows. Let δ_1 and δ_3 equal one and consider a specific time t_0. Assume that $\Lambda_A(t_0) = 0.2$, and that $\Lambda_B(t_0)$ is proportional to the value of a covariate s; for simplicity we put $\Lambda_B(t_0) = s$. (The covariate could be the number of cigarettes smoked or some other factor with an adverse effect on the likelihood of event B.) The term in large parentheses in equation (3.7), which we shall term the hazard ratio, is given by

$$\frac{1}{2.2} + \frac{1}{2.2 + s} \qquad (3.8)$$

This function is plotted in Fig. 3.3. The decrease in the hazard of event A when the risk factor s increases is clearly a false protectivity phenomenon.

3.3.4 Discussion

The examples clearly show that epidemiological relative risk measures are vulnerable to the frailty phenomenon. Now, what is the practical importance of this? Apparently, there are not yet many documented real-life examples of, say, crossover phenomena, although there are some possible examples like the 'black/white mortality crossover' discussed by Manton and Stallard (1981). There are also 'paradoxical' phenomena in

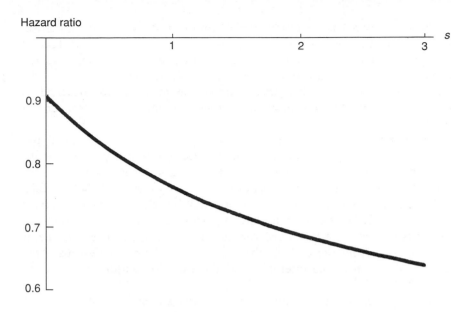

Fig. 3.3 Plot of the hazard ratio showing the effect of false protectivity; see equation (3.8)

medicine that may possibly be explained as crossovers. For instance, Langer *et al.* (1989, 1991) found that for very old men survival improved with increasing diastolic blood pressure.

As regards false protectivity, a medical example is given by Di Serio (1997). There is also medical evidence showing that cigarette smoking has a protective effect against Parkinson's disease and Alzheimer's disease. It has been suggested that this is an example of false protectivity, but the issue is not at all clear. In fact, a recent paper suggests that the phenomenon may be real (Morens *et al.*, 1996).

The point of demonstrations like the ones given here is to become aware of possibilities, so that one is actively looking for possible frailty explanations. Certainly, frailty or heterogeneity must usually be present and cannot be ignored.

3.4　Multivariate survival data

3.4.1　Examples

Data in survival analysis are usually assumed to be univariate, with one, possibly censored, lifetime for each individual. All the standard methodology, including Kaplan–Meier plots and Cox analysis, is geared to tackling this situation. However, multivariate data also arise naturally in many contexts and frailty models are ideally suited for analysing those.

There are two basic ways in which multivariate survival data arise. One, which may be termed the *repeated event model*, is when several successive events are registered for each individual, for instance repeated occurrences of ear infection. The other, which may be termed the *multiple unit model*, is when several units that may fail are attached to each individual, for instance the possible failure of several dental fillings.

An example of the repeated event model may be taken from Aalen and Husebye (1991), who analysed the cyclic pattern of motility (spontaneous movements) of the small bowel in humans. This phenomenon is very important for digestion. In the mentioned paper we studied the so-called MMC complex which travels down the small bowel at irregular intervals (these intervals lasting from minutes up to several hours). Several such intervals in a row are registered for each person, with a censored one at the end, signifying the end of observation. The task is to estimate the average duration of the intervals, and the variation within and between individuals.

An example of the multiple unit model is supplied by Aalen *et al.* (1995), who studied the duration of amalgam fillings in teeth. Each patient has a number of fillings that may fail, and one can imagine that some patients have a larger risk of failure than others owing to varying dental hygiene and other factors.

3.4.2   Likelihood

The basic question is how to model the dependence between the survival data observed for a single individual. It turns out that the proportional frailty model is the answer. This idea was developed in a number of papers, for instance Clayton (1978), Clayton and Cuzick (1985), Hougaard (1986b) and Oakes (1989).

It is assumed that to all survival times coming from a given individual there corresponds one fixed value of the frailty variable Z. Hence frailty measures the individual specific risk level. Otherwise the proportional frailty model as described in equation (3.1) is assumed. On the basis of this assumption the likelihood function is easily derived. The present model is often called the *shared frailty* model. A more sophisticated analysis may in some cases be carried out by a *correlated frailty* model resembling the one studied above for competing risks, see Yashin and Iachine (1995) or Pickles *et al.* (1994).

For individual i, let $X_{ij}, j = 1, \ldots, n_i$, denote the observation times for the n_i units or repeated intervals. The total cumulative hazard for individual i is defined as $V_i = \sum_j \Lambda(X_{ij})$. Furthermore, let $K_{ij}, j = 1, \ldots, n_i$, be binary variables that are equal to one if observation time (i, j) is uncensored and equal to zero if it is censored. Let $R_i = \sum_j K_{ij}$ denote the number of uncensored observations for individual i. The following log likelihood contribution from individual i is easily derived (see, for example, section 4.2 of Aalen and Husebye, 1991):

$$\left(\sum_{j=1}^{n_i} K_{ij} \ln(\lambda(X_{ij})) \right) + \ln\left[(-1)^{R_i} L^{(R_i)}(V_i) \right] \qquad (3.9)$$

with $L^{(k)}(a)$ denoting the kth derivative. These contributions are summed over the index i to yield the full log likelihood.

An important feature of the above likelihood is that it involves derivatives of the Laplace transform of, possibly, high order. Hence, nice frailty distributions would have Laplace transforms for which derivatives of arbitrarily high order can be given explicitly. The gamma distribution again is a prime example with simple explicit derivatives of arbitrary order. A more complex class is given by the generalized inverse Gaussian distributions which are discussed in the Appendix.

3.4.3 Empirical Bayes estimates

As in other variance component models one may be interested in estimating the level of the random factor, which is here the frailty Z, for each individual. The following formula gives the conditional expectation of Z for individual i given the observed history for this individual. The formula is a slight extension of one in Aalen and Husebye (1991):

$$E[Z|H] = -\frac{L^{(R_i+1)}(V_i)}{L^{(R_i)}(V_i)}$$

3.4.4 Duration of dental fillings

Amalgam fillings in teeth have a varying lifetime. Aalen *et al.* (1995) studied the duration of such fillings based on observation of 32 patients in dental practices in Norway. Data concerning fillings inserted over a period of more than 10 years were collected. The patients had between 4 and 38 fillings inserted during the observation period. A number of fillings were observed to fail, but also many fillings remained intact during the whole observation period and hence constituted censored data.

Note the high dimensionality of the data (up to 38 observations for an individual), and the lack of balance (the smallest number of observations for an individual being four). This, together with a large number of censored observations, makes for a situation where one has to model the dependence in just the right way in order to manage the analysis. The multivariate frailty approach described above tackles the situation elegantly.

The basic hazard rate $\lambda(t)$ is assumed to be of Weibull shape, that is of the form bt^k, with t measured in years from insertion of the specific filling. Note, here, that the time scale relates to individual fillings, so that time 0 for different fillings of a certain patient may be at widely differing ages for that patient.

For the frailty distribution we use the gamma, the Laplace transform of which can be differentiated an arbitrary number of times without difficulty. The more general family discussed in the Appendix was also tried but did not yield any improvement in this particular case.

The likelihood function for an individual i is a special case of equation (3.9) with the Laplace transform of equation (3.2). The full likelihood for m individuals is given by

$$L(b, k, \delta) = \sum_{i=1}^{m} \left[\sum_{j=1}^{n_i} K_{ij} \left\{ \ln(b) + k \ln(X_{ij}) + \ln \left[1 + \delta \left(\sum_{r=1}^{j} K_{ir} - 1 \right) \right] \right\} \right]$$

$$- \sum_{i=1}^{m} \left\{ \left(\delta^{-1} + \sum_{j=1}^{n_i} K_{ij} \right) \ln \left[1 + \frac{\delta b}{k+1} \left(\sum_{j=1}^{n_i} X_{ij}^{k+1} \right) \right] \right\}$$

The estimates are found by maximizing this log likelihood. Here, we used the program system GAUSS (Aptech, Inc.).

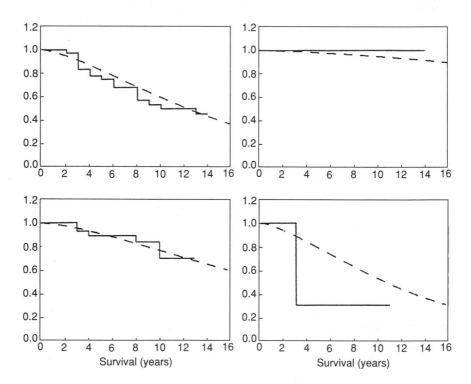

Fig. 3.4 Survival of amalgam fillings for four selected patients. The step functions are individual Kaplan–Meier survival curves. These are compared with smooth estimated survival functions computed from the frailty model

The estimates of the parameters, with SE in parentheses, are: $\hat{b} = 0.015\,(0.004)$, $\hat{k} = 0.43\,(0.10)$ and $\hat{\delta} = 0.85\,(0.31)$. There was a clearly significant frailty effect.

In order to demonstrate the results of the model, survival curves for the fillings of four selected patients are shown in Fig. 3.4. The step functions in the plots are Kaplan–Meier survival curves computed from the fillings for each individual patient. These are compared with smooth survival functions computed as follows. For each patient an empirical Bayesian estimate of the frailty, denoted $\hat{Z}$, is computed. The individual survival curve for this patient is then estimated by the Weibull survival function $\exp\{-\hat{Z}[\hat{b}/(\hat{k}+1)]t^{\hat{k}+1}\}$.

The two left-hand plots in Fig. 3.4 show the results for patients with large numbers of fillings inserted (37 and 26 respectively for the upper and lower plots). Apparently, the fit is good. The two right-hand plots of Fig. 3.4 show results for two patients with few fillings inserted (10 and 4 respectively for the upper and lower plots) and few observed failures (0 and 3 respectively). One sees here that the survival curves computed from the parametric model deviate somewhat from the Kaplan–Meier plot, indicating the empirical Bayes shrinkage towards the mean.

The general impression from considering all data was that the simple parametric frailty gave a well-fitting and compact description.

Appendix

As stated above, useful frailty distributions for likelihood analysis of multivariate survival data should have Laplace transforms with explicit derivatives of any order. One important case is the class of generalized inverse Gaussian distributions, with density

$$f(z, \lambda, \psi, \chi) = \frac{(\psi/\chi)^{\lambda/2}}{2K_\lambda(\sqrt{\chi\psi})} z^{\lambda-1} \exp\left[-\frac{1}{2}\left(\frac{\chi}{z} + \psi z\right)\right] \quad z, \psi, \chi \geq 0$$

where $K_\lambda(x)$ is a modified Bessel function of order λ. Such Bessel functions are available numerically in several packages, for instance Mathematica (see Wolfram, 1991, 576). Notice that the family of gamma distributions is a special case, putting $\chi = 0$. Introductions to generalized inverse Gaussian distributions are given by Jørgensen (1980) and Chhikara and Folks (1989).

One advantage in the frailty context is that these distributions may be more skewed than the gamma distributions; some examples are shown in Fig. 3.5.

The Laplace transform is given by

$$L(a, \lambda, \psi, \chi) = [\psi/(2a + \psi)]^{\lambda/2} K_\lambda[\sqrt{\chi(2a + \psi)}]/K_\lambda(\sqrt{\chi\psi})$$

for which the kth derivative with respect to a is

Density

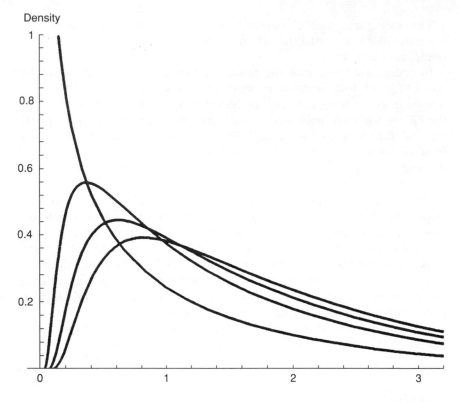

Fig. 3.5 Densities of generalized inverse Gaussian distributions ($f(z, 0.5, \psi, 1.0)$, with ψ equal to 0.001, 0.5, 1.0 and 1.5, respectively

$$(-1)^k(\chi/\psi)^{k/2}[\psi/(2a+\psi)]^{k+\lambda/2}K_{k+\lambda}[\sqrt{\chi(2a+\psi)}]/K_\lambda(\sqrt{\chi\psi})$$

This may be proved by induction from standard properties of the modified Bessel function.

References

Aalen, O. O. 1988: Heterogeneity in survival analysis. *Statistics in Medicine* **7**, 1121–37.

Aalen, O. O. 1992: Modelling heterogeneity in survival analysis by the compound Poisson distribution. *Annals of Applied Probability* **2**, 951–72.

Aalen, O. O. 1994: Effects of frailty in survival analysis. *Statistical Methods in Medical Research* **3**, 227–43.

Aalen, O. O., Bjertness, E. and Sønju, T. 1995: Analysis of dependent survival data applied to lifetimes of amalgam fillings. *Statistics in Medicine* **14**, 1819–29.

Aalen, O. O. and Husebye, E. 1991: Statistical analysis of repeated events forming renewal processes. *Statistics in Medicine* **10**, 1227–40.

Barinaga, M. 1992: Mortality: overturning received wisdom. *Science* **258**, 398–99.

Blumen, I., Kogan, M. and MacCarthy, P. 1955: *Industrial mobility of labor as a probability process.* Ithaca, NY: Cornell University Press.

Carey, J. R., Liedo, P., Orozco, D. and Vaupel, J. W. 1992: Slowing of mortality rates at older ages in large medfly cohorts. *Science* **258**, 457–61.

Chhikara, R. S. and Folks, J. L. 1989: *The inverse Gaussian distribution*. New York: Marcel Dekker.

Clayton, D. 1978: A model for association in bivariate life tables and its applications in epidemiological studies of familial tendency in chronic disease incidence. *Biometrika* **65**, 141–51.

Clayton, D. and Cuzick, J. 1985: Multivariate generalizations of the proportional hazards model (with discussion). *Journal of the Royal Statistical Society (A)* **148**, 82–117.

Di Serio, C. 1997: The problem of protectivity of a risk factor in the presence of competing risks events: an example from bone marrow transplantation study. *Lifetime Data Analysis* **3**, 91–122.

Feller, W. 1971: *An introduction to probability theory and it applications*. New York: John Wiley.

Ginsberg, R. B. 1971: Semi-Markov processes and mobility. *Journal of Mathematical Sociology* **1**, 233–62.

Heckman, J. J. and Singer, B. 1982: Population heterogeneity in demographic models. In Land, K. and Rogers, A. (eds), *Multidimensional mathematical demography*. Orlando, FL: Academic Press.

Hougaard, P. 1984: Life table methods for heterogeneous populations: distributions describing the heterogeneity. *Biometrika* **71**, 75–83.

Hougaard, P. 1986a: Survival models for heterogeneous populations derived from stable distributions. *Biometrika* **73**, 387–96.

Hougaard, P. 1986b: A class of multivariate failure time distributions. *Biometrika* **73**, 671–8.

Jørgensen, B. 1980: Statistical properties of the generalized inverse Gaussian distribution. *Lecture notes in statistics*, vol. 9. New York: Springer.

Langer, R. D., Ganiats, T. G. and Barrett-Connor, E. 1989: Paradoxical survival of elderly men with high blood pressure. *British Medical Journal* **298**, 1356–7.

Langer, R. D., Ganiats, T. G. and Barrett-Connor, E. 1991: Factors associated with paradoxical survival at higher blood pressures in the very old. *American Journal of Epidemiology* **134**, 29–38.

Little, M. P., Muirhead, C. R. and Stiller, C. A. 1996: Modelling lymphocytic leukaemia incidence in England and Wales using generalizations of the two-mutation model of carcinogenesis of Moolgavkar, Venzon and Knudson. *Statistics in Medicine* **15**, 1003–22.

Manton, K. G. and Stallard, E. 1981: Methods for evaluating the heterogeneity of aging processes in human populations using vital statistics data: explaining the black/white mortality crossover by a model of mortality selection. *Human Biology* **53**, 47–67.

Moolgavkar, S. H. and Knudson, A. G. 1981: Mutation and cancer: a model for human carcinogenesis. *Journal of the National Cancer Institute* **66**, 1037–52.

Morens, D. M., Grandinetti, A., Davis, J. W., Ross, G. W., White, L. R. and Reed, D. 1996: Evidence against the operation of selective mortality in explaining the association between cigarette smoking and reduced occurrence of idiopathic Parkinson disease. *American Journal of Epidemiology* **144**, 400–4.

Oakes, D. 1989: Bivariate survival models induced by frailties. *Journal of the American Statistical Association* **84**, 487–93.

Pickles, A., Crouchley, R., Simonoff, E., Eaves, L., Meyer, J., Rutter, M., Hewitt, J. and Silberg, J. 1994: Survival models for developmental genetic data: age at onset of puberty and antisocial behavior in twins. *Genetic Epidemiology* **11**, 155–70.

Strehler, B. L. and Mildvan, A. S. 1960: General theory of mortality and aging. *Science* **132**, 14–21.

Vaupel, J. W., Manton, K. G. and Stallard, E. 1979: The impact of heterogeneity in individual frailty on the dynamics of mortality. *Demography* **16**, 439–54.

Vaupel, J. W. and Yashin, A. I. 1985: The deviant dynamics of death in heterogeneous populations. *Sociological Methodology*. San Francisco: Jossey-Bass, 179–211.

Wolfram, S. 1991: *Mathematica: a system for doing mathematics by computer*, 2nd edn. Menlo Park, CA: Addison-Wesley.

Yashin, A. I. and Iachine, I. 1995: How long can humans live? Lower bound for biological limit of human longevity calculated from Danish twin data using correlated frailty model. *Mechanisms of Ageing and Development* **80**, 147–69.

Zahl, P.-H. 1997: Frailty modelling for the excess hazard. *Statistics in Medicine* **16**, 1573–85.

Zajicek, G. 1983: On the improving chances of the cancer patient. *Medical Hypotheses* **12**, 369–76.

4 Risk set sampling designs for proportional hazards models

Ørnulf Borgan and Bryan Langholz

4.1 Introduction

Cox's regression model (Cox, 1972) and similar proportional hazards models are central to modern survival analysis, and they are the methods of choice when one wants to assess the influence of risk factors and other covariates on mortality or morbidity. Estimation in such proportional hazards models is based on Cox's partial likelihood (see (4.2) below), which at each observed death or disease occurrence (failure) compares the covariate values of the failing individual with those of all individuals at risk at the time of the failure. In large epidemiological cohort studies of a rare disease, (standard) use of proportional hazards models requires collection of covariate information on all individuals in the cohort even though only a small fraction of these actually get diseased. This may be very expensive, or even logistically impossible. Cohort sampling techniques, where covariate information is collected for all failing individuals (cases), but only for a sample of the non-failing individuals (controls), then offer useful alternatives which may drastically reduce the resources that need to be allocated to a study. Further, as most of the statistical information is contained in the cases, such studies may still be sufficient to give reliable answers to the questions of interest.

The most common cohort sampling design is nested case–control sampling, where for each case a small number of controls are selected at random from those at risk at the case's failure time, and where a new sample of controls is selected for each case. This risk set sampling technique was first suggested by Thomas (1977), who proposed to base inference on a modification of Cox's partial likelihood. This suggestion was supported by the work of Prentice and Breslow (1978), who derived the same expression as a conditional likelihood for time-matched case–control sampling from an infinite population. A more decisive, but still heuristic, argument was provided by Oakes (1981), who showed that one indeed gets a partial likelihood when the sampling of controls is performed within the actual finite cohort. It took more than 10 years, however, before Goldstein and Langholz (1992) proved rigorously that the estimator of the regression coefficients based on Oakes' partial likelihood enjoys similar large sample properties as ordinary maximum likelihood estimators.

Goldstein and Langholz's paper initiated further work on risk set sampling methodology, and important progress has been achieved during the last few years both with respect to its theoretical foundation and the development of new methodology of practical importance. The key to this progress has been to model jointly the occurrence of failures and the sampling of controls as a marked point process (Borgan *et al.*, 1995). This marked point process formulation not only gives a more direct proof of Goldstein and Langholz's result; it also solves the problem of how to estimate the baseline hazard rate from nested case–control data, and it makes it simple to study other useful sampling schemes for the controls. In particular Borgan and Langholz (1993) discussed baseline hazard estimation for Cox's model for the relative mortality, while Langholz and Borgan (1995) studied a stratified version of nested case–control sampling, which they denoted counter matching, using this machinery. (Counter matching was first proposed and studied by Langholz in a technical report using the approach of Goldstein and Langholz, 1992.)

The purpose of this chapter is to give a fairly non-technical review of this development. We do want to give the readers a flavour of the general theory, however, so we present heuristic arguments for many of our results – arguments which may be made rigorous using marked point processes, counting processes and martingales (see Borgan *et al.* (1995) for a detailed study of Cox's regression model). The outline of the chapter is as follows. In Section 4.2 we first introduce a proportional hazards model with a general relative risk function and give some specific examples of such models including Cox's regression model. Then we describe the type of failure time data we consider for the cohort and remind the readers about the usual methods of inference for cohort data. In Section 4.3 the sampling of controls is discussed. We first review nested case–control sampling, and in particular point out how this design may be described by a uniform sampling distribution over the sets of potential controls. Then we describe in detail counter-matched (or stratified) sampling of the controls, and here as well we specify the sampling design in terms of its sampling distribution over sets of potential controls. Finally in this section, we introduce a general framework for the sampling of controls including nested case–control sampling and counter-matched sampling as special cases. In Section 4.4 we derive a partial likelihood, generalizing Oakes' (1981) partial likelihood, for estimation of the regression coefficients. Section 4.5 is concerned with estimation of cumulative hazard rates from case–control data. We review how the cumulative baseline hazard rate may be estimated, and show how this forms the basis for estimation of cumulative hazard rates for individuals with given covariate histories. In Sections 4.2–4.5 we consider for simplicity proportional hazards models with a common baseline hazard rate for all individuals. In Section 4.6 this is relaxed by allowing the baseline hazard to differ between population strata. It is discussed how such stratified models are related to matching in epidemiological studies, and how one at the analysis stage may 'pool' baseline hazard estimates across population strata when a matched design has been used but turned out not to be really necessary. Sections 4.7 and 4.8 provide illustrations and extensions of the theory reviewed in earlier sections. In Section 4.7 the methods are illustrated by studying the effect of radon exposure and smoking on the risk of lung cancer deaths among a cohort of uranium miners from the Colorado Plateau, while in Section 4.8 we discuss a new design using neighbourhood-stratified counter matching. In the final Section 4.9 we compare the application of the methods in our two examples.

4.2 Model and inference for cohort data

We consider a cohort of n individuals and denote by $\lambda_i(t) = \lambda(t; \mathbf{z}_i(t))$ the hazard rate at time t for an individual i with vector of covariates $\mathbf{z}_i(t) = (z_{i1}(t), \ldots, z_{ip}(t))'$. Here the time variable t may be age, time since employment, or some other time scale relevant to the problem at hand. The covariates may be time fixed (like gender) or time dependent (like cumulative exposure), and they may be indicators for categorical covariates (like the exposure groups 'non-exposed', 'low', 'medium', and 'high') or numeric (as when actual amount of exposure is recorded). We assume that the covariates of individual i are related to its hazard rate by the proportional hazards model

$$\lambda_i(t) = \lambda_0(t) r(\boldsymbol{\beta}, \mathbf{z}_i(t)) \tag{4.1}$$

Here $r(\boldsymbol{\beta}, \mathbf{z}_i(t))$ is a relative risk function, $\boldsymbol{\beta} = (\beta_1, \ldots, \beta_p)'$ is a vector of regression coefficients describing the effect of the covariates, while the baseline hazard rate $\lambda_0(t)$ is left unspecified. We normalize the relative risk function by assuming $r(\boldsymbol{\beta}, \mathbf{0}) = 1$. Thus $\lambda_0(t)$ corresponds to the hazard rate of an individual with all covariates identically equal to zero. For the exponential relative risk function $r(\boldsymbol{\beta}, \mathbf{z}_i(t)) = \exp(\boldsymbol{\beta}' \mathbf{z}_i(t))$, formula (4.1) gives the usual Cox regression model. Other possibilities include the linear relative risk function $r(\boldsymbol{\beta}, \mathbf{z}_i(t)) = 1 + \boldsymbol{\beta}' \mathbf{z}_i(t)$ and the excess relative risk model $r(\boldsymbol{\beta}, \mathbf{z}_i(t)) = \prod_{j=1}^{p}[1 + \beta_j z_{ij}(t)]$. Even though it is not made explicit in our notation, we will also allow for an 'offset' in the model, that is a covariate for which no regression parameter is estimated. One such example is Cox's regression model for the relative mortality (Andersen *et al.*, 1985, Borgan and Langholz, 1993).

The individuals in the cohort may be followed over different periods of time, that is, our observations may be subject to left truncation and/or right censoring. The risk set $\mathcal{R}(t)$ is the collection of all individuals who are under observation just before time t, and $n(t) = |\mathcal{R}(t)|$ is the number at risk at that time. We let $t_1 < t_2 < \ldots$ be the times when failures are observed and, assuming that there are no tied failures, denote by i_j the index of the individual who fails at t_j (a few ties may be broken at random). We assume throughout that truncation and censoring are independent in the sense that the additional knowledge of which individuals have entered the study or have been censored before any time t do not carry information on the risks of failure at t (see sections III.2–3 in Andersen *et al.* (1993), for a general discussion). Then the vector of regression parameters in (4.1) is estimated by $\hat{\beta}$, the value of β maximizing Cox's partial likelihood

$$L_c(\beta) = \prod_{t_j} \frac{r(\beta, \mathbf{z}_{i_j}(t_j))}{\sum_{l \in \mathcal{R}(t_j)} r(\beta, \mathbf{z}_l(t_j))} \tag{4.2}$$

The cumulative baseline hazard rate $\Lambda_0(t) = \int_0^t \lambda_0(u)\mathrm{d}u$ is estimated by the Breslow estimator

$$\hat{\Lambda}_0(t) = \sum_{t_j \le t} \frac{1}{\sum_{l \in \mathcal{R}(t_j)} r(\hat{\beta}, \mathbf{z}_l(t_j))} \tag{4.3}$$

It is well known that $\hat{\beta}$ enjoys similar large sample properties as an ordinary maximum likelihood estimator, while the Breslow estimator (properly normalized) is asymptotically distributed as a Gaussian process (e.g. Andersen *et al.*, 1993, section VII.2). In particular $\hat{\Lambda}_0(t)$ is asymptotically normally distributed for any given value of t.

4.3   Sampling of controls

From (4.2) and (4.3) it is seen, as already indicated in the introduction, that covariate information is needed for all individuals at risk in order to apply the usual inference methods for cohort data. A similar methodology is available when we only have covariate information for the failing individuals (cases) and control individuals sampled from those at risk at the times of the failures. We will review this methodology in Sections 4.4 and 4.5. But before we do that, we need to describe more precisely how the controls are selected. We will first consider the nested case–control design and counter-matched sampling, which are the two most important risk set sampling techniques. Then we will describe a general framework for the sampling of controls which contain these two as special cases.

4.3.1   Nested case–control sampling

Consider the 'classical' nested case–control design due to Thomas (1977). Here, if an individual i fails at time t, one selects $m - 1$ controls by simple

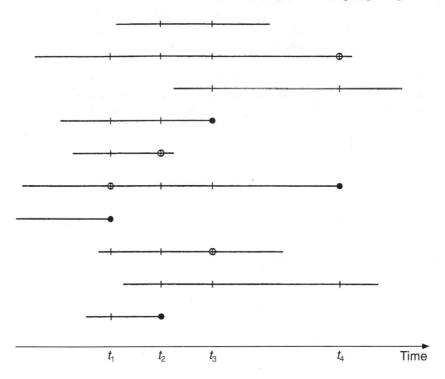

Fig. 4.1 Illustration of risk set sampling, with one control per case, from a hypothetical cohort of 10 individuals. Each individual is represented by a line starting at an entry time and ending at an exit time corresponding to censoring or failure. Failure times are indicated by full circles (•), non-failing individuals at risk at the failure times are indicated by bars (|) and the sampled controls are indicated by open circles (o)

random sampling (without replacement) from the $n(t) - 1$ non-failing individuals in the risk set $\mathcal{R}(t)$. The set $\tilde{\mathcal{R}}(t)$ consisting of the case i and these $m - 1$ controls is denoted the sampled risk set. Note that sampling is done independently across risk sets so that subjects may serve as controls for multiple cases and cases may serve as controls for other cases that failed when the case was at risk.

Figure 4.1 illustrates the basic features of a nested case–control study for a small hypothetical cohort of 10 individuals with one control selected per case (i.e. $m = 2$). Each individual in the cohort is represented by a horizontal line starting at some entry time and ending at some exit time. If the exit time corresponds to a failure, this is represented by a '•' in the figure. In the hypothetical cohort considered, four individuals are observed to fail. The potential controls for these four cases are indicated by a '|' in the figure, and are given as all non-failing individuals at risk at the times of the failures. Among the potential controls one is selected at random as indicated by a 'o' in the figure. The four sampled risk sets are then represented by the four •, o pairs in Fig. 4.1.

In what follows we will not only need to know which individuals were actually selected as controls. For the inference procedures discussed in Sections 4.4 and 4.5, it is crucial also to know the probability of selecting certain sets of individuals as our controls. It turns out to be convenient to describe the sampling scheme for the controls by the conditional probability of selecting a given set $\mathbf{r}$ as our sampled risk set $\tilde{\mathcal{R}}(t)$, given that an individual i fails at time t and given the risk set $\mathcal{R}(t)$. Since the $m-1$ controls are selected at random among the $n(t)-1$ non-failing individuals at risk, we have

$$\Pr\big(\tilde{\mathcal{R}}(t) = \mathbf{r} \mid i \text{ fails at } t, \mathcal{R}(t)\big) = \binom{n(t)-1}{m-1}^{-1} = \binom{n(t)}{m}^{-1}\frac{n(t)}{m} \quad (4.4)$$

for any set $\mathbf{r} \subset \mathcal{R}(t)$ which contains i and is of size $|\mathbf{r}| = m$. Here the last equality follows since

$$\binom{n(t)}{m} = \binom{n(t)-1}{m-1}\frac{n(t)}{m}$$

Note that the rightmost expression in (4.4) gives a factorization into a probability distribution

$$\pi_t(\mathbf{r}) = \binom{n(t)}{m}^{-1} I(|\mathbf{r}| = m) \quad (4.5)$$

over sets $\mathbf{r} \subset \mathcal{R}(t)$ and a weight

$$w_i(t) = \frac{n(t)}{m} I(i \in \mathbf{r}) \quad (4.6)$$

This factorization will be useful below.

4.3.2 Counter matching

To select a nested case–control sample, only the at-risk status of the individuals in the cohort is needed. Often, however, some additional information is available for all cohort members, for example a surrogate measure of exposure, like type of work or duration of employment, may be available for everyone. Langholz and Borgan (1995) have developed a stratified version of the nested case–control design which makes it possible to incorporate such information into the sampling process in order to obtain a more informative sample of controls. For this design, called counter matching, one applies the additional information on the cohort subjects to classify each individual at risk into one of, say, L strata. We denote by $\mathcal{R}_l(t)$ the subset of the risk set $\mathcal{R}(t)$ which belongs to stratum l, and let $n_l(t) = |\mathcal{R}_l(t)|$ be the number at risk in this stratum just before time t. If a failure occurs at t, we want to sample our controls such that the sampled risk set will contain m_l individuals from each stratum $l = 1, \ldots, L$. This is obtained as follows. Assume that an individual i who belongs to stratum $s(i)$ fails at t. Then for $l \neq s(i)$ one samples randomly without replacement m_l controls from $\mathcal{R}_l(t)$. From the case's stratum $s(i)$ only $m_{s(i)} - 1$ controls are sampled. The failing individual i is, however, included in the sampled risk set $\tilde{\mathcal{R}}(t)$, so this contains a total of m_l from each stratum. Even though it is not made explicit in the notation, we note that the classification into strata may be time dependent. A crucial assumption, however, is that the information on which the stratification is based has to be known just before time t.

In probabilistic terms, counter-matched sampling may be described as follows. For any given set $\mathbf{r} \subset \mathcal{R}(t)$ which contains i and satisfies $|\mathbf{r} \cap \mathcal{R}_l(t)| = m_l$ for $l = 1, \ldots, L$, we have

$$\Pr\left(\tilde{\mathcal{R}}(t) = \mathbf{r} \mid i \text{ fails at } t, \mathcal{R}_l(t); l = 1, \ldots, L\right)$$

$$= \left[\binom{n_{s(i)}(t) - 1}{m_{s(i)} - 1} \prod_{l \neq s(i)} \binom{n_l(t)}{m_l}\right]^{-1} = \left[\prod_{l=1}^{L} \binom{n_l(t)}{m_l}\right]^{-1} \frac{n_{s(i)}(t)}{m_{s(i)}} \quad (4.7)$$

Note that the last expression gives a factorization into a probability distribution

$$\pi_t(\mathbf{r}) = \left[\prod_{l=1}^{L} \binom{n_l(t)}{m_l}\right]^{-1} I(|\mathbf{r} \cap \mathcal{R}_l(t)| = m_l; l = 1, \ldots, L) \quad (4.8)$$

over sets $\mathbf{r} \subset \mathcal{R}(t)$ and a weight

$$w_i(t) = \frac{n_{s(i)}(t)}{m_{s(i)}} I(i \in \mathbf{r}) \quad (4.9)$$

By counter matching, one may be able to increase the variation in the value of the covariate of main interest within each sampled risk set, and this will increase the statistical efficiency for estimating the corresponding regression coefficient. In particular, if this covariate is binary, and we select one control per case, concordant pairs (i.e. the case and its control have the same value of the covariate) do not give any information in estimating the effect of the covariate. For a counter-matched design with $L = 2$ and $m_1 = m_2 = 1$, and where stratification is based on a surrogate correlated with the covariate of interest, the single control is selected from the opposite stratum of the case. This will reduce the number of concordant pairs, and thereby increase the information contained in the matched pairs of cases and controls. The situation with two strata and one control per case also gives a motivation for the name counter matching. As the name suggests, it is essentially the opposite of matching, where the case and its control are from the same stratum (cf. Section 4.6).

4.3.3 General sampling designs

In order to describe a general model for the sampling of controls, we first need to introduce 'the history' $\mathcal{F}_{t-}$, which contains information about events (entries, exits, changes in covariate values) in the cohort as well as on the sampling of controls, up to, but not including, time t. Only part of this information, like the numbers at risk in different strata, will be available to the researcher in a case–control study. Based on the information which actually is available just before time t, one decides on a sampling strategy for the controls. This may be described in probabilistic terms as follows. If an individual i fails at time t, the set $\mathbf{r} \subset \mathcal{R}(t)$ is selected as our sampled risk set $\tilde{\mathcal{R}}(t)$ with probability $\pi_t(\mathbf{r} \mid i)$. The sampled risk set consists of the case and its controls, so we let $\pi_t(\mathbf{r} \mid i) = 0$ when $i \notin \mathbf{r}$. With this convention $\pi_t(\cdot \mid i)$ is a probability distribution over all sets $\mathbf{r} \subset \mathcal{R}(t)$. Note that for nested case–control sampling and counter-matched sampling, $\pi_t(\mathbf{r} \mid i)$ is given by (4.4) and (4.7), respectively. The full cohort study is also a special case of this general framework in which the full risk set is sampled with probability 1, that is $\pi_t(\mathbf{r} \mid i) = I(\mathbf{r} = \mathcal{R}(t))$ for all $i \in \mathcal{R}(t)$. Other designs (quota sampling and counter matching with additionally randomly sampled controls) are discussed by Borgan *et al.* (1995) and Langholz and Goldstein (1996). We note that the sampling of controls may depend in an arbitrary way on events in the past (which are known to the researcher), that is on events which are contained in $\mathcal{F}_{t-}$. It may, however, not depend on events in the future. For example, one may not exclude as potential controls for a current case individuals that subsequently fail.

In connection with (4.4) and (4.7), we introduced a factorization of the relevant $\pi_t(\mathbf{r} \mid i)$ into a sampling distribution $\pi_t(\mathbf{r})$ over sets $\mathbf{r} \subset \mathcal{R}(t)$ and a weight $w_i(t)$. A similar factorization is possible for the general case as well. To this end we introduce

$$\pi_t(\mathbf{r}) = n(t)^{-1} \sum_{l=1}^{n} \pi_t(\mathbf{r} \mid l) \tag{4.10}$$

which is a probability distribution over all sets $\mathbf{r} \subset \mathcal{R}(t)$. The formulae (4.5) and (4.8) are special cases of (4.10). We also introduce the weights

$$w_i(t) = \frac{\pi_t(\mathbf{r} \mid i)}{n(t)^{-1} \sum_{l=1}^{n} \pi_t(\mathbf{r} \mid l)} \tag{4.11}$$

and note that (4.6) and (4.9) are special cases of this formula. (It should be realized that the general weights (4.11), as well as the special cases (4.6) and (4.9), do depend on the set $\mathbf{r}$. We have, however, chosen not to make this explicit in the notation.) Corresponding to (4.4) and (4.7), we then have the factorization

$$\Pr(\tilde{\mathcal{R}}(t) = \mathbf{r} \mid i \text{ fails at } t, \mathcal{F}_{t-}) = \pi_t(\mathbf{r} \mid i) = \pi_t(\mathbf{r})w_i(t) \tag{4.12}$$

for sets $\mathbf{r} \subset \mathcal{R}(t)$.

For all the sampling designs, we assume that the selection of controls is done independently at the different failure times, so that an individual may be a member of more than one sampled risk set. Further, a basic assumption throughout is that not only the truncation and censoring, but also the sampling of controls, are independent in the sense that the additional knowledge of which individuals have entered the study, have been censored or have been selected as controls before any time t does not carry information on the risks of failure at t. This assumption will be violated if, for example, in a prevention trial, individuals selected as controls change their behaviour in such a way that their risk of failure is different from similar individuals who have not been selected as controls. If we introduce [dt) as a shorthand notation for the small time interval $[t, t + \mathrm{d}t)$, the above independence assumption and (4.1) imply that

$$\Pr(i \text{ fails in } [\mathrm{d}t) \mid \mathcal{F}_{t-}) = r(\boldsymbol{\beta}, \mathbf{z}_i(t))\lambda_0(t)\mathrm{d}t \qquad (4.13)$$

when $i \in \mathcal{R}(t)$.

4.4 Partial likelihood and estimation of the regression coefficients

Estimation of the regression coefficients in (4.1) is based on a partial likelihood which may be derived in a similar manner as Cox's partial likelihood (4.2) for the full cohort. Heuristically the argument goes as follows. Consider a set $\mathbf{r} \subset \mathcal{R}(t)$ and an individual $i \in \mathbf{r}$. Then by (4.12) and (4.13)

$$\Pr(i \text{ fails in } [\mathrm{d}t), \tilde{\mathcal{R}}(t) = \mathbf{r} \mid \mathcal{F}_{t-})$$
$$= \Pr(i \text{ fails in } [\mathrm{d}t) \mid \mathcal{F}_{t-}) \times \Pr(\tilde{\mathcal{R}}(t) = \mathbf{r} \mid i \text{ fails at } t, \mathcal{F}_{t-})$$
$$= r(\boldsymbol{\beta}, \mathbf{z}_i(t))\lambda_0(t)\mathrm{d}t \times \pi_t(\mathbf{r} \mid i) = r(\boldsymbol{\beta}, \mathbf{z}_i(t))w_i(t)\pi_t(\mathbf{r})\lambda_0(t)\mathrm{d}t \qquad (4.14)$$

Now the sampled risk set equals $\mathbf{r}$ if one of the individuals in $\mathbf{r}$ fails, and the remaining ones are selected as controls. Therefore

$$\Pr(\text{one failure in } \mathbf{r} \text{ in } [\mathrm{d}t), \tilde{\mathcal{R}}(t) = \mathbf{r} \mid \mathcal{F}_{t-}) = \sum_{l\in\mathbf{r}} r(\boldsymbol{\beta}, \mathbf{z}_l(t))w_l(t)\pi_t(\mathbf{r})\lambda_0(t)\mathrm{d}t$$

$$(4.15)$$

Dividing (4.14) by (4.15), it follows that

$$\Pr(i \text{ fails at } t \mid \text{one failure in } \mathbf{r} \text{ at } t, \tilde{\mathcal{R}}(t) = \mathbf{r}, \mathcal{F}_{t-}) = \frac{r(\boldsymbol{\beta}, \mathbf{z}_i(t))w_i(t)}{\sum_{l\in\mathbf{r}} r(\boldsymbol{\beta}, \mathbf{z}_l(t))w_l(t)}$$

$$(4.16)$$

We then multiply together conditional probabilities of the form (4.16) for all observed failure times t_j, cases i_j, and sampled risk sets $\tilde{\mathcal{R}}(t_j)$, and obtain the partial likelihood

$$L_s(\boldsymbol{\beta}) = \prod_{t_j} \frac{r(\boldsymbol{\beta}, \mathbf{z}_{i_j}(t_j))w_{i_j}(t_j)}{\sum_{l\in\tilde{\mathcal{R}}(t_j)} r(\boldsymbol{\beta}, \mathbf{z}_l(t_j))w_l(t_j)} \qquad (4.17)$$

This is similar to the full cohort partial likelihood (4.2), except that the sum in the denominator only is taken over the sampled risk set $\tilde{\mathcal{R}}(t_j)$ and that the contribution of each individual (including the case) has to be weighted by $w_l(t_j)$ to compensate for the differences in the sampling probabilities. In fact, (4.2) is the special case of (4.17) in which the entire risk set is sampled with probability 1 and all weights are unity. Inference concerning $\boldsymbol{\beta}$, using the usual large sample likelihood methods, can be based on the partial likelihood (4.17). In particular the maximum partial likelihood estimator $\hat{\boldsymbol{\beta}}$ is approximately multinormally distributed around the true parameter vector $\boldsymbol{\beta}$ with a covariance matrix that may be estimated as $\mathcal{I}(\hat{\boldsymbol{\beta}})^{-1}$, the inverse of the observed information matrix. Formal proofs, along the lines of Andersen and Gill (1982), are provided by Borgan *et al.* (1995) for Cox's regression model.

Note that for nested case–control sampling, the weights (4.6) are the same for all individuals and hence cancel from (4.17) giving Oakes' (1981) partial likelihood. In fact, the above heuristic derivation of (4.17) is parallel to the one originally given by Oakes for simple random sampling of the controls. Borgan *et al.* (1995) made this argument rigorous and extended it to general sampling designs using a marked point processes formulation.

When we have an exponential relative risk function $r(\boldsymbol{\beta}, \mathbf{z}_i(t)) = \exp(\boldsymbol{\beta}', \mathbf{z}_i(t))$, the partial likelihood (4.17) is formally the same as a weighted conditional logistic regression likelihood used in the analysis of matched case–control studies. Standard software packages which have modules for the analysis of matched case–control studies, such as SAS PHREG, EGRET, EPILOG or EPICURE, may therefore be used to estimate $\boldsymbol{\beta}$. The weights are accommodated by including the weight as a covariate and fixing the parameter associated with it to one. The package EPICURE fits a wide variety of relative risk functions $r(\boldsymbol{\beta}, \mathbf{z}_i(t))$ and was used to estimate parameters from the data of the Colorado Plateau uranium miners in Section 4.7.

4.5   Estimation of cumulative hazard rates

The cumulative baseline hazard rate $\Lambda_0(t) = \int_0^t \lambda_0(u)\mathrm{d}u$ can be estimated by

$$\hat{\Lambda}_0(t; \hat{\boldsymbol{\beta}}) = \sum_{t_j \leq t} \frac{1}{\sum_{l \in \tilde{\mathcal{R}}(t_j)} r(\hat{\boldsymbol{\beta}}, \mathbf{z}_l(t_j)) w_l(t_j)} \tag{4.18}$$

The estimator (4.18) is of the same form as the Breslow estimator (4.3) for cohort data, but with the same modifications as for the partial likelihood (4.17). Here as well the full cohort estimator is obtained as the special case where the entire risk set is sampled with probability 1 and all weights are unity. The estimator (4.18) was first introduced by Borgan and Langholz (1993) for nested case–control studies in the context of Cox's model for the relative mortality. Borgan *et al.* (1995) considered general sampling designs and studied the large sample properties of (4.18) for

Cox's regression model using the theory for counting processes, martingales and stochastic integrals.

The following heuristic argument gives a motivation for the estimator (4.18). Consider the increment over [dt] of $\hat{\Lambda}_0(t; \boldsymbol{\beta})$ defined as in (4.18), but with $\hat{\boldsymbol{\beta}}$ replaced by the true value $\boldsymbol{\beta}$. This increment equals

$$1 \Big/ \sum_{l \in \tilde{\mathcal{R}}(t)} r(\boldsymbol{\beta}, \mathbf{z}_l(t)) w_l(t) \tag{4.19}$$

if a failure occurs at t and the sampled risk set is $\tilde{\mathcal{R}}(t)$, and is zero otherwise. By (4.15), and since (4.10) is a probability distribution over sets $\mathbf{r} \subset \mathcal{R}(t)$, it follows that, given $\mathcal{F}_{t-}$, the expected value of the increment is

$$\sum_{\mathbf{r} \subset \mathcal{R}(t)} \frac{1}{\sum_{l \in \mathbf{r}} r(\boldsymbol{\beta}, \mathbf{z}_l(t)) w_l(t)} \times \mathrm{Pr}\,(\text{one failure in } \mathbf{r} \text{ in } [\mathrm{d}t], \tilde{\mathcal{R}}(t) = \mathbf{r} \mid \mathcal{F}_{t-})$$

$$= \sum_{\mathbf{r} \subset \mathcal{R}(t)} \frac{\sum_{l \in \mathbf{r}} r(\boldsymbol{\beta}, \mathbf{z}_l(t)) w_l(t) \pi_t(\mathbf{r}) \lambda_0(t) \mathrm{d}t}{\sum_{l \in \mathbf{r}} r(\boldsymbol{\beta}, \mathbf{z}_l(t)) w_l(t)}$$

$$= \sum_{\mathbf{r} \subset \mathcal{R}(t)} \pi_t(\mathbf{r}) \lambda_0(t) \mathrm{d}t = \lambda_0(t) \mathrm{d}t$$

that is the increment of $\Lambda_0(t)$ over [dt]. Thus (4.18) is almost unbiased when averaged over all possible failure and sampled risk set occurrences; see Borgan *et al.* (1995) for a rigorous argument using martingales.

Let us then consider estimation of the cumulative hazard rate

$$\Lambda(t; \mathbf{z}_0) = \int_0^t r(\boldsymbol{\beta}_0; \mathbf{z}_0(u)) \lambda_0(u) \mathrm{d}u = \int_0^t r(\boldsymbol{\beta}_0; \mathbf{z}_0(u)) \mathrm{d}\Lambda_0(u)$$

corresponding to an individual with a specified time-dependent covariate history $\mathbf{z}_0(u)$; $0 < u \le t$. By (4.19) this may be estimated by

$$\hat{\Lambda}(t; \mathbf{z}_0) = \sum_{t_j \le t} \frac{r(\hat{\boldsymbol{\beta}}, \mathbf{z}_0(t_j))}{\sum_{l \in \tilde{\mathcal{R}}(t_j)} r(\hat{\boldsymbol{\beta}}, \mathbf{z}_l(t_j)) w_l(t_j)} \tag{4.20}$$

In order to estimate the variance of (4.20), we introduce

$$\hat{\omega}^2(t; \mathbf{z}_0) = \sum_{t_j \le t} \left(\frac{r(\hat{\boldsymbol{\beta}}, \mathbf{z}_0(t_j))}{\sum_{l \in \tilde{\mathcal{R}}(t_j)} r(\hat{\boldsymbol{\beta}}, \mathbf{z}_l(t_j)) w_l(t_j)} \right)^2$$

and

$$\hat{\mathbf{B}}(t; \mathbf{z}_0) = \sum_{t_j \le t} \left(\frac{\dot{r}(\hat{\boldsymbol{\beta}}; \mathbf{z}_0(t_j))}{\sum_{l \in \tilde{\mathcal{R}}(t_j)} r(\hat{\boldsymbol{\beta}}; \mathbf{z}_l(t_j)) w_l(t_j)} - \frac{r(\hat{\boldsymbol{\beta}}; \mathbf{z}_0(t_j)) \sum_{l \in \tilde{\mathcal{R}}(t_j)} \dot{r}(\hat{\boldsymbol{\beta}}; \mathbf{z}_l(t_j)) w_l(t_j)}{\left[\sum_{l \in \tilde{\mathcal{R}}(t_j)} r(\hat{\boldsymbol{\beta}}; \mathbf{z}_l(t_j)) w_l(t_j) \right]^2} \right)$$

with

$$\dot{r}(\boldsymbol{\beta}; \mathbf{z}(u)) = \frac{\partial}{\partial \boldsymbol{\beta}} r(\boldsymbol{\beta}; \mathbf{z}(u))$$

Then $\hat{\Lambda}(t; \mathbf{z}_0)$ is asymptotically normally distributed around its true value $\Lambda(t; \mathbf{z}_0)$ with a variance that may be estimated by

$$\widehat{\mathrm{var}}(\hat{\Lambda}(t; \mathbf{z}_0)) = \hat{\omega}^2(t; \mathbf{z}_0) + \hat{\mathbf{B}}(t; \mathbf{z}_0)'\mathcal{I}(\hat{\beta})^{-1}\hat{\mathbf{B}}(t; \mathbf{z}_0) \qquad (4.21)$$

(Langholz and Borgan, 1997). Here the leading term on the right-hand side is due to the variability in estimating the hazard while the second term accounts for the variability due to the estimation of the relative risk parameters β. Note that the variance estimator for the cumulative baseline hazard rate estimator (4.18) is the special case of (4.21) obtained by letting $\mathbf{z}_0(t) = \mathbf{0}$ for all t. Note also that if the cumulative hazard rate $\Lambda(s, t; \mathbf{z}_0) = \int_s^t r(\beta; \mathbf{z}_0(u))\lambda_0(u)\mathrm{d}u$ over the interval $(s, t]$ is to be estimated, the above formulae still apply provided that the sums are restricted to the failure times t_j falling in this interval.

4.6   Matching and pooling

In order to keep the presentation simple, we have so far considered the proportional hazards model (4.1) where the baseline hazard rate is assumed to be the same for all individuals in the cohort. Sometimes this may not be reasonable; for example, to control for the effect of one or more confounding factors, one may want to adopt a stratified version of (4.1) where the baseline hazards differ between (possibly time-dependent) population strata generated by the confounders. The regression coefficients are, however, assumed to be the same across these strata. Thus the hazard rate of an individual i from population stratum c is assumed to take the form

$$\lambda_i(t) = \lambda_{0c}(t)r(\beta, \mathbf{z}_i(t)) \qquad (4.22)$$

When the stratified proportional hazards model (4.22) applies, the sampling of controls should be restricted to those at risk in the same population stratum as the case. We say that the controls are matched by the stratification variable. In particular for a matched nested case–control study, if an individual in population stratum c fails at time t, one selects at random $m - 1$ controls from the $n_c(t) - 1$ non-failing individuals at risk in this population stratum. Similarly one may combine matching and counter matching by selecting the controls among those in the sampling strata used for counter matching which belong to the population stratum of the case.[1] In general one obtains a matched case–control study by restricting the sampling distributions to those which only give positive probability to sets contained in the population stratum of the case.

---

[1] It is important to distinguish between the population strata which form the basis for stratification in (4.22) and the sampling strata used for counter-matched sampling of the controls. This distinction will be illustrated for the uranium miners' data in the following section. There the population strata will correspond to different calendar periods, while counter matching will be based on cumulative radon exposure.

The general theory of Sections 4.3–4.5 goes through almost unchanged for matched case–control sampling within the framework of the stratified proportional hazards model (4.22) provided one uses the sampling distribution $\pi_t(\mathbf{r})$ and weights $w_i(t_j)$ relevant to the sampling design. For sets $\mathbf{r}$ and individuals i in population stratum c these may be obtained from (4.10) and (4.11) if we replace $n(t)$ by $n_c(t)$, the number at risk in population stratum c just before time t, and restrict the sums to those individuals l who belong to this population stratum. In particular for a matched case–control study using a counter-matched design for control selection, the proper weights are $w_i(t_j) = n_{s(i),c}(t_j)/m_{s(i)}$. Here $s(i)$ denotes the sampling stratum of individual i, while $n_{s(i),c}(t_j)$ is the number of individuals at risk in sampling stratum $s(i)$ who also belong to the population stratum c of the case.

It follows that the partial likelihood (4.17) applies without modification for a matched case–control study provided one uses the proper weights as just described. Further, when there is only a small number of strata, the stratum-specific cumulative baseline hazard rates $\Lambda_{0c}(t) = \int_0^t \lambda_{0c}(u)du$ may be estimated using these weights by a slight modification of (4.18). All that is required is that the sum is restricted to those failure times t_j when a failure in the actual population stratum occurs. When there are many population strata, however, there may be too little information in each stratum to make estimation of the stratum-specific cumulative baseline hazard rates meaningful.

If the estimates for the stratum-specific cumulative baseline hazard rates turn out to be quite similar (so that matching was not really necessary in the first place), one may at the analysis stage want to 'pool' over the population strata to get a common estimator for the cumulative baseline hazard rate. Such a procedure is a special case of the results of Section 4.5. For assuming the model (4.1) with a common baseline hazard across the population strata, the general theory applies with the sampling probability distribution (4.12) giving zero probability to all sets $\mathbf{r}$ not contained in the population stratum of the case. It follows that the common cumulative baseline hazard may be estimated by (4.18), with variance estimator obtained from (4.21), using weights $w_i(t_j)$ which for population stratum c equal those used in the matched analysis times $n(t_j)/n_c(t_j)$. In particular for counter-matched sampling of the controls within each population stratum, the weights equal $w_i(t_j) = (n_{s(i),c}(t_j)/m_{s(i)}) \times (n(t_j)/n_c(t_j))$.

4.7 Lung cancer deaths among uranium miners

Our first illustration uses data from a cohort of uranium miners from the Colorado Plateau and repeats to some extent material earlier published by Langholz and Goldstein (1996) and Langholz and Borgan (1997).

4.7.1   Data and model

The cohort of the Colorado Plateau uranium miners was assembled to study the effects of radon exposure and smoking on mortality rates and has been described in detail in earlier publications (e.g. Lundin *et al.*, 1971, Hornung and Meinhardt, 1987). We will focus on lung cancer mortality. The cohort consists of 3347 Caucasian male miners recruited between 1950 and 1960 and was traced for mortality outcomes to 31 December 1982, by which time 258 lung cancer deaths were observed. Exposure data included radon exposure, in working level months (WLMs) (Committee on the Biological Effects of Ionizing Radiation, 1988, 27), and smoking histories, in number of packs of cigarettes (20 cigarettes per pack) smoked per day.

We consider age as the basic time scale and, as there has been a well-known secular trend in lung cancer rates in the general US population, calendar time was treated as a matching factor with levels defined as the six five-year periods 1950–4, 1955–9, . . . ,1975–9 and 1980–4. Although covariate information is available on all cohort subjects, in order to illustrate the methods we selected nested case–control and counter-matched samples with one and three controls per case from the risk sets formed by the case's age and his five-year calendar period at death. These data sets are denoted 1:1 and 1:3 nested case–control and counter-matched samples, respectively. The 23 tied failure times were broken randomly so that there was only one case per risk set. Following Langholz and Goldstein (1996), counter matching was based on radon exposure grouped into two or four strata according to the quartiles of the cumulative radon exposure for the cases, and one control was sampled at random from each stratum except the one of the case. Details are provided in Section 4.5 in the paper by Langholz and Goldstein; cf. in particular their table 2. Such a counter-matched design is useful for situations where exposure data (here radon) are available for everyone, while confounder information (here smoking) has to be collected from the case–control data, the goal being to assess the effect of the exposure after controlling for the confounder. If data on the exposure of main interest (here radon) are not available for everyone, one option is to counter-match on duration of employment used as a surrogate for exposure, and then collect precise exposure and confounder information for the sampled data (Steenland and Deddens, 1997).

We summarized the radon and smoking data into cumulative exposure up to two years prior to the age of death of the case. Thus, we consider as covariates $\mathbf{z}(t) = (R(t), S(t))$, where $R(t)$ is cumulative radon exposure measured in working level months (WLMs) up to two years prior to age t, and $S(t)$ is cumulative smoking in number of packs smoked up to two years prior to t. As has been the case in previous analyses of these data (Whittemore and McMillan, 1983, Lubin *et al.*, 1994, Thomas *et al.*, 1994), the excess relative risk model was used. Thus the hazard rate is assumed to take the form $\lambda(t) = \lambda_{0c}(t)[1 + \beta_R R(t)][1 + \beta_S S(t)]$ for the cth calendar period; cf. (4.22).

4.7.2　Relative and absolute risk

The regression parameter estimates are given in Table 4.1 for the different sampling designs. It is seen that both radon and smoking have a significant effect on the risk of lung cancer death when adjusted for the effect of the other, and that both the nested case–control designs and the counter-matched designs give estimates quite close to those obtained from the full cohort. The radon excess relative risk is about 0.4 per 100 WLMs cumulative radon exposure for all designs, while the smoking excess relative risk is about 0.2 per 1000 packs of cigarettes smoked. As expected the 1:1 nested case–control design has the largest standard errors, about twice the size of those from the full cohort. Counter matching gives a substantial improvement in the precision of the estimates of the radon excess relative risk; for example, the 1:1 counter-matched sample gives a more precise estimate of β_R than the 1:3 sample with simple random sampling of the controls. Usually counter matching will reduce the precision of estimates of parameters of less importance (Langholz and Borgan, 1995, Langholz and Goldstein, 1996). Here, however, the estimates of β_S based on simple and stratified sampling of the controls have the same precision. This may be due to the commonness of smoking in the cohort and the fact that it is relatively uncorrelated to radon (Langholz and Clayton, 1994, table 4).

We first estimated the cumulative baseline hazard separately for each calendar period. As these turned out to be quite similar, we decided to pool the estimates as described in Section 4.6 to get an estimate for the cumulative baseline hazard valid for all calendar periods. These 'pooled' estimates are shown in Fig. 4.2 for cohort data and the four case–control data sets. The sampled data give cumulative baseline hazard estimates which are somewhat lower than the full cohort. Not surprisingly, the 1:3

Table 4.1 Estimated regression coefficients (with standard errors) per 100 WLMs cumulative radon exposure and per 1000 packs of cigarettes smoked for the stratified excess relative risk model $\lambda(t) = \lambda_{0c}(t)[1 + \beta_R R(t)][1 + \beta_S S(t)]$ for various risk set sampling designs

Sampling design	Radon (β_R)	Smoke (β_S)
1:1 nested case–control	0.42 (0.20)	0.23 (0.10)
1:1 counter-matched	0.39 (0.14)	0.25 (0.10)
1:3 nested case–control	0.43 (0.16)	0.20 (0.07)
1:3 counter-matched	0.41 (0.13)	0.19 (0.07)
Cohort	0.38 (0.11)	0.17 (0.05)

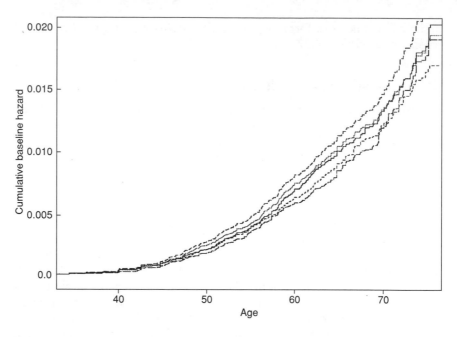

Fig. 4.2 Estimated cumulative baseline hazard $\int_0^t \lambda_0(u)du$ of lung cancer deaths as a function of age from the excess relative risk model $\lambda(t) = \lambda_0(t)(1 + \beta_R R(t))(1 + \beta_S S(t))$ with common baseline hazard for all calendar periods (given from the lowest to the highest at age 60 years): 1:1 nested case–control (— — — —); 1:1 counter-matched (- - - - - - -); 1:3 nested case–control (————); 1:3 counter-matched (············); cohort (– – – –)

case–control data sets give estimates closer to the full cohort than the 1:1 sampled data, and for a given number of controls counter matching gives a slight improvement compared with nested case–control sampling. The differences between the estimates are not big, however, and even the two 1:1 case–control data sets give fairly reliable estimates of the cumulative baseline hazard. This is further illustrated in Table 4.2 where the first line of each panel (no radon, no smoking) gives the increment of the cumulative baseline hazard estimates over the age intervals 40–9, 50–9 and 60–9 years for cohort data and the two 1:1 case–control data sets.

We then computed the cumulative hazard for a given radon exposure history with constant exposure intensity described by the age a at start of exposure, the duration d of exposure, and total exposure. Thus, the two-year lagged cumulative radon exposure $R(t)$ is zero for $t < a + 2$, then increases linearly up to the total exposure at $t = a + d + 2$, and is constant at the total exposure thereafter. Smoking was described by the number of packs per day, and we assumed that smoking began at age 20 and continued throughout life at the same level. The increments of such cumulative hazard rate estimates over the age intervals 40–9, 50–9, and 60–9 years are given in Table 4.2 for cohort data and the two 1:1 case–control data sets with 95% confidence intervals based on the log-

Table 4.2 Risk (95% confidence interval), in per cent, of lung cancer death with specific radon and smoking histories during ages 40–9, 50–9, and 60–9

Age interval	Total dose* (WLMs)	Smoking (packs/day)	Full cohort	1:1 simple	1:1 counter matched
40–9	0	0	0.24 (0.13–0.44)	0.16 (0.06–0.42)	0.19 (0.07–0.48)
	480	0.5	1.0 (0.7–1.4)	0.8 (0.6–1.2)	1.0 (0.7–1.4)
	960	1.0	2.3 (1.7–3.1)	2.0 (1.4–2.9)	2.4 (1.7–3.3)
50–9	0	0	0.5 (0.3–1.0)	0.4 (0.2–1.0)	0.4 (0.2–1.1)
	480	0.5	3.2 (2.5–3.9)	2.9 (2.3–3.8)	3.0 (2.4–3.9)
	960	1.0	7.9 (6.4–9.6)	7.7 (5.7–10.5)	8.0 (6.2–10.4)
60–9	0	0	0.7 (0.4–1.3)	0.6 (0.2–1.6)	0.6 (0.2–1.5)
	480	0.5	4.5 (3.5–5.9)	5.2 (3.9–7.0)	5.0 (3.8–6.6)
	960	1.0	11.7 (9.2–15.0)	14.3 (10.1–20.2)	13.7 (10.1–18.6)

* Assuming a constant rate of radon exposure for a period of 30 years starting at age 20

transform. The estimates can be interpreted as estimating the absolute risk of lung cancer deaths in those for whom the only reason they would have died during the age interval would be because of lung cancer.[2] There are only small differences in the risk estimates for the two 1:1 sampled data sets, and both of them provide estimates (and standard errors) quite close to what one obtains from the full cohort.

4.8 Neighbourhood-stratified counter matching

Our second example illustrates another, though quite different, application of the idea of counter matching. We first review the problem which motivated the development of this particular design. Then the design is described in detail, and we discuss how it fits into our general framework. Some power calculations are also reviewed.

4.8.1 Background

Motivated by the results of a field study that suggested that the homes of children who developed cancer were found unduly often near electric lines carrying high currents, Wertheimer and Leeper (1979) undertook an epidemiological study to investigate the possibility that electromagnetic fields (EMFs), generated by power lines, are associated with childhood

---

[2] The estimates based on the cumulative hazard estimator give a slight overestimate of risk. However, the difference between these and exact estimates based on a Kaplan–Meier-type estimator are of little importance in the situation we consider (Langholz and Borgan, 1997).

cancer. They introduced a classification of residences based on 'wire codes' as surrogate measures for residential exposure to magnetic fields. The wire code categories are based on the assumption that outdoor power lines and grounding systems are a dominant source of long term magnetic field exposure throughout the residence and are ranked according to the theorized magnetic field strength. In their case–control study, Wertheimer and Leeper found a gradient in the rate of cancer with increasing wire code. While this finding has not been reproduced in all subsequent studies,[3] two important case–control studies found similar patterns of relative risks as the Wertheimer–Leeper study, with the largest wire code association observed with childhood leukaemia (Savitz et al., 1988, London et al., 1991). The highest category defined in the wire code classification scheme used in these studies is 'very high current configuration' (VHCC) and the largest increase in risk of childhood leukaemia is observed in this category. In fact, even pooling all the other categories and classifying homes as VHCC+ and VHCC−, the observed rate of childhood leukaemia in the VHCC+ is about twice that of the VHCC−. While each of these studies may be subject to various types of selection or information bias, the findings find some support in a population-based Swedish study which did not use the wire code classifications used in the American studies but classified homes primarily according to 'transmission line exposure'. This study found an association and is apparently devoid of such biases (Feychting and Ahlbom, 1995). The wire code–childhood leukaemia association is especially intriguing given that there is relatively little variation in the rates of childhood leukaemia over geography, gender and ethnicity, and that, aside from ionizing radiation and Down's syndrome, there are no known risk factors. Since VHCCness per se cannot cause childhood leukaemia, it must be correlated with some factor, presumed to be EMF, that does. And, unless very highly correlated, this factor must be much more highly associated with childhood leukaemia than VHCC status. Thus, it would be expected that the relative risks associated with direct measurements of EMFs, which motivated the categorization of homes with respect to power lines in the first place, would be much higher than those found with VHCC status. However, case–control studies in which extensive EMF measurements were made in the homes of participating subjects have, thus far, failed to show much of an association with childhood leukaemia. One possibility is that power line configuration is a better indicator of long term EMF exposure than the short term measurements made in the homes in these studies. A second possibility is that EMF is not causing childhood leukaemia and that the observed association is due to the correlation of power line configuration with another factor that is aetiologically relevant. It is primarily the

---

[3] A recently released study by the United States National Institutes of Health found no gradient with wire code (Linet et al., 1997).

investigation of the latter possibility that motivates the use of a 'neighbourhood-stratified counter-matched design'.

4.8.2 The design

The study design was developed in collaboration with H. Wachtel and R. Pearson of Radian Corporation, K. Ebi of the Electric Power Research Institute, and D. Thomas of the University of Southern California. We wanted the design to be 'highly valid', by which we mean that there should be little chance that the results could be due to selection and information bias. Further, childhood leukaemia is a very rare disease so each case should be used efficiently in the study. To this end, we wanted to exploit the ability to wire-code large numbers of homes at relatively low cost using computerized geographical information system methods. In this situation, wire code is the 'exposure' variable and we wish to investigate other factors that might explain the wire code–childhood leukaemia association. As we discussed in the context of the uranium miners' cohort, counter matching would be an advantageous design for this problem. However, we do not have a well-defined cohort from which to draw our sample. The solution is to define a neighbourhood-stratified cohort, wire code those neighbourhoods that have cases, and select counter-matched controls based on the within-neighbourhood risk sets determined by the case. Ignoring many of the practical aspects of organizing and implementing an epidemiologic study, the resulting neighbourhood-stratified counter-matched study can be broken down into the following design-related steps:

1. Identify incident case through the cancer registry.

2. Wire code a defined neighbourhood[4] (VHCC+ vs. VHCC−) surrounding the case's residence at diagnosis. If there is no variation in VHCC status across the entire neighbourhood (this may be the situation in newer developments where all wiring is buried), the case–neighbourhood set will be uninformative and so will be dropped from the study.

3. For neighbourhoods with variation in VHCC status, survey the neighbourhood to find the addresses of all eligible controls (children of a 'similar' age, i.e. in the risk set, approximately matched on year of birth).

4. From each neighbourhood, form counter-matched sets of one VHCC+ and two VHCC− subjects. That is, if the case is VHCC+ then

---

[4] The definition of the neighbourhood is a topic worthy of further discussion. But, here, we will assume that some sensible method of forming the neighbourhood would be used.

randomly sample two VHCC— controls from all those eligible. If the case is VHCC—, then randomly sample one VHCC— and one VHCC+ control. The two VHCC—, one VHCC+ configuration was chosen based on power considerations described below.

5. The counter-matched sampled subjects would then be enrolled in the study and information on potential explanatory factors would be collected for the case and its two controls.

Note that the study provides two data sets: (i) the *case–neighbourhood* data set consisting of the cases and their neighbourhood controls (selected according to 3), and (ii) the *neighbourhood-stratified counter-matched* data set consisting of the cases and their two counter-matched controls (selected according to 4). Within the framework of cohort sampling, the case–neighbourhood data set represents the risk set data from a full cohort with one stratum for each neighbourhood. In particular, VHCC status is known (from step 2) for each subject in these risk sets at the failure time so that the full cohort partial likelihood analysis of VHCC is possible (see below). The neighbourhood-stratified counter-matched data set is sampled from the cohort risk sets as described in Sections 4.3.2 and 4.6. So, after collecting potential explanatory factor information in step 5, the counter-matched sampled risk sets consist of one case and two controls, two of the set VHCC— and one VHCC+, with all the information needed for the partial likelihood analysis of VHCC status and potential explanatory factors.

The availability of, quality of, and data collection expense associated with a particular covariate depend on many factors such as the availability of a centralized resource, whether field measurements are needed, or whether the subject's participation is required. The overall design has some flexibility to exploit low cost information and efficiently collect high cost information. For instance, in the case–neighbourhood data set, the information on VHCC status could be supplemented by information on other factors that vary across neighbourhoods and are inexpensive to collect for entire neighbourhoods (e.g. it may be possible to calculate traffic density measures for each address from existing computerized records). If information on a covariate is too expensive to collect for the case–neighbourhood set, but does not require actual contact with study subjects (e.g. air and soil samples to assess the presence of environmental pollutants), this may be done on the entire counter-matched sample. Finally, if contact with study subjects is required (e.g. to assess parents' occupations and smoking status), then the counter-matched set would be used but would typically consist of fewer sets because of refusals to participate in the study. Unlike the case–neighbourhood and counter-matched sets that do not require subject participation, this latter counter-matched set would be subject to potential biases if these refusals differ systematically between cases and controls with regard to VHCC or other factors of interest. This is true for any study where interviews are required. But, because the case–neighbourhood set defines the entire study group (risk set), it is possible to assess the extent of such a bias, at least with respect to VHCC status.

4.8.3 Analysis

From the perspective of Section 4.2, the cohort under study is the entire childhood population serviced by the cancer registry. This cohort is followed for the period of time that the study enrols cases. This period then determines the entry and exit times for subjects in this amorphous cohort. The underlying hazard model is stratified, as in (4.22) of Section 4.6, with a separate baseline hazard for each neighbourhood and interval of years of birth. The analysis of relative risk from the case–neighbourhood data set and the neighbourhood-stratified counter-matched sample use the partial likelihood methods for the full cohort and risk set sampled data, respectively. Because the cohort is highly stratified, the estimation of the stratum-specific cumulative hazards is not meaningful. In addition, the pooled cumulative hazard, as described in Section 4.6, cannot be estimated because the number of subjects in the unstratified risk set (i.e. all potential controls in the registry coverage area) is not known.

From the characterization of the case–neighbourhood data as the risk sets from the neighbourhood (and year of birth) stratified cohort study over the registry coverage area, it is clear that (a stratified version of) the cohort partial likelihood (4.2) applies. Because neighbourhoods with no cases do not contribute to the partial likelihood, only the covariates for the cases and the controls in the surrounding neighbourhood are needed for analysis. Further, because childhood leukaemia is a rare disease, there will only be one case (a single risk set) from each stratum so that these data are conveniently analysed using the same conditional logistic software as the sampled data, with weights equal to one.

The neighbourhood-stratified counter-matched sample is analysed in the manner described in Sections 4.3.2, 4.4 and 4.6. Since we are proposing to have matched sets with two VHCC– and one VHCC+ subject, we have that $s(i)$ indicates VHCC status for the i subject in the neighbourhood, with, say, $n_{\text{VHCC}-}(t)$ the number of VHCC– subjects and $n_{\text{VHCC}+}(t)$ the number of VHCC+ subjects of age t. Further, the numbers selected from the sampling strata are $m_{\text{VHCC}-} = 2$ and $m_{\text{VHCC}+} = 1$. Thus, the appropriate weights $w_i(t)$ (4.9) for a given set are $n_{\text{VHCC}-}(t)/2$ and $n_{\text{VHCC}+}(t)$ for the VHCC– subjects and VHCC+ subjects, respectively. Again, as the weights are determined by the VHCC status only, the case is treated in the same way as controls.

4.8.4 Power calculations

Although discussion of the asymptotic behaviour of estimators from sampled risk set data is beyond the scope of this chapter, the asymptotic variance formulae for counter-matched studies (Langholz and Borgan,

1995, Borgan *et al.*, 1995) have an important role in estimating the size of the study needed and the best choice of design parameters. For instance, the decision to use one VHCC+, two VHCC− counter-matched sets was based on a comparison of the power associated with various configurations. Here, we focus on the power of counter-matched sets with this configuration.

The primary goal of these analyses is to identify factors that could explain the association between VHCC status and childhood leukaemia. To this end, we consider the power of the study to detect this association after controlling for the potential explanatory factor. The hypothesis to be tested is whether there is a VHCC association after controlling for another factor given the observed VHCC association when one does not control for the other factor.

A bit more formally, and to explain how the power calculations were done, we start with the 'observed relative risk for VHCC+ vs. VHCC−', ϕ, univariately without accounting for any other factors.[5] Now, we want to see if another dichotomous factor Z explains the observed VHCC association. The null hypothesis to be tested is that, after controlling for Z, the relative risk for VHCC is one (i.e. Z explains VHCC). The alternative hypothesis is that, after controlling for Z, the relative risk for VHCC is still ϕ (i.e. Z does not explain VHCC at all; either Z is uncorrelated to VHCC or the relative risk for Z after controlling for VHCC is one).

If Z is to explain VHCC it must be both correlated to VHCC and univariately associated with the disease. We have expressed the correlation between VHCC and Z as the odds ratio

$$\theta = \Pr(VHCC+, Z+)\Pr(VHCC-, Z-)/\Pr(VHCC+, Z-)\Pr(VHCC-, Z+)$$

We used $\theta = 4$ and 8 for moderate and high correlation between VHCC and presence of the factor ($Z+$). These may approximately be interpreted as saying that a $Z+$ subject is four or eight times as likely to be VHCC+ than a $Z-$ subject. For a given θ, and assuming that the relative risk for VHCC is one after controlling for Z, the relative risk for Z is determined by the marginal VHCC relative risk ϕ. These are given for various other parameter possibilities in the third column of Table 4.3.

The powers for counter-matched studies with 200 or 300 cases under some combinations of parameters are given in the fourth and fifth columns of Table 4.3. Assuming that the proportion of VHCC+ subjects in the neighbourhoods is not too low,[6] 200 1:2 counter-matched sets will have

---

[5] This corresponds to setting $r(\phi, \mathbf{z}_i) = 1$ for $z_i = $ VHCC− and $r(\phi, \mathbf{z}_i) = \phi$ for $z_i = $ VHCC+ in (4.22).

[6] We note that the relative risks for VHCC of 1.75 and 2.0 are realistic given the results of past studies. The proportion of VHCC+ of 10% is probably quite conservative, given that wire code homogeneous neighbourhoods are discarded so that these power figures are probably low.

Table 4.3 Power by sample size (N = number of cases), prevalence of the factor that might potentially explain the VHCC effect (Z) (assumed dichotomous) and odds ratio θ between VHCC status and Z. Also given is the relative risk (RR) associated with Z if it explains the VHCC association. The proportion VHCC+ in the neighbourhoods was taken to be 10%

Proportion Z positive (%)	θ	RR for Z	1:2 counter matching* $N = 200$	$N = 300$	1:2 case–control** $N = 300$
Observed relative risk for VHCC $\phi = 1.75$:					
10	4	7.3	67	86	63
10	8	4.0	66	84	66
25	4	6.2	71	88	65
25	8	3.4	70	86	68
Observed relative risk for VHCC $\phi = 2.0$:					
10	4	11.1	85	97	80
10	8	5.2	85	97	84
25	4	12.0	88	98	82
25	8	4.8	86	97	86

Two-sided $\alpha = 0.05$ level test
* One VHCC+ subject and two VHCC− subjects
** The case and two controls randomly sampled from the neighbourhood

sufficient power, 300 sets would be sufficient in the 'worst case'. For comparison, the powers for a case–control study where two controls are randomly sampled from *all* potential controls in the case–neighbourhood risk sets are given in the sixth column of the table. These powers are about the same as 200 counter-matched sets. Because the rarity of childhood leukaemia occurrence[7] is a major limitation for epidemiological studies of this disease, this increased efficiency greatly reduces the study duration.

A key component in both the cost and validity of the proposed study design is the survey of the neighbourhoods in order to locate all potential controls in the neighbourhood. Using successively more intensive survey methods, the efficacy of 'neighbourhood walk' methods, in which 'walkers' survey a neighbourhood by enquiring door to door about children who live in the neighbourhood (as well as leave letters at homes where this cannot be determined) is currently being investigated under a pilot project grant by the United States National Institute of Environmental Safety and Health Center. If this method is successful, this design promises to be a useful tool for unravelling the power line–childhood leukaemia mystery and, perhaps, will have application to other settings.

[7] For instance, there are about 100 cases per year in Los Angeles County, total population 8 000 000.

4.9   Concluding comments

The conceptual link between epidemiological case–control studies and the 'study base' (cohort) from which it is drawn has been discussed in many textbooks on epidemiological methods. However, while this connection is discussed in order to address the potential sources of bias in case–control studies, the link is not invoked in the presentation of the analytic methods for cohort and case–control studies. The risk set sampling approach we presented here formalizes this connection and unifies the analytic methods, at least with respect to 'matched' case–control studies.

Our examples illustrate application of the risk set sampling approach in two very different cohorts. In the uranium miners' example, cohort members are individually identified and followed for a long period of time. The risk sets (either calendar period stratified or unstratified) can be exactly set up and sampled. Additional information could then be obtained on this sample. In addition to the estimation of relative risk parameters, because the number at risk is known for each risk set, absolute risks can be estimated from the sample using methods that parallel those for the full cohort. In contrast, in the childhood leukaemia example, the cohort is an entire coverage region for a cancer registry and its members are followed for a short period of time. The only cohort members identified are those in the neighbourhood-stratified risk sets formed by the cases that occur over the study period. But this is enough information to (counter-match) sample the risk sets and carry out the appropriate partial likelihood estimation of relative risk parameters. Because the cohort is so highly stratified and the numbers in the unstratified risk sets are not known, absolute risk estimation is not possible.

The general analytic framework makes it possible to explore new case–control designs that are adapted to the particular sampling problem. We have illustrated the application of a new procedure, the counter matching method of case–control (risk set) sampling, in both of our examples. This method exploits information available on the cohort risk sets to obtain a sample that is more efficient, with respect to exposure, than random sampling. We have elsewhere described other designs, such as quota sampling (Borgan *et al.*, 1995) and an efficient two-stage case–control study design (Langholz and Goldstein, 1996), that have promise as solutions to the epidemiological study design problems they were developed to address. We have found that a formal understanding of case–control methodology as sampled risk set data has been tremendously helpful in developing potentially useful new case–control methods.

Acknowledgements

We thank Kristie Ebi and Duncan Thomas for suggestions that greatly improved the chapter. This work was supported by National Cancer

Institute grant CA42949 and Electric Power Research Institute contract 4305-02.

References

Andersen, P. K., Borch-Johnsen, K., Deckert, T., Green, A., Hougaard, P., Keiding, N. and Kreiner, S. 1985: A Cox regression model for the relative mortality and its application to diabetes mellitus survival data. *Biometrics* **41**, 921–32.

Andersen, P. K., Borgan, Ø., Gill, R. D. and Keiding, N. 1993: *Statistical models based on counting processes.* New York: Springer.

Andersen, P. K. and Gill, R. D. 1982: Cox's regression model for counting processes: a large sample study. *Annals of Statistics* **10**, 1100–20.

Borgan, Ø., Goldstein, L. and Langholz, B. 1995: Methods for the analysis of sampled cohort data in the Cox proportional hazards model. *Annals of Statistics* **23**, 1749–78.

Borgan, Ø. and Langholz, B. 1993: Non-parametric estimation of relative mortality from nested case-control studies. *Biometrics* **49**, 593–602.

Borgan, Ø. and Langholz, B. 1997: Estimation of excess risk from case-control data using Aalen's linear regression model. *Biometrics* **53**, 690–7.

Committee on the Biological Effects of Ionizing Radiation 1988: *Health risks of radon and other internally deposited alpha-emitters, BEIR IV.* Washington DC: National Academy Press.

Cox, D. R. 1972: Regression models and life-tables (with discussion). *Journal of the Royal Statistical Society (B)* **34**, 187–220.

Feychting, M. and Ahlbom, A. 1995: Childhood leukemia and residential exposure to weak extremely low frequency magnetic fields. *Environmental Health Perspectives* **103** (suppl. 2), 59–62.

Goldstein, L. and Langholz, B. 1992: Asymptotic theory for nested case-control sampling in the Cox regression model. *Annals of Statistics* **20**, 1903–28.

Hornung, R. and Meinhardt, T. 1987: Quantitative risk assessment of lung cancer in U.S. uranium miners. *Health Physics* **52**, 417–30.

Langholz, B. and Borgan, Ø. 1995: Counter-matching: a stratified nested case-control sampling method. *Biometrika* **82**, 69–79.

Langholz, B. and Borgan, Ø. 1997: Estimation of absolute risk from nested case-control data. *Biometrics* **53**, 767–74.

Langholz, B. and Clayton, D. 1994: Sampling strategies in nested case-control studies. *Environmental Health Perspectives* **102** (suppl. 8), 47–51.

Langholz, B. and Goldstein, L. 1996: Risk set sampling in epidemiologic cohort studies. *Statistical Science* **11**, 35–53.

Linet, M. *et al.* 1997: Residential exposure to magnetic fields and acute lymphoblastic leukemia in children. *New England Journal of Medicine* **337**, 1–7.

London, S., Thomas, D., Bowman, J., Sobel, E., Cheng, T.-C. and Peters, J. 1991: Exposure to residential electric and magnetic fields and risk of childhood leukemia. *American Journal of Epidemiology* **134**, 923–37.

Lubin, J. *et al.* 1994: Radon and lung cancer risk: a joint analysis of 11 underground miners studies. *NIH Publication* 94-3644, US Department of

Health and Human Services, Public Health Service, National Institutes of Health, Bethesda, MD.

Lundin, F., Wagoner, J. and Archer, V. 1971: Radon daughter exposure and respiratory cancer, quantitative and temporal aspects. *Joint Monograph* 1, US Public Health Service, Washington, DC.

Oakes, D. 1981: Survival times: aspects of partial likelihood (with discussion). *International Statistical Review* **49**, 235–64.

Prentice, R. L. and Breslow, N. E. 1978: Retrospective studies and failure time models. *Biometrika* **65**, 153–8.

Savitz, D., Wachtel, H., Barnes, F., John, E. and Tvrdik, J. 1988: Case-control study of childhood cancer and exposure to 60-Hz magnetic fields. *American Journal of Epidemiology* **128**, 21–38.

Steenland, K. and Deddens, J. A. 1997: Increased precision using countermatching in nested case–control studies. *Epidemiology* **8**, 238–42.

Thomas, D. C. 1977: Addendum to: Methods of cohort analysis: appraisal by application to asbestos mining. By F. D. K. Liddell, J. C. McDonald and D. C. Thomas. *Journal of the Royal Statistical Society* (*A*) **140**, 469–91.

Thomas, D., Pogoda, J., Langholz, B. and Mack, W. 1994: Temporal modifiers of the radon-smoking interaction. *Health Physics* **66**, 257–62.

Wertheimer, N. and Leeper, E. 1979: Electrical wiring configurations and childhood cancer. *American Journal of Epidemiology* **109**, 273–84.

Whittemore, A. and McMillan, A. 1983: Lung cancer mortality among U.S. uranium miners: a reappraisal. *Journal of the National Cancer Institute* **71**, 489–99.

5 Tree-structured survival analysis in medical research

Mark R. Segal

5.1 Introduction

Tree-structured or recursive partitioning methods have lately enjoyed widespread usage. This popularity derives from the conceptual appeal and compelling examples as presented in the definitive monograph *Classification and Regression Trees* (hereafter CART) by Breiman *et al.* (1984) along with the availability of companion software. Additionally, Clark and Pregibon (1992) have devised an elegant and interactive set of tree tools within Splus. Augmenting this software development are a number of methodological extensions to the basic CART 'engineering' that have facilitated applications in several new settings.

I recently overviewed and illustrated several of these extensions, especially those having a biomedical emphasis (Segal, 1995). One common theme to the extensions has been the quest to handle an expanded array of outcome types, beyond the continuous (regression trees) and categorical (classification trees) treated in CART. Thus, extensions to both survival and longitudinal data have been devised, both having obvious biomedical relevance. In this chapter the focus will be on survival data where, perhaps, the development has come furthest, and for which tree concepts seem particularly suited. In addition to detailing the methodology itself, including strengths and limitations, a description of public domain software will be provided. The availability of such software is essential for facilitating applications. Some illustrative examples conclude.

5.2 Motivation

The central thrust of tree techniques is the elicitation of subgroups. Within these subgroups covariates are homogeneous and between subgroups outcomes are distinct. So, in clinical settings with survival outcomes, interpretation in terms of prognostic group identification is frequently possible. Creation of the subgroups according to a tree structure (binary recursion) mimics, at least simplistically, medical decision making: if the patient is female, and if she has a family history of breast cancer, and if she is over 40, and if the year is even, then annual mammograms are recommended. Similarly, given a survival tree, it is straightforward to classify a new patient to a prognostic group by simply answering the sequence of binary questions (*splits*) that give rise to each subgroup (*node*).

It is reasonable to assess whether this goal of subgroup extraction requires new methodology. Could not, for example, the Cox (1972) proportional hazards model be employed for this purpose? Suppose, without loss of generality, that in fitting a proportional hazards model with three continuous covariates we obtain positive coefficients for each. That is, each variable is adverse, increased values of each being associated with elevated risk. Thus, we might try to create a high risk group by combining individuals who have high values for all three covariates. However, this approach may fail if no patients possess such a covariate profile. Alternatively, we could compute a risk score for each member of the sample based on substitution of the actual covariate profiles into the log-linear model using the fitted coefficients. Then a high risk stratum could be obtained by selecting the desired percentile of the sample risk scores. The difficulty here is that individuals with potentially disparate covariate values are combined and hence the resultant risk group is hard to label or interpret.

In addition to identifying important prognostic groups, which can be thought of as local interactions, survival tree techniques can also be informative about individual covariates. This derives from single splitting (subdivision) being revealing about threshold effects for time-independent covariates, or change-points in the case of time-dependent covariates. Also, repeated splitting on a given covariate can be revealing about more complex non-linearities. However, use of (smoothed) martingale residual plots (Therneau *et al.*, 1990) is arguably a more direct way for determining appropriate functional form. Further, tree methods in general are not geared towards making global assessments of a covariate's importance. This is for a variety of reasons. Firstly, if a covariate is used (to define a split) in just one branch of the tree, then it is problematic to gauge its overall importance. Secondly, *masking* (CART, section 5.3.4), whereby a covariate selected as (the best) split variable precludes another, almost as good, covariate from emerging, complicates covariate evaluation. We will define the splitting criterion below and, accordingly, what constitutes the best split variable. Finally, covariate splits are selected as the result of optimizing this criterion, and are therefore highly adaptive. While some corresponding distributional results have been obtained (Miller and Siegmund, 1982, Lausen and Schumacher, 1992), there are still difficulties in assigning significances to a sequence of splits, and hence to formally appraising covariate importance. Indeed, Segal and Bloch (1989) contend that subgroup elicitation and covariate evaluation are complementary tasks, making survival tree techniques and (say) proportional hazards models complementary approaches.

5.3 Tree-structured regression methodology

I briefly overview the basic CART prescription for tree construction and indicate the modifications needed to handle survival data. There are four constituent components:

1. A set of questions, or *splits*, phrased in terms of the covariates that serve to partition the covariate space. A tree structure derives from the recursive application of these questions and a binary tree results if the questions are binary (yes/no). The subsamples created by assigning cases according to these splits are termed *nodes*.

2. A *split function* $\phi(s, t)$ that can be evaluated for any split s of any node t. The split function is used to assess the worth of the competing splits.

3. A means for determining appropriate tree size.

4. Statistical summaries for the nodes of the tree.

5.3.1 Allowable splits

The first element defines what sort of subdivisions (splits) are allowed. These are the same for survival and standard regression trees. The CART prescription utilizes binary splits. A general binary question has the form 'Is observation or case $\mathbf{x}_i \in A$?' where A is a region of the covariate space.

Answering such a question induces a partition, or split, of the covariate space: cases for which the answer is *yes* are assigned to region A while those for which the answer is *no* are assigned to A complement. As stated, with A unrestricted, things are impractically vague. The CART implementation proceeds by constraining that:

(a) Each split depends upon the value of only a *single* covariate.

(b) For ordered (continuous or categorical) covariates, X_j, only splits resulting from questions of the form 'Is $X_j \leq c$?' for $c \in \text{domain}(X_j)$ are considered. Thus ordering is preserved.

(c) For categorical predictors all possible splits into disjoint subsets of the categories are allowed.

It may appear that the reduction in possible splits resulting from the above constraints is insufficient. Certainly (a) restricts to examining covariates univariately and (b) restricts to dividing a given covariate X_j into two (semi-infinite) intervals. However, there are seemingly an uncountably infinite number of such intervals as c ranges over the domain of X_j. The point is that the covariate X_j takes on only a finite number of values in the sample at hand – at most n for the n cases. Hence, we only have to examine those values of c that result in a case switching 'sides' – from the right semi-infinite interval to the left. So there are at most $n - 1$ splits given by $\{\text{'Is } X_j \le c_l?'\}$ where the c_l are taken, by convention, halfway between consecutive distinct observed values of X_j. The c_l are called *split points* or *cut-points*.

For unordered categorical covariates no constraints on possible subdivisions are imposed. If such a covariate has M categories then there are $2^{M-1} - 1$ splits to examine leading to combinatorial explosion for large M. However, using a result from Fisher (1958), CART (section 8.8) reduces this to a feasible M splits.

The merit of formulating allowable splits in this fashion is threefold: *interpretability*, *feasibility* and *flexibility*. Briefly, ease of interpretation derives from the simple yes/no comparisons. The associated schematic tree diagram is readily digested. As mentioned, assignment/classification of new cases to terminal nodes just involves answering the sequence of yes/no questions. The tree diagram can also display statistical summaries of the nodes permitting easy prediction. By way of contrast, the ubiquitous use of linear combinations of covariates may not be interpretable when covariates of differing types are mixed.

Criticism of tree-structured approaches has been levelled on the grounds that they amount to fitting uninterpretable high order interaction terms. This is mitigated by the following considerations. The 'interactions' are local and adaptively selected. They are not the familiar product interactions whose interpretation is contingent on lower order effects. Further, the 'order' will depend on the size of the selected tree. Methods for determining tree size are designed to guard against overfitting. In comparison with other contemporary, adaptive, many-parameter modelling schemes (e.g. neural networks) trees are relatively interpretable yet competitive in terms of prediction.

Computational feasibility for the unrestricted splitting of unordered categorical covariates has been indicated above. Feasibility for the order-preserving splitting of ordered (continuous or categorical) covariates relies upon updating algorithms. These algorithms update the value of the split function corresponding to an update (increment) of the split point c_l.

Finally, the splits afford a flexible means for partitioning the predictor space. No impositions are placed on splits of an unordered categorical variable. No restrictions are placed on the split points for dividing an ordered covariate nor on the number of times a given covariate can be used as a split variable.

However, it is largely the goal of enhancing flexibility in partitioning the covariate space that has motivated changes to the basic CART approach. Using the covariates univariately entails that all splits are orthogonal to the coordinate axes. This may be a highly inefficient means of dividing the covariate space; see CART, sections 2.5.3 and 5.2. The solutions offered include extending the allowable splits to embrace (i) linear combinations of covariates; (ii) Boolean combinations of binary covariates; and (iii) the usage of derived covariates split according to the original rules. The price for this improved flexibility is reduced interpretability and a greater computational burden. Use of linear combination splits in particular can be very computer intensive. Thus, in the regression setting (as opposed to classification where the response variable is categorical), CART (p. 248) does not advocate the use of linear combination splits.

The inefficiency resulting from partitioning into axis-oriented regions will be most apparent when either the regression function has no strong interaction effects or the interactions involve only a few covariates. Linear and additive models are examples of the first of these. One motivation for Friedman's (1991) multivariate adaptive regression spline (MARS) extension of regression trees was to overcome this deficiency. This was achieved by retaining all (parent) nodes for further potential splitting after they have already been split. Placing no restrictions on the choice of parent node enables MARS to produce models involving either high or low interactions, or both. Of course, the retention of parent nodes for further splitting means that the procedure is no longer recursive and hence does not admit a tree representation. A detailed discussion of regression trees and MARS in terms of allowable splits is given in Friedman (1991, section 3.3).

5.3.2 Split functions

A tree is grown as follows. For each subgroup or node:

1. Examine every allowable split on each predictor variable.

2. Select and execute (create left and right daughter nodes) the *best* of these splits.

The initial or *root* node comprises the entire sample. Steps 1 and 2 are then reapplied to each of the daughter nodes, and so on. Tree size determination is described later. The allowable splits have been described above; it remains to define what constitutes a 'best' split.

The best split is determined by the value of the split function $\phi(s, g)$ that can be evaluated for any split s of any node g. For regression CART describes two split functions: least squares (LS) described below and least absolute deviations (LAD).

Let g designate a node of the tree. That is, g contains a subsample of cases $\{(\mathbf{x}'_i, y_i)\}$ where $\mathbf{x}'_i = (x_{i1}, x_{i2}, \ldots, x_{ip})$ is the vector of observed covariate values and y_i is the observed outcome for the ith case. Let N_g

be the total number of cases in g and let $\bar{y}(g) = (1/N_g)\sum_{i\in g} y_i$ be the response average for node g. Then the within-node sum of squares is given by $SS(g) = \sum_{i\in g}[y_i - \bar{y}(g)]^2$. Now suppose a split s partitions g into left and right daughter nodes g_L and g_R. The LS split function is $\phi(s, g) = SS(g) - SS(g_L) - SS(g_R)$ and the best split s^* of g is the split such that $\phi(s^*, g) = \max_{s\in\Omega}\phi(s, g)$, where Ω is the set of all allowable splits s of g. An LS regression tree is constructed by recursively splitting nodes so as to maximize the above ϕ function. The function is such that we create smaller and smaller nodes of progressively increased homogeneity on account of the non-negativity of $\phi : \phi \geq 0$ since $SS(g) \geq SS(g_L) + SS(g_R) \, \forall s$

Split functions must also be readily computable owing to the large number of evaluations needed. To this end updating algorithms have been devised for both LS and LAD (CART, section 8.11) that enable recomputation of the split function corresponding to the switching of a case from the right to the left daughter node.

Modifications to the split function are a primary means for expanding the scope of tree-structured methods. We now describe some such modifications that facilitate tree-structured survival analysis. Several such modifications have been proposed; see Segal (1995) for a review. Here we focus on split functions based on between-node separation. This is quantified by using a two-sample statistic (e.g. the log-rank statistic) as split function. While we directly capture the notion of identifying distinct prognostic groups, new methods for determining tree size are required. The reformulated split functions permit handling of right-censored, left-truncated survival times as well as time-dependent covariates as described next.

5.3.2.1   Handling right-censored survival data

Instead of gearing the split function to optimizing within-node homogeneity as above, we can reward splits that result in large between-node separation. The magnitude of any two-sample statistic affords such a split function. For example, we could replace the LS split function with splitting based on two-sample t statistics. These split functions are essentially equivalent (depending on whether pooled or unpooled variance estimates are used for the t statistic). The reasons for using two-sample statistics as split functions are the advantages conferred by using two-sample *rank* statistics. These include (i) invariance under monotone transformation of the outcome (note: all regression trees are invariant to monotone transformations of the covariates); and (ii) reduced sensitivity to outliers. Foremost, however, is the ability to handle censored survival data.

For this purpose, any member of either the Tarone–Ware (1977) or Harrington–Fleming (1982) class of two-sample statistics can be employed. The former class is obtained by constructing a sequence of

2×2 tables, where for each distinct uncensored response the following table pertains:

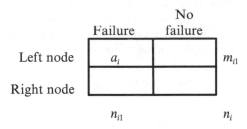

The statistics have the following form:

$$\text{TW} = \frac{\sum_{i=1}^{k} w_i\{a_i - E_0[A_i]\}}{\left(\sum_{i=1}^{k} w_i^2 \, \text{var}_0(A_i)\right)^{1/2}}$$

where A_i is the random variable corresponding to number of deaths in the left node for the ith table; w_i are weights; the sum is over all tables, that is all distinct uncensored observations; and the null hypothesis is that the death rates for the two nodes are equal. For fixed margins the null expectations and variances are hypergeometric:

$$E_0[A_i] = \frac{m_{i1} n_{i1}}{n_i}$$

$$\text{var}_0(A_i) = \left(\frac{m_{i1}(n_i - m_{i1})}{n_i - 1}\right)\left[\left(\frac{n_{i1}}{n_i}\right)\left(1 - \frac{n_{i1}}{n_i}\right)\right]$$

Sensitivity to particular alternatives is governed by the weights w_i, some common specifications for which include the following: $w_i = 1$ gives the log-rank (Peto and Peto, 1972) statistic; $w_i = n_i$ gives the Gehan (1965) statistic; $w_i = n_i^{1/2}$ gives a statistic advocated by Tarone and Ware (1977); $w_i = S_i^*$ gives Prentice's (1978) generalization of the Wilcoxon, where $S_i^* = \prod_{j=1}^{i} n_j/(n_j + 1)$ is almost the Kaplan–Meier survival estimate at the ith uncensored failure time. The Gehan statistic is subject to domination by a small number of early failures (Prentice and Marek, 1979) and hence should be used selectively.

5.3.2.2 Handling left truncation

Left truncation often occurs when subjects are recruited some time after the natural time origin and only if they have not yet experienced the outcome. Cohort studies of HIV where an existing AIDS diagnosis is an exclusion criterion and time to AIDS is the endpoint provide an example. In this situation, each subject has a left truncation time τ_k (possibly zero) corresponding to the time of recruitment and would not have been observed at all if the outcome had occurred at or before this time. Subjects with very short survival times will tend to be excluded from the sample.

Product-limit survival estimates and two-sample statistics of the form given above can easily be calculated by applying the usual formulae but with subjects not considered to be at risk before their recruitment times (Tsai *et al.*, 1987, Ying, 1990). Thus, the counts n_{i1} and n_i are reduced if any subjects were not already recruited by the ith failure time. That is, subjects with $\tau_k \geq t_i$ do not contribute to the 2×2 table for the ith failure time. The resulting modified two-sample statistic can be used as a split function just as with untruncated data.

5.3.2.3   Handling time-dependent covariates

Extending the tree-building procedure to allow for a time-dependent covariate $X_j(t)$ appears to be more difficult. Bacchetti and Segal (1995) proceed as follows. Consider a split based on a question of the form 'Is $X_j(t) \leq c$?' for some specific value c. Subjects k with $x_{jk}(t) \leq c$ at all times clearly go to the left node, while subjects with $x_{jk}(t) > c$ at all times go to the right node, but subjects with $x_{jk}(t) \leq c$ for some failure times and $x_{jk}(t) > c$ at other failure times need to contribute to the left node some of the time and to the right node at other times. To illustrate how this requirement can be properly met, first consider the case where $X_j(t)$ is non-decreasing in t and t^* is the last time when $x_{jk}(t) \leq c$, with $\tau_k < t^* < y_k$. Proper testing of the split requires that subject k be considered part of the left node at failure times t_i such that $\tau_k < t_i \leq t^*$ and part of the right node when $t^* < t_i \leq y_k$. This can be readily incorporated into the tree framework provided left truncation is accommodated. Subject k is simply replaced by two pseudo-subjects k_1 and k_2 as follows: for $\tau_k < t^* < y_k$ define $\tau_{k1} = \tau_k$, $y_{k1} = t^*$, $\delta_{k1} = 0$, $\tau_{k2} = t^*$, $y_{k2} = y_k$ and $\delta_{k2} = \delta_k$. Pseudo-subject k_1 is assigned to the left node, while pseudo-subject k_2 goes to the right. This results in correct calculation of the split statistic, because each subject k contributes to m_{1i} only for t_i such that $t_i \leq t^*$, to n_{1i} only if $y_k = t_i$ and $\delta_i = 1$, and to a_i only if $y_k = t_i$, $\delta_i = 1$ and $y_k \leq t^*$.

If the log-rank statistic is used as the split function, the test is equivalent to fitting a univariate proportional hazards model with time-dependent covariate equal to the indicator $I\{X_j(t) \leq c\}$.

If $X_j(t)$ is non-increasing, the split is handled analogously, with t^* now defined as the last time with $x_{jk}(t) > c$. General time-dependent covariates can be accommodated by splitting observations into more than two pseudo-observations; see Bacchetti and Segal (1995) for details.

One drawback to this method is that the creation of pseudo-observations precludes classifying each individual into one terminal node. This limits the trees' usefulness in assigning individuals to 'prognostic' groups. However, it is possible to assign each individual to a terminal node at any particular time. Given the 'two-dimensional' nature of time-dependent covariates this is the most that can be hoped for. Huang *et al.* (1994) propose a similar generalization that extends the survival tree methodology of LeBlanc and Crowley (1992).

5.3.3 Determining tree size

A crucial aspect of the tree-structured regression is determination of tree size. That is, how many splits should be implemented? There are shortcomings using stopping rules based on either (i) node sizes becoming too small, or (ii) the improvement as measured by the split function ϕ being insufficient. The problems derive from smallness or insufficiency having to be gauged relative to preset thresholds. Misspecification of these thresholds can result in over- or under-fitting. These difficulties are redressed by a pruning algorithm: (1) grow a very large tree initially so as to capture all potentially important splits; (2) collapse this back up – using cost–complexity as defined below – creating a nested sequence of trees; and (3) select an optimal tree from this sequence using cross-validation or an independent test sample.

5.3.3.1 Cost–complexity pruning

In situations where a measure of within-node homogeneity or *cost* is available pruning (step (2)) is accomplished using a *cost–complexity* algorithm. Let $R(g)$ be the cost of node g. For example, for LS splitting we take $R(g) = SS(g)$. Now, define $R(G)$ as the cost of the entire tree G : $R(G) = \sum_{g \in \tilde{G}} R(g)$ where $\tilde{G}$ is the collection of terminal nodes of G. Also, define the *complexity* of G as $|\tilde{G}|$, the number of terminal nodes of G. Then the cost–complexity of G is

$$R_\alpha(G) = R(G) + \alpha|\tilde{G}|$$

where $\alpha \geq 0$ is called the *complexity parameter*. We want to minimize simultaneously both cost and complexity: large trees will have small cost but high complexity and vice versa. Solely minimizing cost will err on the side of overfitting: with $R(g) = SS(g)$ we can achieve zero cost by splitting to the point where each terminal node contains only one observation.

Initially, a large tree G_{max} is grown using the chosen split function. The size of this tree is not critical. For each value of α we find the subtree $G(\alpha)$ of G_{max} that minimizes $R_\alpha(G)$. If α is small the penalty for large $|\tilde{G}|$ will also be small and hence $G(\alpha)$ will be large. As $\alpha \nearrow$, $|\tilde{G}(\alpha)| \searrow$. Finally, for α sufficiently large, $|\tilde{G}(\alpha)| = 1$ and the minimal cost–complexity tree is the root node (the entire original sample) since any splitting will increase the cost–complexity. The determination of the values of α that correspond to a change in $G(\alpha)$, and what that change is, is described in CART, section 3.3.

Thus, the cost–complexity algorithm produces a nested sequence of optimally pruned subtrees. The pruning works by successively lopping branches for which the average (over splits within the branch) improvement is small. Such an algorithm is essential since evaluating cost–complexity for all possible subtrees is computationally infeasible as this number grows exponentially (CART, section 10.1).

Having obtained a nested sequence of pruned subtrees we are left with the problem of selecting a 'best' tree from this sequence. Using resubstitution estimates of cost will result in selection of the largest tree G_{max} due to the familiar overoptimism of resubstitution estimates. Two standard remedies are advocated: test sample estimates and cross-validation estimates. These are described in CART, sections 3.4 and 8.5.

5.3.3.2   Survival tree pruning via split complexity

Split functions that make recourse to measures of between-node separation, such as the two-sample statistic splitting described above, do not lend themselves to cost–complexity pruning methods. The reason is that such split functions often do not admit an associated measure of within-node cost. For such situations, which include survival trees constructed using log-rank statistic splitting, LeBlanc and Crowley (1993) develop an optimal pruning algorithm similar to cost–complexity pruning.

They define the *split–complexity* of a tree G as

$$Q_\alpha(G) = Q(G) - \alpha|S|$$

where S represents the splits in G and $Q(G)$ is the sum of the (standardized) split statistics, $Q(s)$, in G: $Q(G) = \sum_{s \in S} Q(s)$. It is possible to interpret $Q(G)$ as the amount of prognostic structure represented by the tree-based model. This interpretation derives from considering the two-sample split statistic used, say the log-rank statistic, as a standardized distance between empirical hazard functions of adjacent nodes in the tree.

A tree G_1 is an optimally pruned subtree of G for given complexity α if

$$Q_\alpha(G_1) = \max_{G' \preceq G} Q_\alpha(G')$$

where $G' \preceq G$ denotes that G' is a subtree of G. LeBlanc and Crowley's (1993) split–complexity pruning algorithm obtains the best tree (i.e. maximal $Q_\alpha(\cdot)$) for any α. The algorithm repeatedly prunes off branches with, say, smallest average log-rank test statistics. Instead of using cross-validation, selection of an appropriate α, equivalently tree size, is accomplished via bootstrap or permutation testing; see LeBlanc and Crowley (1992, 1993). The role of the permutation testing is to assess significance of the adaptively chosen split. An alternative means for achieving this where a two-sample statistic is employed as the split function is to obtain the distribution for a maximally selected statistic. Lausen and Schumacher (1992) pursue such distributions using asymptotics and simulations for two-sample rank statistics including the log-rank.

5.3.3.3   Survival tree size via graphical methods

Tree techniques are inherently exploratory. They are adept at identifying unanticipated structure and extracting prognostic subgroups. To the extent that exploration is at the forefront, allowing user determination of tree size provides useful augmentation to the above algorithmic approaches and, indeed, is advocated in CART (sections 3.4.2, 6.2). A number of interactive graphical tools have been developed, within Splus, to facilitate this and to allow general investigation of tree-based models. These tools are described in Clark and Pregibon (1992).

The Splus interactive (via graphic input) functions allow for (i) snipping off branches to examine subtrees; (ii) selection of subtrees that, being tree objects themselves, are amenable to all tree display and analysis procedures; (iii) displaying competing splits at each node; and (iv) displaying covariate distributions and summaries according to given splits or terminal nodes. These features, some of which are described further in the next section, permit informal assessment of which aspects of the tree structure are stable, the primary concern when determining tree size.

Further, an additional graphical heuristic for tree size determination follows from some empirical observations given in CART, section 3.4. There it is reported that 'honest' error estimates exhibit a characteristic pattern as a function of tree size. Plots of error estimates versus tree size are characterized by an initial steep decline, followed by a long flat valley, and then a gradual increase as tree size increases. The minimum error or cost occurs in the valley region, but its position within this region is variable. Thus, using plots to identify the 'kink' or 'elbow' corresponding to change in slope after the initial decline provides a means for choosing desirable tree size.

For survival trees this approach is implemented as follows: (1) initially grow a large tree; (2) from the terminal nodes step up this tree assigning to each internal node the maximum split statistic among all splits descendant from this node; (3) place these maxima in increasing order; (4) the first pruned tree corresponds to locating the highest node in the tree and removing all its descendants; (5) the second pruned tree is obtained by reapplying this process to the first pruned tree, and so on. Each pruned tree will have an associated number of terminal nodes and maximal split statistic. It is by treating these quantities as tree size and cost respectively that the graphic described above can be produced. The final tree selected is that corresponding to the position of the 'elbow'. Each internal node of the tree is assigned a cost or error estimate equal to the maximum split statistic among all splits descendant from that node.

5.3.4   Node summaries

As mentioned, node summaries are strongly connected to the split function. For example, in using LS splitting, a natural scalar node summary is just $\bar{y}(g)$. The fact that summaries are not just used for descriptive purposes, but also used for prediction, has resulted in refinements even for such simple split functions. Another reason for requiring more sophisticated summaries is a more complex outcome type such as survival outcomes.

For survival trees Kaplan–Meier curves have been used as summaries for each node and to compare survival in different nodes (Gordon and Olshen, 1985, Segal, 1988, Davis and Anderson, 1989, LeBlanc and Crowley, 1992). This preserves the non-parametric nature of survival trees. The curves are usually unstable only for large times where censoring is typically heaviest. When there is heavy left truncation Kaplan–Meier curves may be unstable at early times. This is a less familiar situation and can distort visual assessment and comparison of curves, particularly because large early jumps influence the height of the curve at all later times. Even if no left truncation is initially present, splits on time-dependent covariates can lead to substantial left truncation for some nodes.

Methods are available (Tsai *et al.*, 1987) for calculating Kaplan–Meier curves and standard errors in the presence of left truncation. To achieve improved stability smoothed non-parametric hazard function estimates can be used as node summaries. The improved stability results from uncertainties at either early or late times not unduly affecting the more accurately estimated parts of these curves. Smoothing can be accomplished using a roughness penalty approach where, for example, the penalty is such that the ultrasmooth case belongs to the Weibull family (Bacchetti and Segal, 1995). Other methods for estimating smooth hazard functions are given by Anderson and Senthilselvan (1980) and Whittemore and Keller (1986). O'Sullivan (1988) describes automatic selection of the amount of smoothness for smoothed log-hazard estimators.

5.4   Software

Public domain software, co-written with Carrie Wager, is available for performing tree-structured survival analysis. A sharfile called `tssa` can be directly downloaded from the statlib S archive (http://lib.stat.cmu.edu/S/tssa). This distribution contains extensive documentation, installation instructions and code. While standalone (C) code is provided, the emphasis is on an Splus interface. This is intended to inherit as much functionality from Splus tree functions, including the above-mentioned interactive graphics tools, as possible. Thus, an extensive suite of methods for producing, exploring and displaying survival trees is available. The package has been tested in Splus Versions 3.1, 3.2, and 3.3 on a variety of platforms and UNIX environments. Brian Ripley has provided a port to Windows (http: www.stats.ox.ac.uk/pub/SWin/tssa.zip).

The principal user-level function is `tssa()` which creates a survival tree (tssa) object. It takes some of the same arguments as its counterpart (regression or classification) tree function (`tree()`), namely, a `formula` object specifying the survival outcome and the covariates to be (potentially) used as split variables, and a `data.frame`. Additional arguments specify which two-sample statistic to use as the split statistic (default is log-rank), and the minimum proportion of uncensored observations within a node required to try splitting that node. The resulting object can be operated on by a variety of generic user-level methods including `plot()`, `summary()`, `print()`, and `text()`.

Many of the functions and methods for class 'tree' also work on tssa objects. Among the former are some interactive graphics tools that facilitate exploratory analyses. Input involves selections (typically of nodes or splits) via mouse from a displayed tree structure (dendrogram). Sample functions include `hist.tree()` which displays side-by-side histograms for specified covariates corresponding to resultant left and right daughter nodes of the indicated parent node, `select.tree()` and `snip.tree()` that allow selection of subtrees of a displayed tree and operations thereon, and `path.tree()` and the generic function `identify()` which respectively display the sequence of splits leading to a selected node, and the case composition of that node.

New, specialized functions have been created to handle survival-specific aspects. These include `km.tssa()` which displays Kaplan–Meier curves corresponding to a given node or split or set thereof and can also be used interactively. Also, `prune.tssa()` produces a subplot of maximal subtree split statistics versus subtree size, enabling pruning to be effected according 'elbow' identification as described previously. Subjective pruning is facilitated by constructing the dendrogram arm lengths connecting parent and daughter nodes to be proportional to the corresponding split statistic. Finally, `post.tssa()` provides for presentation graphics of a survival tree (tssa) object. Node and split information is depicted on a tree schematic that can be sent directly to a PostScript printer. Details and examples of these and other functions are provided in the documentation accompanying the distribution and on-line help is also available.

5.5   Examples

Two illustrative examples are described. The first pertains to a cohort study examining breast cancer incidence and associated risk factors. A covariate of central interest was cytological finding in breast fluid obtained by nipple aspiration. The presentation of results from a tree-structured survival analysis of these data provides a glimpse of some of the (non-interactive) graphical features of the software discussed above.

The second example is concerned with HIV disease progression. The latency or incubation period for AIDS (time from HIV infection to AIDS diagnosis) is both long, with the median latency of approximately 10 years (Muñoz *et al.*, 1989, Bacchetti and Moss, 1989), and variable. In order to try and explain this variability in terms of immune function decay, markers of immune function are regularly measured on longitudinally followed cohorts of HIV seropositive and seroconverting individuals. A tree-structured survival analysis provides some putative prognostic subgroups defined in terms of these immune function markers.

5.5.1   Breast cancer cohort study

A cohort of 2089 white women aged between 30 and 79, living in the San Francisco Bay area, who were neither pregnant nor lactating, and who were breast cancer free, were recruited between 1973 and 1980. Nipple aspirates of breast fluid were collected using a modified breast pump (Petrakis *et al.*, 1981). Each breast fluid specimen was cytologically classified according to the most severe epithelial change present (King *et al.*, 1983). This yielded an ordered categorical variable with the following levels: $0 \equiv$ no breast fluid; $1 \equiv$ unsatisfactory specimen; $2 \equiv$ normal specimen; $3 \equiv$ hyperplasia; $4 \equiv$ hyperplasia and atypia; $5 \equiv$ severe atypia. It is important to note that the coding of levels for such ordered categorical covariates is immaterial for tree methods: tree topologies (i.e. split variables and associated cut-points) are invariant to monotone transformations of the covariates. Cohort follow-up occurred between June 1988 and April 1991. Details on ascertainment and incident breast cancer validation are given by Wrensch *et al.* (1992). The survival time of interest is time to breast cancer from enrolment.

Here we analyse data provided by all women. By not restricting to the subset of parous women we can examine parity (nulli/parous) as a covariate but are precluded from using variables such as age at first pregnancy and breast feeding. Other covariates included in the tree-structured survival analysis were age (continuous), menopausal status (pre/post), family (mother/sister/daughter) history of breast cancer (yes/no), age at menarche (four ordered levels), education (three ordered levels), place of examination (UCSF/other), and Quetelet's index (continuous). Further variable and cohort information, as well as results from Cox proportional hazards modelling, is provided by Wrensch *et al.* (1993). Excluding cases with missing data reduced the sample to 1639 women. The ability to utilize cases with missing covariate information is one of the strengths of CART. However, the technique for handling missings via *surrogate* splits (CART, section 5.3.2) has yet to be implemented for survival trees.

Survival tree results are depicted in Figs 5.1–5.3. These figures are 'snapshots' of the screen – prettier output can be obtained using `post.tssa`. The graphics window is partitioned into upper and lower plotting regions using `tssa.screens()`. The corresponding top panel of Fig. 5.1 displays the large tree prior to pruning obtained using the sequence `fit <- tssa( . . . )`, `plot(fit)`, `text(fit)`. This tree was grown using the log-rank statistic as the split function, although very similar topologies result from using other two-sample censored data rank

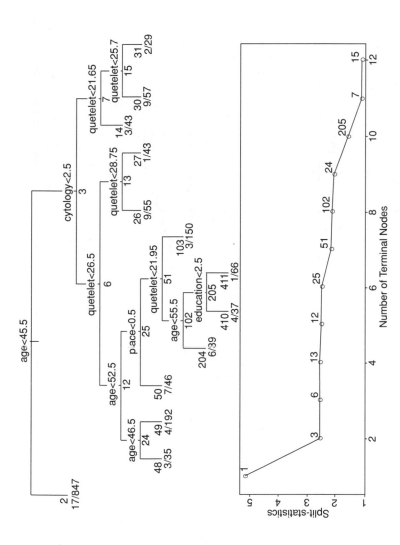

Fig. 5.1 Upper panel: survival tree for the breast cancer cohort study grown using all covariates and the log-rank split statistic. The tree schematic displays the initial large tree prior to pruning (see text). Lower panel: plot of maximal subtree split statistics versus tree size (number of terminal nodes) showing characteristic 'elbow' (see text)

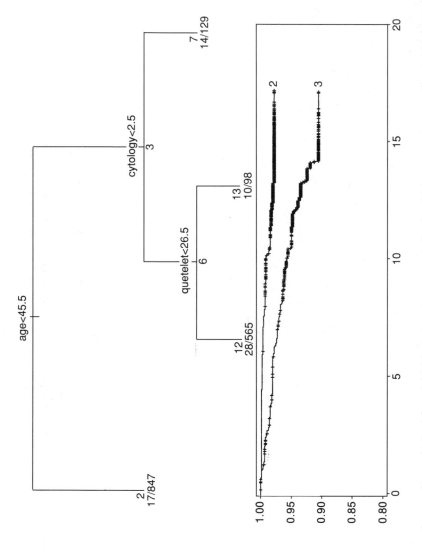

Fig. 5.2 Upper panel: pruned tree obtained from initial large tree. Lower panel: Kaplan–Meier curves corresponding to the first split on age with cut-point 45.5 years

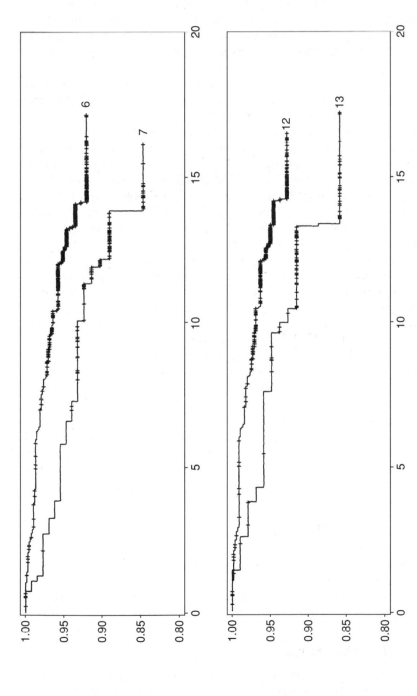

Fig. 5.3 Upper panel: Kaplan–Meier curves corresponding to the second split on cytology finding with cut-point 2.5. Lower panel: Kaplan–Meier curves corresponding to the third split on Quetelet's index with cut-point 26.5

statistics. Two additional user-specified parameters control the extent of the tree: the first specifies the minimum node size required in order to entertain splitting (here 30) and the second specifies the minimum proportion of uncensored observations within a node required in order to entertain splitting. This was set at 3%, less than the overall uncensored rate of 4.2%. As described, these settings are not critical provided that a suitably large tree results.

Above each non-terminal node number the covariate and cut-point defining the split is given. Thus, node 1 is split on age with those women aged < 45.5 assigned to node 2 and those aged > 45.5 assigned to node 3. Age was given in (integer) years so this is unambiguous. Below each terminal node is a summary ratio of number of events (breast cancers) to number of subjects in that node. For example, node 2 consists of the 847 women aged < 45.5 of whom 17 were diagnosed with breast cancer during follow-up. This anticipated low event rate (2%) explains why this large node is not further subdivided, in contrast with the older women for whom the event rate is 6.6%. The Kaplan–Meier survival curves associated with this age split are given in the bottom panel of Fig. 5.2.

The bottom panel of Fig. 5.1 displays subtree maximal split (log-rank) statistics plotted against subtree size (number of terminal nodes) and indexed by subtree root. As discussed, the characteristic 'elbow' is evident. Selection of a pruned tree at or just beyond the elbow is recommended. Interactive pruning (using `prune.tssa(fit)`) based on this plot yields a selected tree as displayed in the top panel of Fig. 5.2.

The node 3 older (> 45.5) women resulting from the age split described above are further subdivided on the basis of cytology. The cut-point of 2.5 means that those women who have (favourable) cytological findings (levels 0, 1 and 2) are separated from those with abnormal cytological findings (levels 3, 4 and 5). We anticipate that this latter subgroup of older women with abnormal cytology (node 7) would constitute the prognostic subgroup with poorest survival. However, the older women with normal cytological findings (node 6) are further split on the basis of Quetelet's index, a measure of obesity. Examining the survival curves given in Fig. 5.3 it appears that the more obese subgroup (node 13) have comparable survival with the older women with abnormal cytology. Thus, in addition to eliciting an anticipated prognostic subgroup with poor survival, the exploratory survival tree analysis has identified another prognostic subgroup with similarly high risk. The Kaplan–Meier curves in Figs 5.2 and 5.3 were obtained using `km.tssa(...)` which allows for interactive selection using the mouse to indicate splits in a displayed dendrogram, or by specifying node numbers as arguments.

5.5.2   HIV cohort study

The natural history of HIV disease is still not fully understood. Following infection with HIV, subjects progress to opportunistic infections, malignancies or neurological disease, defining AIDS, and then to death. These complications result from deterioration of immune function. It is of considerable clinical and epidemiological importance to understand the nature of this immune function decay since this will facilitate improvements in the timing and evaluation of therapies and in projecting the course of the epidemic. As mentioned, immune function markers such as CD4 T-lymphocytes (Lange *et al.*, 1992, and references therein) are used both to follow the course of immune function loss and to predict time to AIDS or death. More recently, direct measures of HIV viral burden have also been used for these purposes (Mellors *et al.*, 1996).

Here we consider a particular marker, delayed-type hypersensitivity (DTH) skin tests, as a supplement to the most established marker, namely CD4. CD4 cells are lost as part of the immunopathogenesis of HIV infection and CD4 counts have been a useful, but not entirely satisfactory, disease marker. Quantitation of peripheral blood CD4 depletion under-estimates the severity of the HIV-induced loss of antigen-specific cellular immunity and provides no guide as to which antigen-specific responses have been lost. More sensitive measures of antigen-specific cellular immunity are therefore required as an adjunct to the monitoring of CD4 counts. Testing of cutaneous DTH responses to recall antigens provides a direct measure of cell-mediated antigen-specific responses *in vivo*.

Assessment of these markers made recourse to the Western Australian HIV (WAHIV) database. Patients in Western Australia with HIV infection have been managed at a single specialist referral centre since the first AIDS case was confirmed in August, 1983. Both HIV-infected ($N = 545$) and at-risk individuals ($N = 191$) have been followed regularly. The closely scheduled (bimonthly) visits and early inception of the cohort provide a good opportunity for marker evaluation. Further details on the cohort, markers, handling seroprevalent (HIV positive at enrolment) subjects in the context of survival analysis, treating markers as time-dependent covariates, and complementary Cox proportional hazards results are given in Segal *et al.* (1995).

Here we present results from a tree-structured survival analysis of time to AIDS. The log-rank statistic was used a split function, although results were insensitive to this choice. The covariates used were age, CD4 and DTH, all measured at enrolment. CD4 is expressed as the percentage of T-lymphocytes that are CD4 positive, called CD4 per cent. This is in accord with Taylor *et al.* (1989) who, while noting strong correlations between this and other measures (CD4 count, CD4/CD8 ratio), found that CD4 per cent was most prognostic for time to AIDS and exhibited the smallest variability on repeated determinations.

The survival tree itself is displayed in Fig. 5.4. Restricting to complete cases yields a sample of 336 individuals, 76 of whom progressed to AIDS. This sample (here labelled as Node 0) is subdivided on the basis of CD4 per cent, the optimal cut-point being 11.5%. As displayed in Fig. 5.5, the survival (time to AIDS) of those 45 individuals with low CD4 per cent

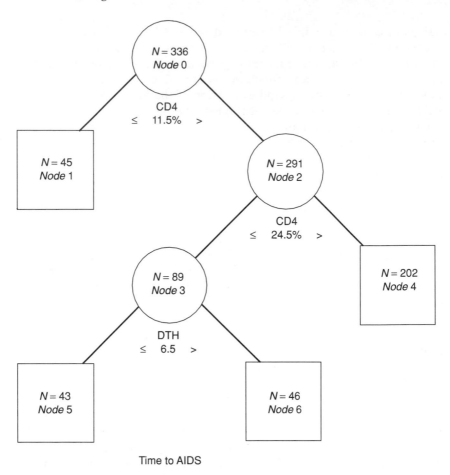

Fig. 5.4 Pruned survival tree for the HIV cohort study grown using covariates age, CD4%, DTH. The log-rank split statistic was used

(Node 1) is very poor. The 291 individuals with CD4 per cent exceeding 11.5% (Node 2) are also subdivided on the basis of CD4 per cent. Again, as anticipated, the 202 individuals with relatively high CD4 per cent (greater than 24.5%) have relatively good survival prospects (Fig. 5.6). The 75th percentile survival for these Node 4 individuals of 4.9 years is almost double that for the individuals whose CD4 per cent is less than 24.5% but greater than 11.5% (Node 3) – their 75th percentile is 2.5 years. The 89 Node 3 individuals are further partitioned, this time on the basis of DTH. The optimal cut-point is at DTH values of 6.5 mm. Figure 5.7 reveals appreciable survival differences for those in the two DTH defined subgroups. Thus, it is possible that DTH can serve to augment CD4 per cent as a marker for HIV progression: for individuals whose CD4 per cent values are intermediary, rather than extreme, additional prognostic information may be obtained from their DTH values.

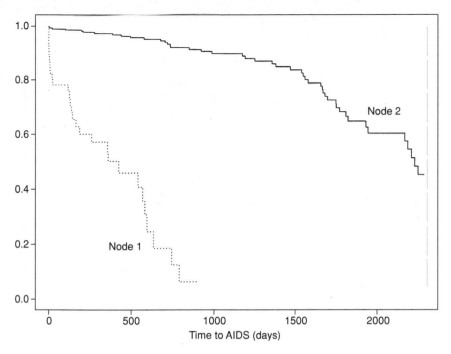

Fig. 5.5 Kaplan–Meier curves corresponding to the first split on CD4% with cut-point 11.5%

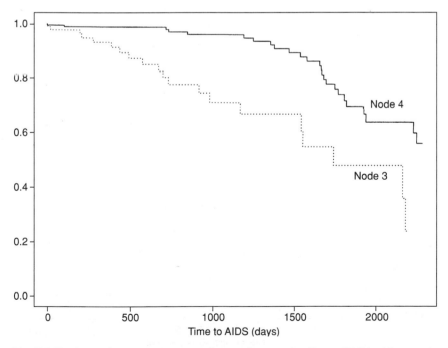

Fig. 5.6 Kaplan–Meier curves corresponding to the second split on CD4% with cut-point 24.5%

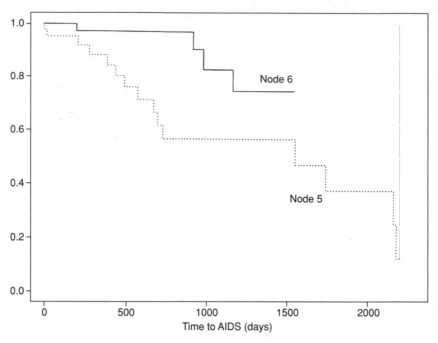

Fig. 5.7 Kaplan–Meier curves corresponding to the third split on DTH with cut-point 6.5 mm

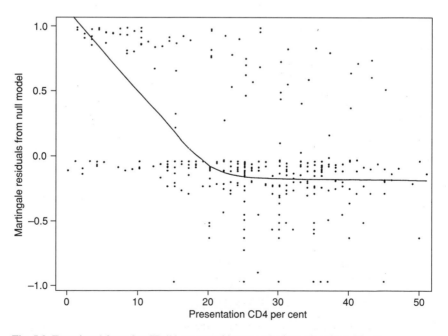

Fig. 5.8 Functional form for CD4% suggested by smoothed martingale residuals

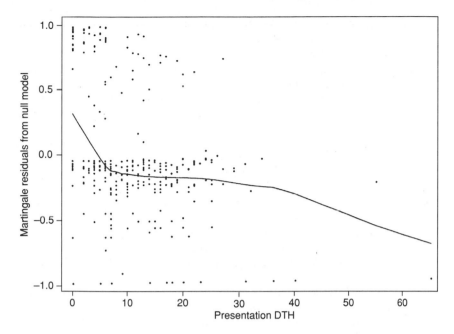

Fig. 5.9 Functional form for DTH suggested by smoothed martingale residual

It is interesting to contrast the splits with smoothed martingale residual plots obtained from a null Cox proportional hazards model that are useful for suggesting appropriate covariate functional form (Therneau *et al.*, 1990). Firstly, with regard the two successive CD4 per cent splits, it should be noted that the resultant trichotomy so obtained can be very different from trichotomies resulting from (computationally prohibitive) approaches based on either optimal ternary splitting (e.g. maximizing the three-sample version of the log-rank statistic), or less 'greedy' binary splitting employing lookahead (Elder, 1994). However, here the resultant CD4 per cent trichotomy (≤ 11.5, $11.5 < \text{CD4}\% \leq 24.5$, >24.5) conforms qualitatively with a three-piece step function approximation to the smoothed martingale residual plot for CD4 per cent (Fig. 5.8). Secondly, the cut-point of 6.5 mm for DTH conforms with clinical practice where dichotomies based on a threshold of 5 mm have been employed and is again consistent with a step function approximation of smoothed martingale residuals for DTH (Fig. 5.9).

References

Anderson, J. A. and Senthilselvan, A. 1980: Smooth estimates for the hazard function. *Journal of the Royal Statistical Society (B)* **42**: 322–7.

Bacchetti, P. and Moss, A. R. 1989: Incubation period of AIDS in San Francisco. *Nature* **338**, 251–3.

Bacchetti, P. and Segal, M. R. 1995: Survival trees with time-dependent covariates: application to estimating changes in the incubation period of AIDS. *Lifetime Data Analysis* **1**, 35–47.

Breiman, L., Friedman, J. H., Olshen, R. A. and Stone, C. J. 1984: *Classification and regression trees*. Belmont, CA: Wadsworth.

Clark, L. A. and Pregibon, D. 1992: Tree-based models. In Chambers, J. M. and Hastie, T. J. (eds), *Statistical models in S*. Pacific Grove, CA: Wadsworth.

Cox, D. R. 1972: Regression models and life-tables (with discussion). *Journal of the Royal Statistical Society (B)* **34**, 187–220.

Davis, R. and Anderson, J. 1989: Exponential survival trees. *Statistics in Medicine* **8**, 947–62.

Elder, J. F. 1994: Growing decision trees less greedily. *Proceedings of Interface 94: The 26th Symposium on the Interface*.

Fisher, W. D. 1958: On grouping for maximum heterogeneity. *Journal of the American Statistical Association* **53**, 789–98.

Friedman, J. H. 1991: Multiple adaptive regression splines. *Annals of Statistics* **19**, 1–67.

Gehan, E. A. 1965: A generalized Wilcoxon test for comparing arbitrarily singly-censored samples. *Biometrika* **52**, 203–23.

Gordon, L. and Olshen, R. 1985: Tree-structured survival analysis. *Cancer Treatment Reports* **69**, 1065–9.

Harrington, D. and Fleming, T. 1982: A class of rank test procedures for censored survival data. *Biometrika* **69**, 553–66.

Huang, X., Chen, S. and Soong, S.-J. 1994: Piecewise proportional hazards survival trees with time-dependent covariates. *Proceedings of Interface 94: The 26th Symposium on the Interface*.

King, E. B. *et al.* 1983: Nipple aspirate cytology for the study of breast cancer precursors. *Journal of the National Cancer Institute* **71**, 1115–21.

Lange, N., Carlin, B. P. and Gelfand, A. 1992: Hierarchical Bayes models for the progression of HIV infection using longitudinal CD4 T-cell numbers. *Journal of the American Statistical Association* **87**, 615–32.

Lausen, B. and Schumacher, M. 1992: Maximally selected rank statistics. *Biometrics* **48**, 73–85.

LeBlanc, M. and Crowley, J. 1992: Relative risk regression trees for censored survival data. *Biometrics* **48**, 411–25.

LeBlanc, M. and Crowley, J. 1993: Survival trees by goodness of split. *Journal of the American Statistical Association* **88**, 457–67.

Mellors, J. W., Rinaldo, C. R., Gupta, P., White, R. M., Todd, J. A. and Kingsley, J. A. 1996: Prognosis in HIV-1 infection predicted by the quantity of virus in plasma. *Science* **272**, 1167–70.

Miller, R. G. and Siegmund, D. 1982: Maximally selected chi square statistics. *Biometrics* **38**, 1011–16.

Muñoz, A. *et al.* 1989: AIDS free time after HIV seroconversion in homosexual men. *American Journal of Epidemiology* **130**, 530–9.

O'Sullivan, F. 1988: Fast computation of fully automated log-density and log-hazard estimators. *SIAM Journal of Scientific and Statistical Computing* **9**, 363–79.

Peto, R. and Peto, J. 1972: Asymptotically efficient rank-invariant test procedures. *Journal of the Royal Statistical Society (A)* **135**, 185–98.

Petrakis, N. L. *et al.* 1981: Epidemiology of breast fluid secretion: association with breast cancer risk factors and cerumen type. *Journal of the National Cancer Institute* **67**, 277–84.

Prentice, R. L. 1978: Linear rank tests with right-censored data. *Biometrika* **65**, 167–79.

Prentice, R. L. and Marek, P. 1979: A qualitative discrepancy between censored data rank tests. *Biometrics* **35**, 861–7.

Segal, M. R. 1988: Regression trees for censored data. *Biometrics* **44**, 35–47.

Segal, M. R. 1995: Extending the elements of tree-structured regression. *Statistical Methods in Medical Research* **4**, 219–36.

Segal, M. R. and Bloch, D. A. 1989: A comparison of proportional hazards and regression trees for censored data. *Statistics in Medicine* **8**, 539–50.

Segal, M. R., James, I. R., French, M. A. H. and Mallal, S. 1995: Statistical issues in the evaluation of markers of HIV progression. *International Statistical Review* **63**, 179–97.

Tarone, R. E. and Ware, J. 1977: On distribution-free tests for equality of survival distributions. *Biometrika* **64**, 156–60.

Taylor, J. M. G., Fahey, J. L., Detels, R. and Giorgi, J. V. 1989: CD4 percentage, CD4 number, and CD4:CD8 ratio in HIV infection: which to choose and how to use. *Journal of Acquired Immune Deficiency Syndromes* **2**, 114–24.

Therneau, T. M., Grambsch, P. M. and Fleming, T. R. 1990: Martingale-based residuals for survival models. *Biometrika* **77**, 147–60.

Tsai, W.-Y., Jewell, N. P. and Wang, M.-C. 1987: A note on the product-limit estimator under right censoring and left truncation. *Biometrika* **74**, 883–6.

Whittemore, A. S. and Keller, J. B. 1986: Survival estimates using splines. *Biometrics* **42**, 495–506.

Wrensch, M. R. *et al.* 1992: Breast cancer incidence in women with abnormal cytology in nipple aspirates of breast fluid. *American Journal of Epidemiology* **135**, 130–41.

Wrensch, M. R. *et al.* 1993: Breast cancer risk associated with abnormal cytology in nipple aspirates of breast fluid and prior history of breast biopsy. *American Journal of Epidemiology* **137**, 829–33.

Ying, Z. 1990: Linear rank statistics for truncated data. *Biometrika* **77**, 909–14.

6 Mixed and multi-level models for longitudinal data: growth curve models of language development

Alan Taylor, Kevin Pickering, Catherine Lord and Andrew Pickles

6.1 Introduction

Although methods of analysis for estimating population means and average effects dominate medical statistics, there are important areas in which the variability among individuals in these quantities is also of considerable importance. The analysis of cognitive development is one such area. This chapter will illustrate the application of *mixed* models (Goldstein, 1986) to analyse the development of language in young clinically referred children, in particular focusing on so-called *growth curve* models (Bryk and Raudenbush, 1987, Breslow and Clayton, 1993, Goldstein, 1995, Plewis, 1996). Methods for the analysis of growth have become more easily applicable with the development of software for multi-level models, such as MLn (Rasbash and Woodhouse, 1995) and HLM (Bryk *et al.*, 1993), and other programs for random effects modelling of unbalanced data (BMDP, 1990). These programs require neither the number of observations nor the intervals of time between observations to be the same for all sample units, making them applicable to a much wider range of clinical and epidemiological studies than their less flexible predecessors. We demonstrate this flexibility by means of an example investigating the structure and variability in the growth of language, using data from a longitudinal study of children suspected of having autism. In addition to standard univariate and multivariate growth models, we illustrate how left and right *censored* observations can be tackled, these being common in psychological testing where they are more usually referred to as *ceiling* or *floor* effects.

6.2   Language ability in autism

The data used in our examples are taken from a study on the early diagnosis of autism (the EDX study) carried out in North Carolina. The sample consisted of referrals to clinics taking part in TEACCH, a state-wide programme for children with autism. Those selected for inclusion in the sample were children below the age of 3, who had been referred to a clinic because of the possibility that they had autism or an autistic spectrum disorder or had other developmental delay. Autistic problems typically first become apparent before age 3 but it is often difficult to obtain a confident diagnosis until later. The selected children were followed up to the age of 5, and were seen for a total of three occasions over the length of the study. The median ages at each observation were 2.6, 3.6 and 4.7 years of age. Final diagnoses were obtained at age 5 when three groups were identified: (1) a group who were given a diagnosis of autism ($n = 64$); (2) a group who were diagnosed as having pervasive developmental disorder (PDD; $n = 31$); and (3) a group who were not diagnosed as either autistic or PDD – the non-spectrum group ($n = 29$). In these preliminary analyses eight cases have been excluded owing to missing covariate data. A major research interest of the study was to assess the extent of potentially distinctive developmental profiles among these three groups.

In our examples we will focus on the development of language as this is often much impaired in children with autism. Measures of language development were obtained at each occasion from parents and also by using standard psychometric tests. The parent measures used were the expressive and receptive language subscales of the Vineland adaptive behaviour scales (Sparrow *et al.*, 1984). On occasions 1 and 2 the standard psychometric measure used was the Mullen scales of early learning (Mullen, 1989). On occasion 3, when the children were between 4 and 5 years of age, some children were likely to have abilities that exceeded the upper limit of the Mullen scales. Thus on this occasion children received either the Mullen or the differential ability scales (DAS) (Elliott, 1990) or both. On the first occasion the Bayley developmental quotient (DQ) was also obtained for each child (Bayley, 1969, 1993). This is a standard measure of developmental level. In all analyses age-equivalent scores, with months as the units, have been used to simplify interpretation. For age-equivalent scores a value of k is equal to the normative language ability score at age k months.

The marginal distributions of the four language measures are given in Fig. 6.1. This shows spikeplots (Tukey, 1977) which give the frequencies of particular values for each of our measures. The cluster of observations at low values reflects the similarity of the children upon first assessment, nearly all with marked language delay. By the time of their final assessment there is much more variability in their scores as indicated by the larger spread of observations over the higher values of each scale. The

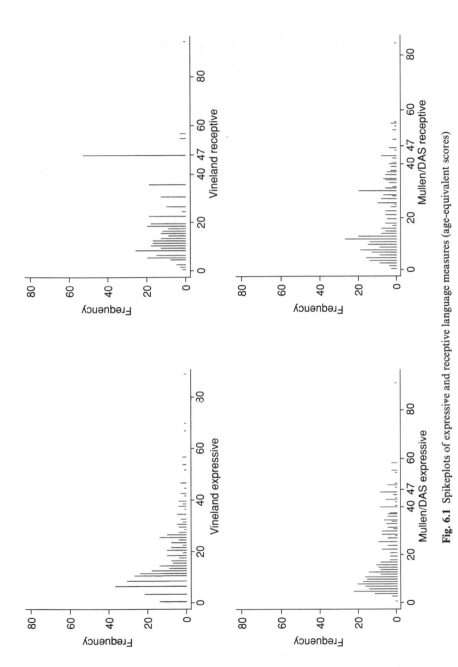

Fig. 6.1 Spikeplots of expressive and receptive language measures (age-equivalent scores)

distribution of the Vineland receptive measure shows an unusual feature: a large number of children with a value of 47, primarily obtained at the last measurement occasion. The reasons for this anomaly, and a method we illustrate for dealing with it, are discussed later. On all measures a single child from the PDD group has very high values on the last occasion but has been retained in our analyses as these elevated measures are in line with the expectation that the PDD group would be very heterogeneous.

6.3   Growth curve models

A major advantage of a growth curve model specified within a mixed modelling framework is that each individual's growth is modelled separately. This allows us to look at mean differences between groups while still retaining the ability to investigate individual differences in growth trajectories. This flexibility is achieved by having two parts to the model: a within-subjects model and a between-subjects model (Bryk and Raudenbush, 1987, 1989, Goldstein, 1995). For the within-subjects part we model each individual's observed measurements as a function of an individual growth trajectory with the addition of random error:

$$y_{it} = \pi_{0i} + \pi_{1i} \cdot Age_{it} + \pi_{2i} \cdot Age_{it}^2 + \cdots + \pi_{ki} \cdot Age_{it}^m + \varepsilon_{it} \qquad (6.1)$$

Here y_{it} is the observed outcome variable for individual i at occasion t and Age_{it} is the age of that individual at the same occasion. In this general model the growth terms can have a maximum polynomial of order m. The ε_{it} is random error and is assumed to have a mean of zero and some specified covariance structure. This covariance can take a wide variety of forms (Sternio *et al.*, 1983, Louis and Spiro, 1984, Ware, 1985, Goldstein, 1995) but since our sample is not that large, and the intervals between observations quite long, we apply the simplest assumption of constant variance and independent errors: $\text{cov}(\varepsilon_{it}, \varepsilon_{jt}) = 0$ where $i \neq j$. The larger the number of observations the more complex the polynomial in age that can be fitted. As we have a maximum of three measurement occasions we will restrict our attention to linear and quadratic growth terms in our examples.

The between-subjects model allows each of the parameters in the within-subjects model to vary over individuals. Interest usually lies in accounting for the between-subjects variability by measured substantive variables. Therefore we can make each growth parameter in equation (6.1) a function of P known variables as shown below:

$$\pi_{ki} = \beta_{k0} + \beta_{k1}X_{k1} + \cdots + \beta_{kP}X_{kP} + u_{ki} \qquad (6.2)$$

where $p = 1, \ldots, P$ are measured variables (X_{kp}), β_{kp} is the effect of X_{kp} on the kth growth parameter and u_{ki} is random error. The random terms (u_{ki}) are assumed to have a mean of zero and a general covariance structure of

$$\text{cov}(u_{hi}, u_{ki}) = \text{cov}(\pi_{hi}, \pi_{ki}|\mathbf{X}_h, \mathbf{X}_k) = \sigma_{hk} \tag{6.3}$$

for $h, k = 0, 1, \ldots, K$ and $p = 1, \ldots, P$ where $\mathbf{X}_h$ and $\mathbf{X}_k$ are the covariates in the between-subjects model for the growth terms h and k. In the language of multi-level models the β_{kp} terms are known as fixed effects and the u_{ki} as random effects.

To illustrate, consider the following simple within-subjects model:

$$y_{it} = \pi_{0i} + \pi_{1i} \cdot Age_{it} + \varepsilon_{it} \tag{6.4}$$

Here the intercept (π_{0i}) and the linear growth term (π_{1i}) are used to model the growth curve of each individual. We then model the between-subjects variability using a single covariate as follows:

$$\begin{aligned}
\pi_{0i} &= \beta_{00} + \beta_{01}X_i + u_{0i} \\
\pi_{1i} &= \beta_{10} + \beta_{11}X_i + u_{1i}
\end{aligned} \tag{6.5}$$

If we write out the full model and collect all the random terms together we have the following specification of the random part of the model for a given subject i at time t:

$$\text{total random part} = u_{0i} + u_{1i} \cdot Age_{it} + \varepsilon_{it} \tag{6.6}$$

We have assumed the within-subjects random term to be constant and independent across subjects. If its value is denoted as σ^2 then the total variance of the random part of the model is given as

$$\text{var}(y_{it}|X_i) = \sigma_{00}^2 + (Age_{it})^2\sigma_{11}^2 + 2Age_{it}\sigma_{01} + \sigma^2 \tag{6.7}$$

where σ_{00}^2 is the variance around the group mean, σ_{11}^2 is the variance around the linear growth term, and σ_{01} is the covariance between the mean and growth terms. This shows that the random variation in these models is a function of time (or age), which is sensible as subjects are assumed to grow at different rates. It is also worth noting that our models assume that each subject's observations are correlated over time. The covariance for subject i between two observations at t and t' under our current model is

$$\text{cov}(y_{it}, y_{it'}|X_i) = \sigma_{00}^2 + (Age_{it} + Age_{it'})\sigma_{01} + Age_{it}Age_{it'}\sigma_{11}^2 \tag{6.8}$$

This implies that the temporal correlation depends on the spacing of the observations, the magnitude of the variances of the linear growth and intercept terms, and the covariance between them.

In our examples we have applied an alternative parameterization to that given above, one which can be easier to interpret when the main covariate is a set of dummy variables for different clinical groups as it allows for distinct mean and growth terms for each group. In the example below the study-group-specific parameters are labelled as follows: non-spectrum (n); PDD (p); and autistic (a). A simple within-subjects model with intercept and linear growth terms in our parameterization is then given as

$$y_{it} = \pi_{0i}^n + \pi_{1i}^n \cdot Age_{it}^n$$
$$+ \pi_{0i}^p + \pi_{1i}^p \cdot Age_{it}^p$$
$$+ \pi_{0i}^a + \pi_{1i}^a \cdot Age_{it}^a$$
$$+ \varepsilon_{it} \tag{6.9}$$

where all the π parameters are now defined solely for members of each group using dummy variables for the intercept and with age terms specific to each group.

We then extend this model using the Bayley DQ measure as a covariate but only allowing it to impact on the between-subjects variability for the intercept terms. For simplicity we constrained the effect of the Bayley DQ to be constant over the three study groups rather than letting it vary across them. Our between-subjects model for the intercepts then becomes

$$\pi_{0i}^n = \beta_{00}^n + \beta_{01} DQ_i + u_{0i}^n$$
$$\pi_{0i}^p = \beta_{00}^p + \beta_{01} DQ_i + u_{0i}^p \tag{6.10}$$
$$\pi_{0i}^a = \beta_{00}^a + \beta_{01} DQ_i + u_{0i}^a$$

where β_{01} is the effect of the Bayley DQ measure. A simple between-subjects model with no added covariates was assumed for the other growth terms. For example, in the basic model (equation (6.9)) the linear growth terms are specified as

$$\pi_{1i}^n = \beta_{10}^n + u_{1i}^n$$
$$\pi_{1i}^p = \beta_{10}^p + u_{1i}^p \tag{6.11}$$
$$\pi_{1i}^a = \beta_{10}^a + u_{1i}^a$$

In this parameterization, u_{0i}^a is the variation in the autistic group around the group mean intercept β_{00}^a and u_{1i}^a is the variation around the group mean growth rate β_{10}^a. As equation (6.3) indicates, we also allow for a covariance term between the slopes and intercepts within each group; this is reasonable as those who start well often continue to do well.

It is important to appreciate the flexibility of these models besides allowing for the investigation of mean differences, differences in variability and in assessing the impact of measured covariates. Firstly, full data are not required for all time points as the estimation procedure takes account of missing values by assuming they are missing at random (Little and Rubin, 1987). Although this is quite a strong assumption it is less restrictive than the requirements of complete case analysis. Secondly, there is no requirement that the data be collected at the same time points or ages for all individuals. Obviously, if there is wide variation in the observation period then this will lead to sparseness of data at certain times, making inference less precise. Thirdly, as indicated above, the within-subjects covariance structure can take a wide variety of forms although the more complex modelling options are best applied to data with many time points per individual. Finally, there are many options for modelling the between-individual variability. For example, these models can accommodate different covariates for each growth parameter.

We used MLn (Rasbash and Woodhouse, 1995) to estimate all the models presented. MLn is a flexible PC package that allows for the estimation of a wide range of mixed models including those for binary and multi-category response data.

6.4   Growth curve model for parent report of expressive language

Table 6.1 gives the results for a model of the Vineland measure of expressive language. In all models age has been centred around the median

Table 6.1 Vineland expressive measure with and without Bayley developmental quotient

Fixed effects	Without Bayley DQ			With Bayley DQ		
	β	SE(β)	P value	β	SE(β)	P value
Mean at 40 months (intercept)						
Non-spectrum	24.00	1.80	<0.001	20.21	1.49	<0.001
PDD	16.56	1.29	<0.001	15.31	0.96	<0.001
Autistic	10.26	0.76	<0.001	10.95	0.63	<0.001
Growth at 40 months						
Non-spectrum	0.90	0.09	<0.001	0.90	0.09	<0.001
PDD	0.68	0.09	<0.001	0.68	0.08	<0.001
Autistic	0.35	0.04	<0.001	0.37	0.04	<0.001
Acceleration						
Non-spectrum	0.013	0.003	<0.001	0.012	0.004	0.003
PDD	0.003	0.003	0.317	0.004	0.003	0.182
Autistic	0.003	0.002	0.134	0.002	0.002	0.317
Bayley DQ	–	–	–	0.17	0.02	<0.001
Random effects	σ^2	SE(σ^2)	P value	σ^2	SE(σ^2)	P value
Mean at 40 months (intercept)						
Non-spectrum	78.68	22.64	0.001	45.11	13.86	0.001
PDD	42.67	12.11	<0.001	18.55	6.08	0.002
Autistic	27.70	5.81	<0.001	15.76	3.76	<0.001
Growth at 40 months						
Non-spectrum	0.18	0.06	0.003	0.17	0.06	0.005
PDD	0.17	0.05	0.001	0.16	0.05	0.001
Autistic	0.06	0.02	0.003	0.05	0.02	0.012
Covariance			Correlation			Correlation
Non-spectrum	3.45	1.04	0.92	2.52	0.79	0.90
PDD	2.30	0.70	0.84	1.64	0.49	0.95
Autistic	1.23	0.27	0.96	0.93	0.20	1.03
Residual variance	11.54	1.58	<0.001	12.77	1.69	<0.001

age over the study period (approximately 40 months). As a result, intercept estimates refer to the language ability at this age in the growth trajectories. The model was fitted with and without the Bayley DQ. As expected, the Bayley DQ is an important covariate for modelling language ability. The within-group random variation around the group intercept (or mean) at age 40 months is reduced when this covariate is included.

In this basic model of Table 6.1, all three groups have mean levels of expressive language at age 40 months below that of the norm of 40. The most severely affected group is the autistic group which has a mean expressive ability of just 25% of the norm for this age. As we are using age-equivalent scores the expected value of the linear growth rate is 1.0; becoming older by one month would normally give a one-month increase in the age-equivalent language ability. Both the PDD group and particularly the autistic group (only 35% of the norm) have a much lower growth rate than this expectation, while the non-spectrum group has a growth rate only slightly below the expected rate. An age-squared term was fitted for each group to detect any acceleration of the growth rate over the study period. This was only significant for the non-spectrum group and was small in magnitude. The growth trajectories of the other groups were adequately described by a linear growth term alone.

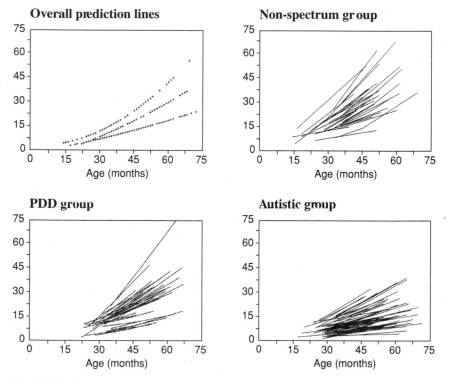

Fig. 6.2 Vineland expressive measure prediction lines

Plots of the overall prediction line and the individual prediction lines for each group give valuable information on the nature of the fitted model. Figure 6.2 gives the prediction lines for the three study groups. The mean prediction lines highlight the fact that the fitted model has the slowest growth rate for the autistic group (the bottom line) with the PDD group (the middle line) and the non-spectrum group (top line) having much higher growth rates. The small acceleration parameter for the non-spectrum group is reflected by the slight upward curve of the top line. The means at age 40 months, shown in Table 6.1, also show that the group of children with autism has a much lower mean expressive language ability than the other groups. The individual prediction lines for the non-spectrum and PDD groups show that there is much more variability in their language ability at 40 months and that their growth rates are more variable than those in the autism group.

6.5   Ceilings and floors: mixed models for censored data

Data from psychometric testing often have additional problems arising from ceiling or floor effects, since typically each test is designed to assess children within a limited age and ability range. Observations that fall up against the boundaries of this range can be considered as censored observations; the actual value for a given subject is not known but it is known to be above the recorded score, in the case of a ceiling, or below the recorded score, in the case of a floor. A model fitted to such data that does not allow for the presence of these ceiling or floor effects can lead to erroneous inference. For example, growth can appear to falter and flatten out as the result of the use of a measuring instrument beyond the point where the ceiling begins to limit recorded scores. A general procedure for taking account of censored observations is to model the censored data by some appropriate cumulative distribution function. If we assume an underlying normal distribution, this can be done by estimating underlying regression coefficients, mean and variance parameters that are common across a normal regression model for the uncensored observations, and a probit regression model for the censored observations (Maddala, 1983).

Consider the case of data with n_1 observations directly observed and n_2 observations right censored. A model for these data can be defined as

$$y_{it} = \beta'x_i + u_i \quad \text{if } y_{it} \text{ is uncensored}$$
$$= c_i \qquad \qquad \text{otherwise} \tag{6.12}$$

where c_i is the censoring value for subject i. Assuming the data are normally distributed the likelihood function for this model has the form

$$L = \prod_{n_2} [1 - \Phi(y_{it} = c_i)] \prod_{n_1} \frac{1}{(2\pi\sigma^2)^{1/2}} \exp[-(1/2\sigma^2)(y_i - \beta'x_i)^2] \tag{6.13}$$

with the log likelihood being defined as

$$\log L = \sum_{n_2} \log[1 - \Phi(y_{it} = c_i)] + \sum_{n_1} \log\left(\frac{1}{(2\pi\sigma^2)^{1/2}}\right) - \sum_{n_1} \frac{1}{2\sigma^2}(y_i - \beta'x_i)^2$$

(6.14)

Note that the log likelihood now has two additive components: one based on the cumulative normal distribution for the censored observations and the other based on the normal density function for the uncensored observations. This model can be estimated using a *composite link function* (CLF) that allows different link functions to be fitted to the censored and uncensored data (Thompson and Baker, 1981) to allow the simultaneous fitting of the normal regression and probit models. Application of this method is relatively straightforward using MLn macros that combine iterative weighted least squares estimation of a generalized linear model (Nelder and Wedderburn, 1972) with a Taylor series linearization for the random effects (Goldstein, 1991, Breslow and Clayton, 1993, Goldstein, 1995).

Consider a GLM with fixed effects collected up in the linear predictor η_f and random effects collected up in η_r, with the expected value given by $f(\eta_f + \eta_r)$. We expand $f(\eta_f + \eta_r)$ about the current estimates of the η, denoted by η^* (that for the random effects being a sum of shrunken random effects residuals), such that to the first order

$$E[Y] = f(\eta_f^* + \eta_r^*) + (\eta_f + \eta_r - \eta_f^* - \eta_r^*)f'(\eta_f^* + \eta_r^*) \qquad (6.15)$$

which can be rearranged such that each multi-level model fit is of the form

$$y - f(\eta_f^* + \eta_r^*) + (\eta_f^* + \eta_r^*)f'(\eta_f^* + \eta_r^*) = \eta_f f'(\eta_f^* + \eta_r^*) + \eta_r f'(\eta_f^* + \eta_r^*) + \varepsilon$$

(6.16)

This provides new estimates of η_f and η_r that are used in the next iteration.

Extension to the case where both left and right censoring are present is also possible, as is interval censoring where one knows the range, but not the actual value, of the observation. In these cases the log likelihood consists of two separate terms for the cumulative normal distribution for the left and right censored data points.

6.6   Ceiling effects in the parent report of receptive language

The Vineland is a parent report measure that is intended to cover almost the whole range of ability. As a result some compromises in its construction are inevitable. The Vineland parent report of receptive language provides an interesting example of what could be termed a 'sticky ceiling'. The spikeplot for the Vineland receptive measure in Fig. 6.1 indicates a large group of values at 47 months. This is a consequence of the scale having a region of sparse items, there being in this sample only one item that discriminates between 35 months and 54 months. Children with a language ability above 35 months are likely to appear to jump first to 47 months and then only once they have reached a language ability well beyond 47 months do they 'break through' this ceiling. We were therefore concerned that for the purposes of this study the scale did not function satisfactorily above a score of 35 months and have investigated the impact of recoding all measurements above 35 months back to this value and treating them as censored at this value. This issue is of particular

Table 6.2 Vineland receptive measure with and without censoring

Fixed effects	Without censoring			With censoring		
	β	SE(β)	*P* value	β	SE(β)	*P* value
Mean at 40 months (intercept)						
Non-spectrum	29.37	1.48	<0.001	27.92	1.46	<0.001
PDD	19.92	1.29	<0.001	19.10	1.12	<0.001
Autistic	13.46	0.83	<0.001	12.90	0.66	<0.001
Growth at 40 months						
Non-spectrum	0.86	0.07	<0.001	0.77	0.07	<0.001
PDD	0.86	0.09	<0.001	0.80	0.09	<0.001
Autistic	0.46	0.06	<0.001	0.42	0.04	<0.001
Acceleration						
Non-spectrum	−0.012	0.004	0.003	−0.010	0.004	0.012
PDD	−0.001	0.005	0.841	−0.001	0.005	0.841
Autistic	0.002	0.003	0.505	0.001	0.002	0.617
Bayley DQ	0.19	0.03	<0.001	0.16	0.02	<0.001

Random effects	σ^2	SE(σ^2)	*P* value	σ^2	SE(σ^2)	*P* value
Mean at 40 months (intercept)						
Non-spectrum	25.77	10.51	0.014	34.50	12.65	0.006
PDD	31.17	10.63	0.003	27.17	8.66	0.002
Autistic	22.88	6.12	<0.001	17.13	4.12	<0.001
Growth at 40 months						
Non-spectrum	0.04	0.03	0.182	0.05	0.03	0.096
PDD	0.14	0.06	0.020	0.18	0.07	0.010
Autistic	0.11	0.03	<0.001	0.07	0.02	<0.001
Covariance			Correlation			Correlation
Non-spectrum	0.74	0.43	0.70	1.05	0.54	0.80
PDD	1.69	0.61	0.81	1.55	0.61	0.70
Autistic	1.45	0.36	0.93	1.01	0.24	0.93
Residual variance	28.17	3.49	<0.001	13.37	2.01	<0.001

importance for the non-spectrum group as a particularly high proportion of this group (20 out of 29) had a score of 47 on the Vineland receptive scale on the last assessment occasion. Censoring the data in this way reduces the risk of model misspecification but at the possible cost of making less efficient use of the available information.

Table 6.2 gives results for models fitted with and without censoring to the Vineland receptive measure. Eliminating the 'sticky' 47 month score in fact results in a clear decrease in the fixed effect linear growth parameters, the magnitude of the changes being in the expected group ordering (non-spectrum > PDD > autism). Relatively bigger increases are seen for the estimated random effect variances. Overall, allowing for censoring also led to an increase in the standard errors of the estimates.

6.7   Ceiling and floor effects in the choice of measuring instrument

The Mullen and DAS measures are well-constructed tests with different but overlapping measurement ranges. The DAS measure has a floor of around 24 months for standardized scores but provides age-equivalent scores only down to 31 months. The Mullen scales have a ceiling of 60 months. In this study, in common with the use of such tests in most clinics, there was a preferred test (on the third assessment this was the DAS) which was used unless a preliminary informal assessment of the child, or a failure to obtain a score within the calibrated range of the preferred test, meant that an alternative test (the Mullen) was used. Of the 114 children with a third occasion assessment analysed here, only 10 children received age-equivalent test scores in the calibrated range of both tests, 68 received just a Mullen score (40 judged below the DAS floor), 27 children received just a DAS score, and 9 children fell below the 31 month DAS floor (but above the 24 month standardized score floor) but were not tested on the Mullen. How should such information be used?

The first column of Table 6.3 presents results where only valid test responses were included in the analysis. This excluded, for example, the group of 9 children identified above from contributing data for the last test occasion. The results in the second set of columns were obtained by adding additional records reflecting the below floor responses or likely responses on the DAS obtained by 49 less able subjects.

The below floor responses were again analysed by censored data models using the composite link function approach. Table 6.3 indicates increased growth rate estimates, particularly for the non-spectrum group, and much increased random effect variances in the model that adjusts for censoring. This more complete specification comes at a price, however, as can be seen by the inflated standard errors for both the mean and growth terms in the censored data model. For example, the estimated standard error for the comparison group's mean level increases from 1.25 to 1.37.

Table 6.3 Mullen/DAS receptive measures with and without ceiling and floor adjusted by censoring

	Without censoring			With censoring		
Fixed effects	β	SE(β)	P value	β	SE(β)	P value
Mean at 40 months (intercept)						
Non-spectrum	26.54	1.25	<0.001	27.02	1.37	<0.001
PDD	19.32	1.31	<0.001	19.35	1.31	<0.001
Autistic	12.30	0.65	<0.001	12.34	0.67	<0.001
Growth at 40 months						
Non-spectrum	0.79	0.06	<0.001	0.82	0.07	<0.001
PDD	0.70	0.07	<0.001	0.72	0.07	<0.001
Autistic	0.48	0.05	<0.001	0.49	0.05	<0.001
Bayley DQ	0.15	0.02	<0.001	0.14	0.02	<0.001
DAS	0.07	1.15	0.951	−3.10	0.99	0.002
Random effects	σ^2	SE(σ^2)	P value	σ^2	SE(σ^2)	P value
Mean at 40 months (intercept)						
Non-spectrum	26.21	9.30	0.005	36.00	11.51	0.002
PDD	44.92	13.26	0.001	45.83	13.30	0.001
Autistic	19.32	4.71	<0.001	21.26	5.00	<0.001
Growth at 40 months						
Non-spectrum	0.05	0.03	0.096	0.07	0.03	0.020
PDD	0.10	0.04	0.012	0.11	0.04	0.006
Autistic	0.08	0.02	<0.001	0.10	0.03	0.001
Covariance			Correlation			Correlation
Non-spectrum	1.27	0.43	1.09	1.71	0.53	1.07
PDD	2.06	0.63	0.97	2.13	0.64	0.96
Autistic	1.38	0.29	1.08	1.49	0.31	1.03
Residual variance	17.09	2.11	<0.001	16.31	2.02	<0.001

The DAS term in the model identifies the effects of a dummy variable for measurements where the DAS was used. Its presence in the model allowed for the testing of whether the two measures shared a common calibration. The inclusion of censored observations suggested that for the children of this study, the DAS was calibrated more stringently than the Mullen.

6.8   Multivariate growth curve models

Multivariate growth curve models can be applied easily within a mixed model framework and allow us to extend our analyses to investigate cross-measure correlations. This may be of interest for a variety of reasons. For example, the development of language might be less well synchronized for autistic individuals, suggesting that the correlation between their rates of growth of expressive and receptive language might be lower than among other children. Alternatively, our interests might lie in the correspondence of the estimates obtained from using different measurement methods. The example investigated here is of this kind, and concerned the relation between expressive language development as measured through the parental assessment and that through formal psychological testing. We expected that language growth based on the psychometric measure would be superior to that based on the parent measure, with the latter being contaminated by various forms of parental random and systematic bias, and therefore that the correlation between these two measures of growth might not be that high. We used a multivariate growth curve model to estimate this correlation.

In addition to estimating the variances of the random intercepts and random slopes for each measure, together with the covariance of the intercepts and slopes within each measure, four additional covariance terms are now required. These are the cross-measure covariances of intercepts, of slopes, and of intercepts of one measure with the slopes of the other. Different fixed effects can also be applied to each measure although in our simple model the same fixed effects were used for both.

Asymptotically, multivariate models should give estimates with smaller standard errors than their univariate equivalents. Although not shown, in our example the precision of the estimates compared with equivalent univariate models were in this case similar. Table 6.4 gives the estimated covariances and standard errors, and also the implied correlations and their standard errors. These last standard errors are not routine output of the program, but have been derived using the delta method applied to the covariance matrix of the estimated variance and covariance parameters. If the covariance between the variance of the intercept term σ_{00}^2 and the variance of the linear growth term σ_{11}^2 is denoted σ_{01}, then the implied correlation between the intercept and slope random terms is $\rho_{01} = \sigma_{01}/(\sqrt{\sigma_{00}^2 \sigma_{11}^2})$. By the delta method the variance of ρ_{01} is then

Table 6.4 Covariances and correlations for multivariate growth curve model: Vineland and Mullen/DAS expressive measures

Covariance	β	SE(β)	Correlation (ρ)	SE(ρ)
Within measure mean/growth				
Vineland	1.28	0.21	0.80	0.06
Mullen	1.66	0.27	0.82	0.05
Cross-measure				
Mean/mean	25.63	3.71	0.98	0.03
Growth/growth	0.11	0.02	0.91	0.04
Mean/growth	1.18	0.22	0.69	0.07
Growth/mean	1.32	0.24	0.71	0.07

$$\text{var}(\rho_{01}) = \frac{1}{\sigma_{00}^2 \sigma_{11}^2} \text{var}(\sigma_{01}) + \frac{\sigma_{01}^2}{4\sigma_{00}^6 \sigma_{11}^2} \text{var}(\sigma_{00}^2) + \frac{\sigma_{01}^2}{4\sigma_{00}^2 \sigma_{11}^6} \text{var}(\sigma_{11}^2)$$

$$+ 2\left(-\frac{\sigma_{01}}{2\sigma_{00}^4 \sigma_{11}^2} \text{cov}(\sigma_{01}, \sigma_{00}^2) - \frac{\sigma_{01}}{2\sigma_{00}^2 \sigma_{11}^4} \text{cov}(\sigma_{01}, \sigma_{11}^2) \right.$$

$$\left. + \frac{\sigma_{01}^2}{4\sigma_{00}^4 \sigma_{11}^4} \text{cov}(\sigma_{00}^2, \sigma_{11}^2) \right) \tag{6.17}$$

As can be seen the cross-measure correlations are surprisingly high, especially those of main interest, namely the cross-measure correlations of means (0.98) and of linear growth (0.91). There were no significant differences in any of the groups between the estimated mean intercepts and mean slopes for the two methods. Thus there was, for example, little evidence that parents were overemphasizing the progress of their children compared with the objective psychometric measure. This suggests that, for the assessment of expressive language, parental report may often be an adequate alternative to a psychometric assessment.

6.9 Discussion

In this chapter we have shown how the use of mixed models for the analysis of longitudinal data provides an efficient and flexible modelling framework that can handle problems far beyond the range of standard methods such as MANOVA. Mixed models also have the major advantage of estimating and displaying both systematic effects and patterns of variation in those effects. This is valuable in avoiding an exaggerated impression of the homogeneity of groups, but also properly reflects the likely real limits in the range of developmental outcomes of clinical groups of interest.

The software that is now available for estimating these models provides many options and possibilities for exploring the intricacies of model specification. Within the text we have tried to highlight this flexibility and how these models allow appropriate analysis of complex unbalanced data of the type that commonly occur in medical and psychological research. Other applications of mixed models include the analysis of physical growth (Yang and Leung, 1994), accelerated (overlapping) cohort designs (Raudenbush and Chan, 1993), and studies investigating geographical variation of health needs (Carr-Hill *et al.*, 1994). The mixed modelling approach is also useful with longitudinal data from experimental and clinical trials sources.

In this chapter we illustrated estimation only by iterative generalized least squares (IGLS). In the case of general linear models there would seem to be some grounds for preferring the use of restricted maximum likelihood rather than maximum likelihood (Diggle *et al.*, 1994). Use of the IGLS approach in the non-linear case of censored data required an approximate linearization technique, and alternative estimation methods might be preferred. Gibbs sampling would be an obvious contender. Regardless of the estimation method chosen, the mixed modelling method is not without problems. One of these is that the inherent flexibility of the approach can lead to a desire to fit overly complex models, a desire that often needs curbing, particularly in smaller samples.

Acknowledgements

The research reported here was supported by grants MH46865 and MH01196 (to CL) from the US NIMH and grant H519 25 5031 (to AP) from the UK ESRC Analysis of Large and Complex Datasets Programme.

References

Bayley, N. 1969: *Manual for the Bayley scales of infant development*. Psychological Corporation, New York.

Bayley, N. 1993: *Manual for the Bayley scales of infant development*, 2nd edn. Psychological Corporation, San Antonio, TX.

BMDP 1990: *BMDP 1990 Release*. BMDP Statistical Software Inc., Cork.

Breslow, N. E. and Clayton, D. G. 1993: Approximate inference in generalised linear models. *Journal of the American Statistical Association* **88**, 9–25.

Bryk, A. S. and Raudenbush, S. W. 1987: Application of hierarchical linear models to assessing change. *Psychological Bulletin* **101**, 147–58.

Bryk, A. S. and Raudenbush, S. W. 1989: Toward a more appropriate conceptualization of research on school effects: a three level hierarchical model. In Bock, D. R. (ed.), *Multilevel analysis of educational data*. San Diego: Academic Press, 159–204.

Bryk, A. S., Raudenbush, S. W. and Congdon, R. 1993: An introduction to HLM: computer program and user's manual. *Technical Report*, Department of Education, University of Chicago.

Carr-Hill, R. A., Sheldon, T. A., Smith, P., Martin, S., Peacock, S. and Hardman, G. 1994: Allocating resources to health authorities: development of a method for small area analysis of use of patient services. *British Medical Journal* **309**, 1046–9.

Diggle, P. J., Liang, K.-Y. and Zeger, S. L. 1994: *Analysis of longitudinal data*. Oxford Statistical Science. Oxford: Oxford Science Publications.

Elliott, C. D. 1990: *Differential ability scales (DAS)*. Psychological Corporation, San Antonio, TX.

Goldstein, H. 1986: Multilevel mixed linear model analysis using iterative generalised least squares. *Biometrika* **73**, 43–56.

Goldstein, H. 1991: Nonlinear multilevel models with an application to discrete response data. *Biometrika* **78**, 45–51.

Goldstein, H. 1995: *Multilevel statistical models*, 2nd edn. London: Arnold.

Little, R. J. A. and Rubin, D. B. 1987: *Statistical analysis with missing data*. Wiley Series in Probability and Mathematical Statistics. New York: John Wiley.

Louis, T. A. and Spiro, A. III 1984: Fitting first order auto-regressive models with covariates. *Technical Report*, Department of Biostatistics, Harvard University School of Public Health, Cambridge, MA.

Maddala, G. S. 1983: *Limited-dependent and qualitative variables in econometrics*. Cambridge: Cambridge University Press.

Mullen, E. 1989: *Mullen scales of early learning*. TOTAL Child Inc., Cranston, RI.

Nelder, J. A. and Wedderburn, R. W. M. 1972: Generalised linear models. *Journal of the Royal Statistical Society (A)* **135**, 370–84.

Plewis, I. 1996: Reading progress. In Woodhouse, G. (ed.), *Multilevel modelling applications: a guide for users of MLn*. Institute of Education, University of London: Multilevel Models Project, ch. 4.

Rasbash, J. and Woodhouse, G. 1995: *MLn command reference, version 1.0a*. Institute of Education, University of London: Multilevel Models Project.

Raudenbush, S. W. and Chan, W. S. 1993: Application of a hierarchical linear model to the study of adolescent deviance in an overlapping cohort design. *Journal of Consulting and Clinical Psychology* **61**, 941–51.

Sparrow, S., Balla, D. and Cicchetti, D. 1984: *Vineland adaptive behaviour scales*. American Guidance Service, Circle Pines, MN.

Sternio, J. L. F., Weisberg, H. I. and Bryk, A. S. 1983: Empirical Bayes estimation of individual growth curve parameters and their relationship to covariates. *Biometrics* **39**, 71–86.

Thompson, R. and Baker, R. J. 1981: Composite link functions in generalized linear models. *Applied Statistics* **30**, 125–31.

Tukey, J. W. 1977: Exploratory data analysis. Reading, MA: Addison-Wesley, ch. 17.

Ware, J. H. 1985: Linear models for the analysis of longitudinal studies. *Journal of the American Statistical Association* **80**, 95–101.

Yang, M. and Leung, S. S. 1994: Weight and length growth of two Chinese infant groups and the seasonal effects on their growth. *Annals of Human Biology* **21**, 547–62.

7 The analysis of longitudinal studies having non-normal responses

Charles S. Davis

7.1 Introduction

Many types of studies have research designs in which multiple measurements of a response variable are obtained from each experimental unit. Longitudinal studies, in which repeated measures are obtained over time from each subject, are one important and commonly used type of repeated measures study. A longitudinal study is uniquely suited to the study of individual patterns of change over time. In addition, longitudinal designs can provide more efficient estimators of parameters and more powerful tests of hypotheses than cross-sectional designs.

There are two main difficulties in the analysis of data from repeated measure designs. Firstly, the analysis is complicated by the dependence among repeated observations made on the same experimental unit. Secondly, the investigator often cannot control the circumstances for obtaining measurements, so that the data may be unbalanced or partially incomplete.

Longitudinal designs are used in many areas of application and are especially common in biomedical research. One indication of their importance in medical research is that four of the 13 chapters in this volume pertain to longitudinal data. In addition, several recent books written largely or partially from a biostatistical perspective focus on statistical methodology for the analysis of repeated measures; these include Jones (1993), Lindsey (1993), Diggle *et al.* (1994), Davidian and Giltinan (1995), Kshirsagar and Smith (1995), Crowder and Hand (1996), Vonesh and Chinchilli (1996) and Kenward (1997).

Numerous approaches to the analysis of longitudinal data have been studied; see, for example, the Koch *et al.* (1980) review and bibliography of parametric and non-parametric approaches. When the response variable is normally distributed, classical multivariate analysis techniques, repeated measures analysis of variance, growth curve analysis, and mixed effects models can be used. Normal theory methods for longitudinal data are discussed in Chapters 6 and 9 of this volume. The development of methods for the analysis of repeated measures categorical data for binary, polytomous and ordered categorical response variables is also an important area of research. In addition, recently developed approaches of generalized estimating equations based on extensions of generalized linear model methodology can be applied to a wide variety of types of continuous and categorical response variables with marginal (univariate) distributions from the class of generalized linear models. Chapter 8 discusses these approaches.

This chapter discusses the analysis of longitudinal studies having non-normal responses. More specifically, the focus is on distribution-free methods. While the approaches mentioned in the preceding paragraph require assumptions on either the joint or the marginal distributions of the response variable, there are at least three situations in which distribution-free methods may be useful. Firstly, when the response is continuous, the assumption of multivariate normality may not be reasonable or the underlying distribution may be unknown. In this case, the use of standard parametric procedures may not be justified. Secondly, when the response is an ordered categorical variable with a large number of possible outcomes, the general categorical data methods may be inapplicable owing to sample size limitations. In addition, the restrictive proportional odds assumption underlying some of the approaches for analysing ordered categorical repeated measures may not be justified. Apart from these considerations, there are also situations in which it may be desirable to confirm the results of a parametric analysis using distribution-free methods.

Section 7.2 presents the general layout and notation for longitudinal data and also discusses some specific special cases. In Section 7.3, I describe three examples of longitudinal studies with non-normal responses. Section 7.4 reviews and summarizes various statistical methods for analysing non-normal repeated measures. Finally, Section 7.5 applies several of these methods to the examples.

7.2   Layout and notation for longitudinal data

Table 7.1 displays the general layout and notation for a repeated measures design with n subjects (experimental units) and t_i measurement times for the ith subject, $i = 1, \ldots, n$. The response from subject i at time j is y_{ij} and $\mathbf{x}_{ij} = (x_{ij1}, \ldots, x_{ijp})'$ is the corresponding $p \times 1$ vector of covariates. In general, the covariates can be a mixture of time-independent (between-subject) covariates and time-dependent (within-subject) covariates. Since values of the response variable and/or covariates might be missing, it may be convenient to define indicator variables δ_{ij} by

Table 7.1 Layout and notation for a general repeated measures design

Subject	Time point	Missing indicator	Response	Covariates		
1	1	δ_{11}	y_{11}	x_{111}	$\cdots$	x_{11p}
	$\vdots$	$\vdots$	$\vdots$	$\vdots$	$\ddots$	$\vdots$
	j	δ_{1j}	y_{1j}	x_{1j1}	$\cdots$	x_{1jp}
	$\vdots$	$\vdots$	$\vdots$	$\vdots$	$\ddots$	$\vdots$
	t_1	δ_{1t_1}	y_{1t_1}	x_{1t_11}	$\cdots$	x_{1t_1p}
i	1	δ_{i1}	y_{i1}	x_{i11}	$\cdots$	x_{i1p}
	$\vdots$	$\vdots$	$\vdots$	$\vdots$	$\ddots$	$\vdots$
	j	δ_{ij}	y_{ij}	x_{ij1}	$\cdots$	x_{ijp}
	$\vdots$	$\vdots$	$\vdots$	$\vdots$	$\ddots$	$\vdots$
	t_i	δ_{it_i}	y_{it_i}	x_{it_i1}	$\cdots$	x_{it_ip}
n	1	δ_{n1}	y_{n1}	x_{n11}	$\cdots$	x_{n1p}
	$\vdots$	$\vdots$	$\vdots$	$\vdots$	$\ddots$	$\vdots$
	j	δ_{nj}	y_{nj}	x_{nj1}	$\cdots$	x_{njp}
	$\vdots$	$\vdots$	$\vdots$	$\vdots$	$\ddots$	$\vdots$
	t_n	δ_{nt_n}	y_{nt_n}	x_{nt_n1}	$\cdots$	x_{nt_np}

$$\delta_{ij} = \begin{cases} 1 & \text{if } y_{ij} \text{ and } \mathbf{x}_{ij} \text{ are observed} \\ 0 & \text{otherwise} \end{cases}$$

One simplification of the general notation displayed in Table 7.1 is the case when every subject has the same fixed set of measurement times, so that $t_i = t$, for $i = 1, \ldots, n$. The situation is also simplified when there are no missing data. A special case which has been studied extensively from the distribution-free perspective is the multi-sample setting in which repeated measurements are obtained from samples from s subpopulations. The s groups may be defined by the s levels of a single covariate or by the cross-classification of several discrete covariates. In terms of the general notation, the s groups can thus be described in terms of $p = s - 1$ dichotomous, time-independent covariates. In this setting, the notation of Table 7.2 is useful, in which y_{hij} denotes the response at time j from subject i in group h, for $j = 1, \ldots, t$, $i = 1, \ldots, n_h$, and $h = 1, \ldots, s$.

In the case of repeated measurements obtained at t time points from each of n subjects from a single sample, the data can be displayed even more simply in an $n \times t$ matrix, as shown in Table 7.3. As before, missing value indicators can be defined by

$$\delta_{ij} = \begin{cases} 1 & \text{if } y_{ij} \text{ is observed} \\ 0 & \text{otherwise} \end{cases}$$

In the one-sample situation, interest often focuses on assessing whether, and how, the distribution of the response variable changes over time.

Table 7.2 Layout and notation for a multi-sample repeated measures design

Group	Subject	Time point 1	$\cdots$	j	$\cdots$	t
1	1	y_{111}	$\cdots$	y_{11j}	$\cdots$	y_{11t}
	$\vdots$	$\vdots$	$\ddots$	$\vdots$	$\ddots$	$\vdots$
	i	y_{1i1}	$\cdots$	y_{1ij}	$\cdots$	y_{1it}
	$\vdots$	$\vdots$	$\ddots$	$\vdots$	$\ddots$	$\vdots$
	n_1	$y_{1n_1 1}$	$\cdots$	$y_{1n_1 j}$	$\cdots$	$y_{1n_1 t}$
h	1	y_{h11}	$\cdots$	y_{h1j}	$\cdots$	y_{h1t}
	$\vdots$	$\vdots$	$\ddots$	$\vdots$	$\ddots$	$\vdots$
	i	u_{hi1}	$\cdots$	y_{hij}	$\cdots$	y_{hit}
	$\vdots$	$\vdots$	$\ddots$	$\vdots$	$\ddots$	$\vdots$
	n_h	$y_{hn_h 1}$	$\cdots$	$y_{hn_h j}$	$\cdots$	$y_{hn_h t}$
s	1	y_{s11}	$\cdots$	y_{s1j}	$\cdots$	y_{s1t}
	$\vdots$	$\vdots$	$\ddots$	$\vdots$	$\ddots$	$\vdots$
	i	y_{si1}	$\cdots$	y_{sij}	$\cdots$	y_{sit}
	$\vdots$	$\vdots$	$\ddots$	$\vdots$	$\ddots$	$\vdots$
	n_s	$y_{sn_s 1}$	$\cdots$	$y_{sn_s j}$	$\cdots$	$y_{sn_s t}$

Table 7.3 Layout and notation for a one-sample repeated measures design

Subject	Time point 1	$\cdots$	j	$\cdots$	t
1	y_{11}	$\cdots$	y_{1j}	$\cdots$	y_{1t}
$\vdots$	$\vdots$	$\ddots$	$\vdots$	$\ddots$	$\vdots$
i	y_{i1}	$\cdots$	y_{ij}	$\cdots$	y_{it}
$\vdots$	$\vdots$	$\ddots$	$\vdots$	$\ddots$	$\vdots$
n	y_{n1}	$\cdots$	y_{nj}	$\cdots$	y_{nt}

7.3   Examples

7.3.1   A one-sample problem

As part of a protocol at the University of Iowa Mental Health Clinical Research Center, 44 schizophrenic patients participated in a four-week antipsychotic medication washout. The severity of extrapyramidal side effects was assessed just prior to discontinuation of antipsychotic medication and at weeks 1, 2, 3 and 4 during the washout period. Since

Table 7.4 Weekly Simpson–Angus ratings for 44 schizophrenic patients

Patient	Week 0	Week 1	Week 2	Week 3	Week 4
1	1	4	0	0	0
2	4	5	8	9	3
3	1	2	2	1	1
4	8	7	0	5	5
5	1	1	0	1	1
6	3	2	0	0	0
7	4	4	4	–	2
8	–	–	1	9	6
9	6	6	0	0	0
10	3	3	0	0	0
11	6	4	1	0	0
12	0	0	0	0	–
13	3	0	17	5	22
14	8	1	2	2	0
15	0	0	0	0	0
16	0	0	5	1	2
17	1	5	4	5	2
18	2	1	–	–	–
19	0	0	0	0	0
20	0	0	6	8	5
21	0	0	0	0	–
22	11	12	0	0	0
23	10	6	0	0	1
24	3	0	2	1	1
25	1	0	1	1	0
26	0	5	0	?	4
27	0	0	0	–	–
28	3	0	0	0	–
29	7	7	3	4	5
30	12	22	15	24	5
31	3	0	0	0	0
32	0	0	0	0	0
33	1	0	0	0	0
34	0	0	0	0	0
35	7	1	10	7	5
36	2	0	0	1	0
37	10	5	5	8	2
38	2	0	4	0	1
39	5	2	1	3	2
40	0	0	0	–	–
41	1	1	0	1	3
42	0	0	0	0	–
43	0	0	0	0	0
44	1	0	2	1	1

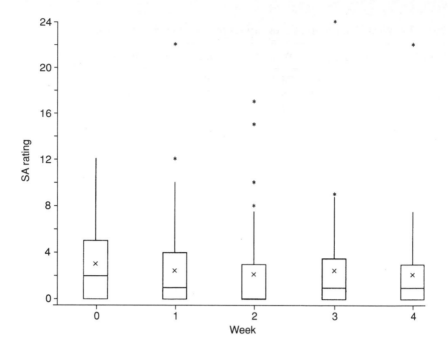

Fig. 7.1 Modified boxplots of weekly Simpson–Angus ratings for 44 schizophrenic patients

these types of side effects frequently accompany the use of antipsychotic medications, the investigators were interested in determining if such symptoms improve during washout.

Table 7.4 displays the resulting ratings on the Simpson–Angus (SA) scale (Simpson and Angus, 1970). The SA scale rates 10 aspects (e.g. elbow rigidity, arm dropping) from 0 to 4 (normal to extremely symptomatic) and yields a total score ranging from 0 to 40. High scores indicate greater symptom severity. A few missing values in Table 7.4 are denoted by –.

Figure 7.1 displays modified boxplots (Moore and McCabe, 1993, 42–3) of the weekly SA ratings. At each time point, the first quartile (25th percentile), median, third quartile (75th percentile) and sample mean (denoted by ×) are displayed. Data points more than 1.5 times the interquartile range beyond the quartiles are displayed individually (∗); otherwise, the upper and lower limits of each plot extend to the largest and smallest observations.

The marginal distributions of the SA ratings are clearly non-normal. At each time point, both the minimum value and the 25th percentile are equal to zero, as is the median at week 2. The median SA ratings at weeks 0–4 are 2, 1, 0, 1 and 1, respectively. The mean ratings of 3.0, 2.5, 2.2, 2.5 and 2.1 also indicate a tendency for SA ratings to decrease following the withdrawal of antipsychotic medications.

7.3.2 A multi-sample problem with complete data

Leppik *et al.* (1987) conducted a clinical trial in 59 epileptic patients. In this study, patients suffering from simple or complex partial seizures were randomized to receive either the antiepileptic drug progabide (31 patients) or a placebo (28 patients). At each of four successive postrandomization visits, the number of seizures occurring during the previous two weeks was reported. The medical question of interest is whether or not progabide reduces the frequency of epileptic seizures.

Table 7.5 displays the seizure counts during the successive two-week periods for patients in each of the two groups; these data were obtained from Thall and Vail (1990). Figure 7.2 displays side-by-side modified boxplots (Moore and McCabe, 1993, 42–3) for the two treatments at each assessment time. The sample means in the progabide and placebo groups are denoted by full and open circles, respectively. During each two-week period, there appears to be a slight tendency for seizure counts to be lower in progabide-treated patients than in placebo-treated patients. The median number of seizures in the progabide group at weeks 2, 4, 6 and 8 is 4, 5, 4 and 4, respectively. The corresponding medians in the placebo group are 5, 4.5, 5 and 5, respectively.

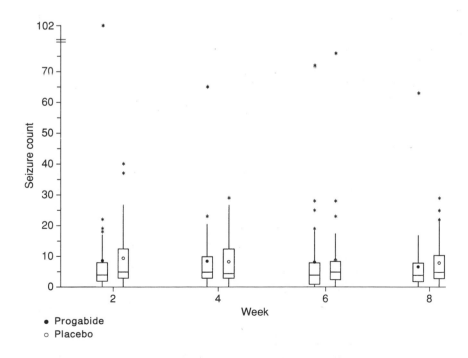

● Progabide
○ Placebo

Fig. 7.2 Modified boxplots of successive two-week seizure counts for 59 epileptic patients

Table 7.5 Successive two-week seizure counts for 59 epileptic patients

Treatment	ID	Week 2	Week 4	Week 6	Week 8
Progabide	101	11	14	9	8
	102	8	7	9	4
	103	0	4	3	0
	108	3	6	1	3
	110	2	6	7	4
	111	4	3	1	3
	112	22	17	19	16
	113	5	4	7	4
	117	2	4	0	4
	121	3	7	7	7
	122	4	18	2	5
	124	2	1	1	0
	128	0	2	4	0
	129	5	4	0	3
	137	11	14	25	15
	139	10	5	3	8
	143	19	7	6	7
	147	1	1	2	3
	203	6	10	8	8
	204	2	1	0	0
	207	102	65	72	63
	208	4	3	2	4
	209	8	6	5	7
	211	1	3	1	5
	214	18	11	28	13
	218	6	3	4	0
	221	3	5	4	3
	225	1	23	19	8
	228	2	3	0	1
	232	0	0	0	0
	236	1	4	3	2
Placebo	104	5	3	3	3
	106	3	5	3	3
	107	2	4	0	5
	114	4	4	1	4
	116	7	18	9	21
	118	5	2	8	7
	123	6	4	0	2
	126	40	20	23	12
	130	5	6	6	5
	135	14	13	6	0
	141	26	12	6	22
	145	12	6	8	4
	201	4	4	6	2
	202	7	9	12	14
	205	16	24	10	9
	206	11	0	0	5
	210	0	0	3	3
	213	37	29	28	29
	215	3	5	2	5
	217	3	0	6	7
	219	3	4	3	4
	220	3	4	3	4
	222	2	3	3	5
	226	8	12	2	8
	227	18	24	76	25
	230	2	1	2	1
	234	3	1	4	2
	238	13	15	13	12

7.3.3 A multi-sample problem with incomplete data

In a clinical trial comparing two treatments for maternal pain relief during labour, 83 women in labour were randomized to receive an experimental pain medication (43 subjects) or placebo (40 subjects). Treatment was initiated when the cervical dilation was 8 cm. At 30 min intervals, the amount of pain was self-reported by placing a mark on a 100 mm line (0 = no pain, 100 = very much pain).

Table 7.6 displays the resulting pain scores. There are numerous missing values; these occur most frequently at the later time points. Figure 7.3 displays side-by-side modified boxplots (Moore and McCabe, 1993, 42–3) for the two treatments at each assessment time. The sample means in the experimental and placebo groups are denoted by full and open circles, respectively. The marginal distributions at each time point are clearly non-normal. At the 30 and 60 min assessments in the placebo group and at all assessments in the experimental group, both the minimum value and the 25th percentile are equal to zero (no pain). While the marginal distributions are positively skewed in the experimental group at all time points, the distributions in the placebo group at minutes 120, 150 and 180 are negatively skewed.

At each of the six assessment times, the distributions in the two groups appear to differ. The median pain scores in the experimental group at

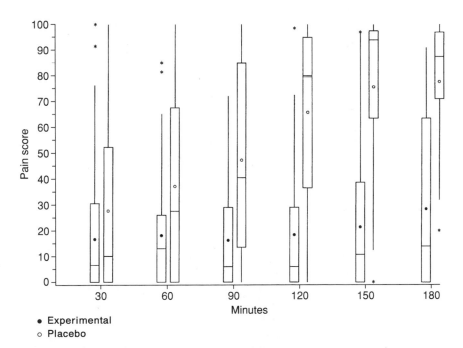

● Experimental
○ Placebo

Fig. 7.3 Modified boxplots of self-reported pain scores at 30 min intervals for 83 women in labour

Table 7.6 Self-reported pain scores at 30 min intervals for 83 women in labour

Treatment	Patient	Minute					
		30	60	90	120	150	180
Active	1	0.0	0.0	0.0	–	–	–
	2	0.0	0.0	0.0	2.5	2.3	14.0
	3	5.0	1.0	1.0	0.0	5.0	–
	4	48.0	85.0	0.0	0.0	–	–
	5	5.0	–	–	–	–	–
	6	0.0	0.0	0.0	–	–	–
	7	42.0	42.0	45.0	–	–	–
	8	0.0	0.0	0.0	0.0	6.0	24.0
	9	35.0	13.0	–	–	–	–
	10	30.5	81.5	67.5	98.5	97.0	–
	11	44.5	55.0	69.0	72.5	39.5	26.0
	12	0.0	0.0	0.0	0.0	0.0	0.0
	13	30.5	26.0	24.0	29.0	45.0	91.0
	14	6.5	7.0	4.0	10.0	–	–
	15	8.5	19.5	16.5	42.5	45.5	48.5
	16	9.5	7.5	5.5	4.5	0.0	7.0
	17	10.0	18.0	32.5	0.0	0.0	0.0
	18	20.5	32.5	37.0	39.0	–	–
	19	91.5	4.5	32.0	10.5	10.5	10.5
	20	0.0	0.0	0.0	13.5	7.0	–
	21	0.0	0.0	1.0	1.5	0.0	0.0
	22	21.0	15.5	10.5	11.5	11.0	9.5
	23	7.0	19.5	22.0	57.5	38.0	68.0
	24	43.0	43.0	41.5	41.5	–	–
	25	0.0	0.0	0.0	0.0	0.0	1.5
	26	0.0	0.0	0.0	0.0	0.0	0.0
	27	0.0	35.0	72.0	–	–	–
	28	19.0	23.0	0.0	37.0	42.0	66.0
	29	0.0	23.0	11.0	3.0	34.5	–
	30	0.0	15.5	6.0	0.0	–	–
	31	100.0	–	–	–	–	–
	32	3.0	–	–	–	–	–
	33	7.0	18.5	–	–	–	–
	34	0.5	0.0	1.0	–	–	–
	35	1.0	0.0	10.0	6.0	11.0	25.0
	36	9.5	14.5	9.5	2.5	23.5	63.5
	37	4.5	–	–	–	–	–
	38	31.0	37.5	–	–	–	–
	39	51.0	49.0	29.0	26.5	68.0	84.0
	40	0.0	0.0	–	–	–	–
	41	0.0	1.5	5.5	19.5	25.5	–
	42	21.0	9.0	9.0	–	–	–
	43	0.0	3.0	0.5	0.0	0.0	0.0

Table 7.6 (*continued*)

Treatment	Patient	Minute					
		30	60	90	120	150	180
Placebo	1	9.0	30.0	75.0	49.0	97.0	–
	2	0.0	1.0	27.5	95.0	100.0	–
	3	6.0	25.0	–	–	–	–
	4	18.0	12.5	–	–	–	–
	5	99.0	100.0	100.0	100.0	100.0	100.0
	6	70.0	81.5	94.5	97.0	–	–
	7	0.0	0.0	1.5	0.0	18.0	71.0
	8	51.5	56.0	–	–	–	–
	9	7.0	7.0	9.0	25.0	36.0	20.0
	10	31.0	41.0	58.0	–	–	–
	11	23.0	45.0	67.0	90.5	–	–
	12	64.0	6.0	–	–	–	–
	13	53.0	88.0	100.0	100.0	–	–
	14	100.0	100.0	100.0	100.0	–	–
	15	36.5	74.0	97.0	100.0	100.0	95.0
	16	0.0	6.0	6.0	–	–	–
	17	79.0	80.5	85.0	90.0	97.5	97.0
	18	27.5	21.0	60.0	80.0	97.0	–
	19	5.5	18.5	20.0	36.5	63.5	81.5
	20	9.0	35.5	39.0	70.0	92.0	98.0
	21	11.0	13.5	31.0	32.5	36.5	87.5
	22	74.0	91.5	–	–	–	–
	23	0.0	0.0	0.5	48.0	–	–
	24	3.5	–	–	–	–	–
	25	2.5	5.0	33.0	52.5	89.0	96.5
	26	4.5	–	–	–	–	–
	27	0.0	10.0	5.0	18.0	–	–
	28	0.0	0.0	13.5	49.5	94.0	80.5
	29	19.0	42.0	18.0	25.0	24.0	36.0
	30	68.5	92.5	100.0	100.0	100.0	100.0
	31	0.0	0.0	28.0	81.5	100.0	–
	32	25.0	45.5	50.0	60.5	65.5	72.5
	33	100.0	–	–	–	–	–
	34	5.0	5.5	5.0	–	–	–
	35	26.0	35.0	42.0	94.0	97.0	97.0
	36	0.0	0.0	0.0	0.0	0.0	32.0
	37	0.0	–	–	–	–	–
	38	0.0	9.0	54.0	81.5	84.5	–
	39	71.0	93.0	94.0	95.0	95.0	–
	40	0.0	61.0	–	–	–	–

minutes 30, 60, 90, 120, 150 and 180 are 6.5, 13, 6, 6, 10.75 and 14, respectively. The corresponding median scores in the placebo group are 10, 27.5, 40.5, 80, 94 and 87.5. Although the pain scores tend to increase in both groups over time, the scores in the experimental group tend to be lower than the scores in the placebo group at each time point. The difference between the two groups also seems to increase over time.

7.4   Distribution-free methods for the analysis of non-normal repeated measures

7.4.1   Univariate methods

The simplest approach to analysing longitudinal data is to reduce the vector of responses from each subject or experimental unit to a single measurement. This avoids the issue of correlation among the repeated measures for each subject. Pocock (1983), Matthews *et al.* (1990), Frison and Pocock (1992) and Dawson (1994) refer to these types of methods as the 'summary statistic approach'. Crowder and Hand (1990) and Diggle *et al.* (1994) call such methods 'response feature analysis' and 'derived variable analysis', respectively. The univariate function of the repeated measures from each subject can then be analysed using distribution-free methods.

For example, in the one-sample setting (Table 7.3), interest may focus on assessing the extent of association between the response variable and the repeated measures factor. If the Spearman rank correlation coefficient between the response variable and the repeated measures variable is used as the summary statistic for each subject, the sign test or the Wilcoxon signed rank test can be used to test if the median of the distribution of the summary statistic is equal to zero. In the multi-sample setting (Table 7.2), similar methods can be used. For example, the Mann–Whitney–Wilcoxon (if $s = 2$) or Kruskal–Wallis ($s > 2$) test can be used to assess if the distribution of the summary statistic is the same across the s groups.

While the summary statistic approach can be useful in certain situations, a shortcoming is that the results may be misleading if the selected univariate summary measure does not adequately describe each subject's data. Ghosh *et al.* (1973) describe multivariate non-parametric methods based on the use of two or more summary statistics for each subject. This extension of the univariate summary statistic approach may be useful when multiple univariate statistics are necessary to summarize each subject's data adequately. Carr *et al.* (1989) describe a different type of multivariate approach based on summary statistics. They consider the situation in which an ordered categorical or interval response variable is measured at multiple time points for each subject in two or more ordered groups. Rank measures of association between group and response are constructed at each time point; the estimated covariance matrix of these summary measures is then used to test hypotheses concerning the rank measures of association.

7.4.2 Multivariate generalizations of univariate distribution-free methods

Standard asymptotically distribution-free tests for multivariate one-sample and multi-sample problems can also be used in the repeated measures setting. These rank-based methods are appropriate for samples from continuous multivariate distributions.

For the one-sample case with complete data, Hettmansperger (1984, ch. 6) and Puri and Sen (1971, ch. 4) study multivariate generalizations of the sign and Wilcoxon signed rank tests. In the repeated measures setting of Table 7.3 with no missing data, let θ_t denote the median of the marginal distribution of the response at time t. By transforming each of the n t-component vectors $\mathbf{y}_i = (y_{i1}, \ldots, y_{it})'$ to a $(t-1)$-component vector of differences $\mathbf{y}_i^* = (y_{i1} - y_{i2}, \ldots, y_{i,t-1} - y_{it})'$, these methods can then be used to test the null hypothesis that $\theta_1 = \cdots = \theta_t$.

Hettmansperger (1984) also considers the two-sample situation with complete data; the test statistic is a multivariate version of the Mann–Whitney–Wilcoxon test. Puri and Sen (1971, ch. 5) discuss multivariate generalizations of the Kruskal–Wallis (1952) and Brown–Mood (1951) tests for the multivariate multi-sample situation with complete data. Based on these results, Schwertman (1982) gives a computer algorithm for two of these tests: the multivariate multi-sample rank sum test and the multivariate multi-sample median test. These methods can be applied to the repeated measures setting of Table 7.2, as follows.

Let $F_h(\mathbf{u})$ denote the t-variate cumulative distribution function (cdf) in group h, for $h = 1, \ldots, s$, where $\mathbf{u} = (u_1, \ldots, u_t)'$. Assume that the cdfs F_h have a common unspecified form with possible differences in their location (or scale) parameters. For example, suppose that $F_h(\mathbf{u}) = F(\mathbf{u} + \boldsymbol{\Delta}_h)$, where $\boldsymbol{\Delta}_h = (\Delta_{h1}, \ldots, \Delta_{ht})'$. The null hypothesis of no difference among groups across all time point tests $H_0\colon \boldsymbol{\Delta}_1 = \cdots = \boldsymbol{\Delta}_s = (0, \ldots, 0)'$. The omnibus alternative hypothesis is that $\boldsymbol{\Delta}_1, \ldots, \boldsymbol{\Delta}_s$ are not all equal.

Consider the $n \times t$ data matrix ($n = n_1 + \cdots + n_s$) of Table 7.2 and let $\mathbf{R}$ denote the $n \times t$ matrix of ranks resulting from ranking each of the t columns of the data matrix (all groups combined) in ascending order. Let R_{ij} denote the (i, j)th element of $\mathbf{R}$, let $E_{ij} = J[R_{ij}/(n+1)]$ for some function J satisfying Puri and Sen's (1971, 95) conditions, and let $\overline{E}_{hj}$ denote the average rank score at the jth time point in the hth sample. Puri and Sen (1971) derive a general test statistic L which is a weighted sum of s quadratic forms in $\overline{\mathbf{E}}_h - \overline{\mathbf{E}}_.$, where $\overline{\mathbf{E}}_h$ is the $t \times 1$ vector of average rank scores from the hth sample and $\overline{\mathbf{E}}_.$ is the vector of average rank scores from all samples combined. They show that the asymptotic null distribution of L is chi-square with $t(s-1)$ degrees of freedom ($\chi^2_{t(s-1)}$) and also note that

L is asymptotically equivalent to the likelihood ratio test based on Hotelling's T^2 statistic.

For each sample at each time point, the multivariate multi-sample rank sum test compares the difference between the sample average rank and the combined data average rank. Let $\mathbf{r}_h$ denote the average rank vector $(t \times 1)$ from the hth group, with elements $r_{hj} = \sum_{i=1}^{n_h} r_{hij}/n_h$, where r_{hij} is the rank of the jth response from the ith subject in sample h. Let $\bar{\mathbf{r}}_{\cdot}$ denote the average rank vector $(t \times 1)$ for the combined samples; the jth component of $\bar{\mathbf{r}}_{\cdot}$ is

$$\bar{r}_{\cdot j} = \sum_{h=1}^{s} \sum_{i=1}^{n_h} r_{hij} \bigg/ \sum_{h=1}^{s} n_h$$

The test statistic is

$$L_{RS} = \sum_{h=1}^{s} n_h (\mathbf{r}_h - \bar{\mathbf{r}}_{\cdot})' \mathbf{V}^{-1} (\mathbf{r}_h - \bar{\mathbf{r}}_{\cdot})$$

where the covariance matrix $\mathbf{V}$ has elements

$$V_{jl} = \left(\sum_{h=1}^{s} \sum_{i=1}^{n_h} r_{hij} r_{hil} \bigg/ \sum_{h=1}^{s} n_h \right) - \bar{r}_{\cdot j} \bar{r}_{\cdot l}$$

The statistic L_{RS} tests the hypothesis of no differences in the multivariate response profiles from the s samples; the asymptotic null distribution of this statistic is $\chi^2_{t(s-1)}$.

Similarly, for each sample at each time point, the multivariate multi-sample median test compares differences between proportions of responses less than or equal to the median to the corresponding combined data proportions. Let $\mathbf{p}_h$ denote the $t \times 1$ vector of proportions from the hth sample which are less than or equal to the median of the combined samples. The jth component of $\mathbf{p}_h$ is $p_{hj} = \sum_{i=1}^{n_h} x_{hij}/n_h$, where

$$x_{hij} = \begin{cases} 1 & \text{if } r_{hij} \leq \sum_{h=1}^{s} n_h/2 \\ 0 & \text{otherwise} \end{cases}$$

Let $\bar{\mathbf{p}}_{\cdot}$ denote the $t \times 1$ vector of proportions of observations from the combined samples that are less than or equal to the combined samples median, with elements

$$\bar{p}_{\cdot j} = \sum_{h=1}^{s} \sum_{i=1}^{n_h} x_{hij} \bigg/ \sum_{h=1}^{s} n_h$$

The test statistic is

$$L_M = \sum_{h=1}^{s} n_h (\mathbf{p}_h - \bar{\mathbf{p}}_{\cdot})' \mathbf{V}^{-1} (\mathbf{p}_h - \bar{\mathbf{p}}_{\cdot})$$

where the covariance matrix $\mathbf{V}$ has elements

$$V_{jl} = \left(\sum_{h=1}^{s} \sum_{i=1}^{n_h} x_{hij} x_{hil} \Big/ \sum_{h=1}^{s} n_h \right) - \overline{p}_{.j} \overline{p}_{.l}$$

The asymptotic null distribution of L_M is $\chi^2_{t(s-1)}$. If $t = 1$, L_M reduces to the Brown–Mood (1951) several-sample median test.

Schwertman (1985) describes this approach in further detail and gives an example of its application to the analysis of repeated measurements.

7.4.3 Randomization tests

In the one-sample repeated measures setting (Table 7.3), randomization tests based on the use of Mantel–Haenszel methods can be used to test the null hypothesis of no association between a repeated measurement factor and a response variable, adjusting for the effect of subject. The randomization model approach applies to categorical or continuous outcome variables y_{ij}, requires no distributional assumptions, and is useful in small samples. Landis *et al.* (1978) give a general overview of the three types of Mantel–Haenszel statistics; Landis *et al.* (1988) and Crowder and Hand (1990, section 8.6) describe the use of these procedures in analysing repeated measures.

The basic idea underlying the Mantel–Haenszel randomization model approach to one-sample repeated measures is to restructure the $n \times t$ data matrix of Table 7.3 as follows. Firstly, let c denote the number of distinct values of the response y_{ij}. If the response variable is categorical with a limited number of possible values, c will be relatively small. At the other extreme, if each of the n subjects has a unique response at each time point, $c = nt$. Now define indicator variables

$$n_{ijk} = \begin{cases} 1 & \text{if subject } i \text{ is classified in response category } k \text{ at time } j \\ 0 & \text{otherwise} \end{cases}$$

for $i = 1, \ldots, n$, $j = 1, \ldots, t$ and $k = 1, \ldots, c$. The data from subject i can then be displayed in a $t \times c$ contingency table, as shown in Table 7.7. Thus, the data from a one-sample repeated measures study can be viewed as a set of n independent $t \times c$ contingency tables.

Table 7.7 Contingency table layout for subject i in the one-sample repeated measures design

Time point	Response category 1	$\cdots$	c	Total
1	n_{i11}	$\cdots$	n_{i1c}	n_{i1+}
$\vdots$	$\vdots$	$\ddots$	$\vdots$	$\vdots$
t	n_{it1}	$\cdots$	n_{itc}	n_{it+}
Total	n_{i+1}	$\cdots$	n_{i+c}	N_i

When the data are complete, that is when the outcome variable is measured at every time point for each subject, the total sample size for each of the n tables is $N_i = t$ and every row marginal total n_{ij+} is equal to one. In this case, each row of Table 7.7 has exactly one n_{ijk} value equal to one and the remaining values are equal to zero. If, however, a particular subject has a missing response at one or more time points, the corresponding row of the subject's table will have each n_{ijk} value, as well as the marginal total n_{ij+}, equal to zero. The total sample size N_i will then equal t minus the number of missing observations.

In the framework of Table 7.7, let $\mathbf{n}_i = (n_{i11}, \ldots, n_{i1c}, \ldots, n_{it1}, \ldots, n_{itc})'$ denote the $tc \times 1$ vector of observed counts from the ith subject. Assume that the marginal totals $\{n_{ij+}\}$ and $\{n_{i+k}\}$ of each table are fixed. Under the null hypothesis that, for each subject, the response variable is distributed at random with respect to the t time points, the vectors $\mathbf{n}_i$, for subjects $i = 1, \ldots, n$, are independent, multiple hypergeometric random variables with probability distributions

$$f(\mathbf{n}_i) = \prod_{j=1}^{t} n_{ij+}! \prod_{k=1}^{c} n_{i+k}! \Big/ N_i! \prod_{j=1}^{t} \prod_{k=1}^{c} n_{ijk}!$$

Let $\mathbf{p}_{i*+} = (p_{i1+}, \ldots, p_{it+})'$, where $p_{ij+} = n_{ij+}/N_i$, and let $\mathbf{p}_{i+*} = (p_{i+1}, \ldots, p_{i+c})'$, where $p_{i+k} = n_{i+k}/N_i$, denote the vectors of row and column marginal proportions for subject i, respectively. One can then show that the mean and variance of $\mathbf{n}_i$ under the null hypothesis are

$$\mathbf{m}_i = E[\mathbf{n}_i] = N_i(\mathbf{p}_{i*} \otimes \mathbf{p}_{i.*})$$

$$\Sigma_i = \mathrm{var}(\mathbf{n}_i) = \frac{N_i^2}{N_i - 1}(\mathbf{Dp}_{i*+} - \mathbf{p}_{i*+}\mathbf{p}'_{i*+}) \otimes (\mathbf{Dp}_{i+*} - \mathbf{p}_{i+*}\mathbf{p}'_{i+*})$$

where $\mathbf{Dp}_{i*+}$ and $\mathbf{Dp}_{i+*}$ are diagonal matrices with the elements of $\mathbf{p}_{i*+}$ and $\mathbf{p}_{i+*}$ on the main diagonal.

Based on the multiple hypergeometric randomization model distribution of the $t \times c$ contingency table for each of the n subjects, Mantel–Haenszel statistics can be used to test the null hypothesis of no association between the row dimension (time) and the column dimension (response), adjusted for subject. As discussed in Landis *et al.* (1978), this null hypothesis is precisely the interchangeability hypothesis of Madansky (1963). In turn, the hypothesis of interchangeability implies marginal homogeneity in the distribution of the response variable across the t time points. Although the interchangeability hypothesis is a somewhat stronger condition than marginal homogeneity, the Mantel–Haenszel general association statistic Q_G (with $(t-1)(c-1)$ degrees of freedom (df)), mean score statistic Q_M (with $t-1$ df), and correlation statistic Q_C (with 1 df) are directed at alternatives that correspond to various types of departures from marginal homogeneity.

The general association statistic Q_G tests the null hypothesis in terms of $(t-1)(c-1)$ linearly independent functions of the observed counts. Thus, both the time variable and the outcome are treated as categorical variables, with t and c levels, respectively. Let $\mathbf{A} = (\mathbf{I}_{t-1}, \mathbf{0}_{t-1}) \otimes (\mathbf{I}_{c-1}, \mathbf{0}_{c-1})$, where $\mathbf{I}_u$ is the $u \times u$ identity matrix and $\mathbf{0}_u$ is the $u \times 1$ vector $(0, \dots, 0)'$. Note that $\mathbf{A}$ is a $(t-1)(c-1) \times tc$ matrix. Let $\mathbf{G}_i = \mathbf{A}(\mathbf{n}_i - \mathbf{m}_i)$ denote the $(t-1)(c-1) \times 1$ vector of differences between the observed and expected frequencies (under the null hypothesis of randomness) in the ith table, where the linear transformation matrix $\mathbf{A}$ eliminates the last row and last column. Let $\mathbf{G} = \sum_{i=1}^{n} \mathbf{G}_i$. Since the n tables are independent,

$$E[\mathbf{G}] = \sum_{i=1}^{n} E[\mathbf{G}_i] = \mathbf{0}_{(t-1)(c-1)}$$

$$\mathrm{var}(\mathbf{G}) = \mathbf{V}_G = \sum_{i=1}^{n} \mathrm{var}(\mathbf{G}_i) = \sum_{i=1}^{n} \mathbf{A}\boldsymbol{\Sigma}_i\mathbf{A}'$$

if H_0 is true. Since $\mathbf{G}$ has an approximate multivariate normal distribution with mean vector $\mathbf{0}_{(t-1)(c-1)}$ and covariance matrix $\mathbf{V}_G$ under H_0, the large sample quadratic form statistic for testing H_0 is $Q_G = \mathbf{G}'\mathbf{V}_G^{-1}\mathbf{G}$. If H_0 is true, Q_G has an approximate $\chi^2_{(t-1)(c-1)}$ distribution. If $c = 2$ and $t = 2$, Q_G is equivalent to McNemar's (1947) test. If $c = 2$ and $t > 2$, Q_G is Cochran's (1950) Q test. If $c > 2$ and $t > 2$, Q_G is equivalent to Birch's (1965) Lagrange multiplier test and Madansky's (1963) interchangeability test.

The Mantel–Haenszel mean score statistic Q_M can be used when the outcome (column variable of each of the n $t \times c$ tables) is ordinal and when it is reasonable to assign scores $b_1, \dots, b_c$ to the c levels of the response. The null hypothesis of no association between the row variable (time) and column variable (response) in any of the n tables is now tested in terms of $(t-1)$ linearly independent functions of the observed mean scores. The alternative hypothesis is that the t mean scores differ, on average, across subjects. In this case, let $\mathbf{A}_i = (\mathbf{I}_{t-1}, \mathbf{0}_{t-1}) \otimes (b_1, \dots, b_c)$ be a $[t-1] \times tc$ transformation matrix, let $\mathbf{M}_i = \mathbf{A}_i(\mathbf{n}_i - \mathbf{m}_i)$ denote the $(t-1) \times 1$ vector of differences between the observed and expected mean scores (under the null hypothesis of randomness) in the ith table, and let $\mathbf{M} = \sum_{i=1}^{n} \mathbf{M}_i$. Since the n tables are independent,

$$E[\mathbf{M}] = \sum_{i=1}^{n} E[\mathbf{M}_i] = \mathbf{0}_{(t-1)}$$

$$\mathrm{var}(\mathbf{M}) = \mathbf{V}_M = \sum_{i=1}^{n} \mathrm{var}(\mathbf{M}_i) = \sum_{i=1}^{n} \mathbf{A}_i\boldsymbol{\Sigma}_i\mathbf{A}_i'$$

if H_0 is true. Since $\mathbf{M}$ is approximately multivariate normal with mean vector $\mathbf{0}_{(t-1)}$ and covariance matrix $\mathbf{V}_M$ under H_0, the large sample quadratic form statistic for testing H_0 is $Q_M = \mathbf{M}'\mathbf{V}_M^{-1}\mathbf{M}$. If H_0 is true, Q_M has an approximate $\chi^2_{(t-1)}$ distribution. The statistic Q_M is directed at location-shift alternatives, the extent to which the mean scores at certain time points consistently exceed (or are exceeded by) the mean scores at other time points.

The Mantel–Haenszel correlation statistic Q_C is appropriate when both the repeated measures factor (row variable) and outcome (column variable) of the n $t \times c$ tables are ordinal. As in the case of the mean score statistic, scores $b_1, \ldots, b_c$ are assigned to the c levels of the response. In addition, scores $a_1, \ldots, a_t$ are now assigned to the t time points. (In the situation of repeated measurements obtained over time, the scores for the time points would generally be set equal to the time values.) The null hypothesis of no association between the row variable (time) and column variable (response) in any of the n tables is now tested versus the alternative that there is a consistent positive (or negative) association between the row scores and the column scores, across tables.

In this case, let $\mathbf{A}_i = (a_1, \ldots, a_t) \otimes (b_1, \ldots, b_c)$ be a row vector with tc components, let $\mathbf{C}_i = \mathbf{A}_i(\mathbf{n}_i - \mathbf{m}_i)$ denote the difference between the observed and expected association scores (under the null hypothesis of randomness) in the ith table, and let $\mathbf{C} = \sum_{i=1}^{n} \mathbf{C}_i$. Since the n tables are independent,

$$E[\mathbf{C}] = \sum_{i=1}^{n} E[\mathbf{C}_i] = 0$$

$$\text{var}(\mathbf{C}) = \mathbf{V}_C = \sum_{i=1}^{n} \text{var}(\mathbf{C}_i) = \sum_{i=1}^{n} \mathbf{A}_i \mathbf{\Sigma}_i \mathbf{A}_i'$$

if H_0 is true. Since $\mathbf{C}$ is approximately normal with mean 0 and variance $\mathbf{V}_C$ under H_0, the large sample quadratic form statistic for testing H_0 is $Q_C = \mathbf{C}^2/\mathbf{V}_C$. If H_0 is true, Q_C has an approximate χ_1^2 distribution. The statistic Q_C is directed at correlation alternatives, the extent to which there is a consistent (across-subjects) positive (or negative) linear association between the row and column scores.

In summary, all three Mantel–Haenszel randomization model statistics are useful in the analysis of longitudinal data from a single sample. The general association statistic Q_G tests marginal homogeneity across time, the mean score statistic Q_M tests equality of means across time, and the correlation statistic Q_C tests for linear association between the response and time. This approach is useful for assessing evidence of association between a response and a repeated measures factor in a relatively assumption-free context; random sampling of subjects from some underlying probabilistic framework is not required. Since the sample size requirements for validity of the asymptotic tests apply to across-strata totals, rather than to within-strata totals, the methodology is often applicable when sample sizes are too small to warrant the use of large sample methods.

One disadvantage of randomization model methods is that they provide hypothesis testing procedures only; estimation of parameters and their standard errors, as well as construction of confidence intervals, are not generally possible. Because the methodology is limited to one-sample problems, it is not useful for modelling the effects of additional covariates on the response. In addition, the scope of inference is restricted to the actual subjects under study, rather than to some broad population which the subjects might conceptually represent. Finally, in the application of randomization model methods to longitudinal data, the tests are insensitive to alternatives in which associations vary in direction across strata (subjects).

Several common non-parametric test procedures are special cases of Mantel–Haenszel randomization model tests. These include the tests of Friedman (1937), Durbin (1951), Benard and van Elteren (1953) and Page (1963), as well as the aligned ranks test introduced by Hodges and Lehmann (1962) and further studied by Koch and Sen (1968). Randomization tests for other types of repeated measures situations have also been studied. For example, Zerbe and Walker (1977) and Zerbe (1979a, 1979b) discuss randomization tests for the multi-sample situation of Table 7.2. These procedures can be used to test the equality of s mean growth curves over a specified time interval.

7.4.4 Distribution-free methods for incomplete repeated measurements from two samples

Wei and Lachin (1984) and Wei and Johnson (1985) study distribution-free methods for the two-sample case (Table 7.2 with $s = 2$) when the data are incomplete. These approaches allow the missing value patterns in the two samples to be different, but require the assumption that the missing value mechanism is independent of the response.

Wei and Lachin (1984) propose and study a family of asymptotically distribution-free tests for equality of two multivariate distributions. Although their methodology was motivated and developed for multivariate censored failure time data, an important application is to repeated measures with missing observations.

Let $F_h(x_1, \ldots, x_t)$ denote the multivariate cumulative distribution function (cdf) of the repeated observations from group h, for $h = 1, 2$. The Wei–Lachin statistic for testing

$$H_0: F_1(x_1, \ldots, x_t) = F_2(x_1, \ldots, x_t)$$

against the general alternative that $F_1 \neq F_2$ is $X_W^2 = \mathbf{W}' \hat{\mathbf{\Sigma}}_W^{-1} \mathbf{W}$, where $\mathbf{W}' = (W_1, \ldots, W_t)$ is a vector of test statistics comparing groups 1 and 2 at each of the t time points, and $\hat{\mathbf{\Sigma}}_W$ is a consistent estimator of var($\mathbf{W}$) given by Theorem 1 of Wei and Lachin (1984). Apart from a scale factor, the jth component of W is

$$W_j = \sum_{i=1}^{n_1} \sum_{i'=1}^{n_2} \delta_{1ij} \delta_{2i'j} \phi(y_{1ij}, y_{2i'j})$$

where

$$\phi(x, y) = \begin{cases} 1 & \text{if } x > y \\ 0 & \text{if } x = y \\ -1 & \text{if } x < y \end{cases} \qquad (7.1)$$

and δ_{hij} is 1 if y_{hij} is observed, 0 otherwise. Thus, at each time point j, comparisons between groups 1 and 2 are made for all i, i' for which y_{1ij} and $y_{2i'j}$ are both observed. The asymptotic null distribution of χ^2_W is χ^2_t.

In many studies, the detection of stochastic ordering of the distributions F_1 and F_2 is of primary interest. For example, the alternative hypothesis H_1 may be that $F_{1j}(x) \le F_{2j}(x)$ for each pair (F_{1j}, F_{2j}) of marginal cdfs, $j = 1, \ldots, t$. Under this alternative, the observations from group 1 tend to be larger than those from group 2 at each time point. For this situation, Wei and Lachin (1984) proposed the statistic

$$z_W = \frac{e'W}{\sqrt{e\hat{\Sigma}_W e}}$$

where e' is the t-component vector $(1, \ldots, 1)$. The asymptotic null distribution of z_W is normal with mean 0 and variance 1 ($N(0, 1)$). If the alternative hypothesis is $F_1 \le F_2$ ($F_1 \ge F_2$), the null hypothesis is rejected when z_W is a large positive (negative) value.

The Wei–Lachin methodology is based on a commonly used random censorship model (Kalbfleisch and Prentice, 1980) and the focus is on an omnibus test of equality versus a general alternative. In contrast, Wei and Johnson (1985) focus primarily on optimal methods of combining dependent tests and propose a class of two-sample non-parametric tests for incomplete repeated measures based on two-sample U statistics. Their motivation is that if a researcher wishes to draw an overall conclusion regarding the superiority of one treatment over another (across time), then a univariate one-sided test that combines the results at individual time points is more appropriate than an omnibus two-sided test of $H_0: F_1(x_1, \ldots, x_t) = F_2(x_1, \ldots, x_t)$.

The Wei–Johnson test statistic at the jth time point is

$$U_j = \sqrt{\frac{n_1 + n_2}{n_1 n_2}} \sum_{i=1}^{n_1} \sum_{i'=1}^{n_2} \delta_{1ij} \delta_{2i'j} \phi(y_{1ij}, y_{2i'j})$$

where $\phi(x, y)$ is a 'kernel' function. Under mild regularity conditions, the elements of the variance–covariance matrix $\hat{\Sigma}_U$ of $U = (U_1, \ldots, U_t)'$ can be estimated consistently by

$$\hat{\sigma}_{jk} = \frac{n_1 + n_2}{n_1} \hat{\sigma}_{1jk} + \frac{n_1 + n_2}{n_2} \hat{\sigma}_{2jk}$$

where

$$\hat{\sigma}_{1jk} = \frac{1}{n_1 n_2 (n_2 - 1)} \sum_{i=1}^{n_1} \sum_{l \neq l'=1}^{n_2} \delta_{1ij} \delta_{1ik} \delta_{2lj} \delta_{2l'k} \phi(y_{1ij}, y_{2lj}) \phi(y_{1ik}, y_{2l'k})$$

$$\hat{\sigma}_{2jk} = \frac{1}{n_2 n_1 (n_1 - 1)} \sum_{l=1}^{n_2} \sum_{i \neq i'=1}^{n_1} \delta_{1ij} \delta_{1i'k} \delta_{2lj} \delta_{2lk} \phi(y_{1ij}, y_{2lj}) \phi(y_{1i'k}, y_{2lk})$$

Since the null distribution of $\mathbf{U}$ is approximately multivariate normal with mean vector $\mathbf{0}_t$ and variance–covariance matrix $\hat{\mathbf{\Sigma}}_U$, the hypothesis $H_0: F_1 = F_2$ can be tested against a general alternative using the statistic $X_U^2 = \mathbf{U}' \hat{\mathbf{\Sigma}}_U^{-1} \mathbf{U}$, which is asymptotically χ_t^2. A univariate one-sided test that combines the results at individual time points can be based on the linear combination $\mathbf{c}' \mathbf{U} = \sum_{j=1}^{t} c_j U_j$, where $\mathbf{c}' = (c_1, \ldots, c_t)$ is a vector of weights. Under H_0, the statistic

$$z_U = \frac{\mathbf{c}' \mathbf{U}}{\sqrt{\mathbf{c}' \hat{\mathbf{\Sigma}}_U \mathbf{c}}}$$

is asymptotically $N(0, 1)$.

The simplest choice for the vector $\mathbf{c}$ is to weight each component equally, that is $\mathbf{c}' = (1, \ldots, 1)$. Another possibility is to weight by the reciprocals of the variances, that is $\mathbf{c}' = (1/\hat{\sigma}_{11}, \ldots, 1/\hat{\sigma}_{tt})$. Under the assumption that the test statistics at the individual time points are estimates of a common effect, the optimal weights are given by $\mathbf{c}' = (1, \ldots, 1) \hat{\mathbf{\Sigma}}_U^{-1}$ (O'Brien, 1984, Ashby *et al.*, 1986). In practice, however, this assumption may not hold. In addition, Bloch and Moses (1988) show that the use of simple weights often results in little loss of efficiency. Note that if the values of the test statistics differ considerably across time points, the weights $\mathbf{c}' = (1, \ldots, 1) \hat{\mathbf{\Sigma}}_U^{-1}$ may give a result which is quite different from that using equal weights or weighting by precision.

Wei and Johnson (1985) suggest several choices for the kernel function $\phi(x, y)$. If equation (7.1) is used, the Wei–Johnson vector of test statistics $\mathbf{U}$ and the Wei–Lachin vector of test statistics $\mathbf{W}$ are equivalent, apart from a scale factor. The consistent estimators of the variances and covariances of the components of the vector of test statistics, however, are different. The two methods will usually give similar results.

Davis (1991, 1994) provides further discussion of these methods and a computer program. Lachin (1992) proposes additional test statistics and provides estimators of the treatment difference, Palesch and Lachin (1994) extend these methods to more than two groups, and Thall and Lachin (1988), Davis and Wei (1988) and Davis (1996) study related methods for special types of situations with incomplete data.

7.4.5 Other methods

Asymptotically distribution-free analogues of general parametric procedures for normally distributed outcome variables have also been studied. Bhapkar (1984) discusses non-parametric counterparts of Hotelling's T^2

statistic and profile analysis. Sen (1984) studies non-parametric analogues of the Potthoff and Roy (1964) growth curve model.

Another potential approach to the analysis of repeated measures when the underlying parametric assumptions are not satisfied is the rank transform method, which consists of replacing observations by their ranks and performing a standard parametric analysis on the ranks (Conover and Iman, 1981). Unfortunately, the rank transform method has been shown to be inappropriate for many common hypotheses (Akritas 1991, 1993). Thompson (1991) and Akritas and Arnold (1994) provide valid asymptotic tests based on the rank transform for selected hypotheses of interest in several repeated measures models. Kepner and Robinson (1988) consider the one-sample situation of Table 7.3 under the assumption that the repeated measurements y_{ij} from the ith subject are equally correlated. They show the relationships between the rank transform method and the rank tests of Agresti and Pendergast (1986) and Koch (1969) for testing the null hypothesis of no time effect, expressed as $H_0: F(x_1, \ldots, x_t) = F(x_{\alpha(1)}, \ldots, x_{\alpha(t)})$, where $F(x_1, \ldots, x_t)$ is the t-variate distribution of the data vectors $\mathbf{y}_1, \ldots, \mathbf{y}_n$ and $[\alpha(1), \ldots, \alpha(t)]$ is any permutation of the first t positive integers.

Müller (1988), Diggle *et al.* (1994, ch. 3) and Kshirsagar and Smith (1995, ch. 10) discuss non-parametric regression methods for the analysis of repeated measurements, including kernel estimation, weighted local least squares estimation, and smoothing splines. Hart and Wehrly (1986) study the theoretical properties of kernel regression estimation for repeated measures and show how the case of correlated errors changes the behaviour of a kernel estimator; Altman (1990) demonstrates that the standard techniques for bandwidth selection perform poorly when the errors are correlated. Raz (1989) describes an analysis procedure for repeated measurements that combines non-parametric regression methods and the randomization tests of Zerbe (1979a).

7.5   Applications to the examples

7.5.1   A one-sample problem

In Example 7.3.1, the summary statistic approach is one possible method of testing if there is an association between SA ratings and measurement week. When the Spearman rank correlation coefficient between SA rating and week is computed for each subject, the correlation coefficients range from -1 to 0.8. Of the 32 non-zero correlations, 8 are positive and 24 are negative. Based on the sign test, the exact two-sided P value is 0.007. Using the Wilcoxon signed rank test, the sum of the ranks corresponding to positive correlations is 103 and the sum of the ranks of negative correlations is 425. The normal approximation to the distribution of the

Wilcoxon statistic yields $P = 0.003$. Both tests indicate the tendency of SA ratings to decrease over time.

The randomization model approach using the Mantel–Haenszel mean score and correlation statistics is also applicable. Using within-subject rank scores for the SA rating, the Mantel–Haenszel mean score chi-square statistic Q_M is 13.674 with 4 df ($P = 0.008$); thus, there is substantial evidence that the distributions are not the same at the five measurement times. Using rank scores for the SA rating and the scores 0, 1, 2, 3 and 4 for the five measurement times, the Mantel–Haenszel correlation statistic Q_C is 10.375 with 1 df ($P = 0.001$). This result indicates that there is a consistent monotonic association between SA rating and week across subjects. Both of these methods use all available data from each subject.

7.5.2   A multi-sample problem with complete data

The objective of the study described in Section 7.3.2 was to determine whether or not progabide reduces the frequency of epileptic seizures. One possible approach is to reduce the vector of four observations from each subject (weeks 2, 4, 6 and 8) to a single measurement. The total seizure count is one potential summary statistic. The median of the four measurements from each subject is another choice; this summary statistic will be less affected by extreme observations.

The distributions of the total seizure counts are extremely non-normal in both treatment groups; the P values from the Shapiro–Wilk (1965) test of normality are less than 0.001. The median total seizure counts in the progabide and placebo groups are 15 and 16, respectively. Using the Mann–Whitney–Wilcoxon test, there is insufficient evidence to conclude that progabide reduces the total seizure count; the two-sided P value is 0.19.

The distributions of the median two-week seizure counts are also extremely non-normal in both treatment groups; the P values from the Shapiro–Wilk test of normality are again less than 0.001. The median of the two-week median count in the progabide group is 3.5; the corresponding median in the placebo group is 4.25. Using the Mann–Whitney–Wilcoxon test, there is insufficient evidence to conclude that progabide reduces the median two-week seizure count; the two-sided P value is 0.27.

The two groups can also be compared using the multivariate non-parametric tests of Puri and Sen (1971). Using the multivariate multi-sample rank sum test, the chi-square statistic is 5.47 with 4 df ($P = 0.24$). The multivariate multi-sample median test gives an even less significant result (chi-square $= 3.46$, df $= 4$, $P = 0.48$).

Although the Wei–Lachin (1984) and Wei–Johnson (1985) procedures were developed for the two-sample case with incomplete data, these procedures can also be applied. The Wei–Lachin vector of test statistics at the four time points is $\mathbf{W}' = (-0.4700, -0.0375, -0.2008, -0.3685)$ with estimated covariance matrix

$$\hat{\Sigma}_W = \begin{pmatrix} 0.078\,842 & 0.052\,873 & 0.046\,046 & 0.050\,903 \\ 0.052\,873 & 0.080\,367 & 0.053\,850 & 0.055\,578 \\ 0.046\,046 & 0.053\,850 & 0.078\,895 & 0.050\,123 \\ 0.050\,903 & 0.055\,578 & 0.050\,123 & 0.077\,457 \end{pmatrix}$$

The Wei–Lachin omnibus chi-square statistic for testing equality of distributions is $\mathbf{W}'\hat{\Sigma}_W^{-1}\mathbf{W} = 5.661$ with 4 df ($P = 0.23$). The Wei–Johnson procedure using the 'kernel' function

$$\phi(x, y) = \begin{cases} 1 & \text{if } x > y \\ 0 & \text{if } x = y \\ -1 & \text{if } x < y \end{cases}$$

gives a vector $\mathbf{U}$ of test statistics equivalent (apart from a scale factor) to the Wei–Lachin $\mathbf{W}$, but uses a different estimator of the covariance matrix. Weighting each time point equally, the Wei–Johnson univariate statistic $\mathbf{c}'\mathbf{U}/\sqrt{\mathbf{c}'\hat{\Sigma}_U\mathbf{c}}$, with $\mathbf{c}' = (1, \ldots, 1)$, is equal to -1.09. With reference to the $N(0, 1)$ distribution, the two-sided P value is 0.14.

7.5.3 A multi-sample problem with incomplete data

Since the repeated pain scores described in Section 7.3.3 are both non-normal and incomplete, it seems appropriate to compare the two groups using the Wei–Lachin or the Wei–Johnson procedure. Based on the data from minutes 30, 60, 90, 120, 150 and 180, the Wei–Lachin vector of test statistics is $\mathbf{W}' = (-0.394\,09, -0.601\,72, -0.755\,13, -0.728\,68, -0.497\,25, -0.297\,55)$ with estimated covariance matrix

$$\hat{\Sigma}_W = \begin{pmatrix} 0.079355 & 0.047\,911 & 0.028\,357 & 0.017\,829 & 0.011\,357 & 0.005\,749 \\ 0.047\,911 & 0.058\,464 & 0.031\,605 & 0.020\,765 & 0.015\,458 & 0.006\,445 \\ 0.028\,357 & 0.031\,605 & 0.036\,803 & 0.019\,749 & 0.011\,149 & 0.003\,628 \\ 0.017\,829 & 0.020\,765 & 0.019\,749 & 0.026\,539 & 0.014\,794 & 0.005\,351 \\ 0.011\,357 & 0.015\,458 & 0.011\,149 & 0.014\,794 & 0.013\,187 & 0.005\,691 \\ 0.005\,749 & 0.006\,445 & 0.003\,628 & 0.005\,351 & 0.005\,691 & 0.005\,249 \end{pmatrix}$$

The Wei–Johnson procedure using the 'kernel' function

$$\phi(x, y) = \begin{cases} 1 & \text{if } x > y \\ 0 & \text{if } x = y \\ -1 & \text{if } x < y \end{cases}$$

gives the vector of test statistics $\mathbf{U}' = (-1.5784, -2.4100, -3.0245, -2.9185, -1.9916, -1.1918)$ with estimated covariance matrix

$$\hat{\Sigma}_U = \begin{pmatrix} 1.132\,98 & 0.926\,83 & 0.655\,67 & 0.418\,22 & 0.242\,87 & 0.143\,34 \\ 0.926\,83 & 1.112\,00 & 0.778\,26 & 0.557\,65 & 0.362\,51 & 0.211\,44 \\ 0.655\,67 & 0.778\,26 & 0.933\,73 & 0.751\,14 & 0.498\,50 & 0.255\,48 \\ 0.418\,22 & 0.557\,65 & 0.751\,14 & 0.779\,04 & 0.501\,55 & 0.252\,77 \\ 0.242\,87 & 0.362\,51 & 0.498\,50 & 0.501\,55 & 0.418\,88 & 0.223\,44 \\ 0.143\,34 & 0.211\,44 & 0.255\,48 & 0.252\,77 & 0.223\,44 & 0.181\,91 \end{pmatrix}$$

Table 7.8 Wci–Lachin and Wei–Johnson analyses of labour pain clinical trial

	Standardized test statistic	
	Wei–Lachin	Wei–Johnson
Time point (min)		
30	−1.40	−1.37
60	−2.49	−2.28
90	−3.94	−3.13
120	−4.47	−3.31
150	−4.33	−3.08
180	−4.11	−2.79
Linear combinations		
Equal weights	−3.88	−3.06
Reciprocals of variances	−4.85	−3.28
Optimal	−4.42	−2.11

Table 7.8 gives the standardized test statistics (statistic/standard error) for the Wei–Lachin and Wei–Johnson methods at each of the six time points. The signs of the test statistics indicate that, at each time point, the pain scores are lower (better) in the experimental group than in the placebo group. Although the two methods yield similar conclusions, the Wei–Lachin standardized statistic is larger in absolute value (more significant) than the Wei–Johnson statistic at every time point. The Wei–Lachin omnibus chi-square statistic for testing equality of distributions is highly significant ($\mathbf{W'\hat{\Sigma}_W^{-1}W} = 30.1$ with 6 df, $P < 0.001$), while the omnibus Wei–Johnson statistic is marginally significant ($\mathbf{U'\hat{\Sigma}_U^{-1}U} = 11.9$ with 6 df, $P = 0.065$). Table 7.8 also displays standardized values of three linear combinations of the statistics calculated at the separate time points. For both methods, all three linear combination statistics indicate a significant difference between the two groups (with respect to the $N(0, 1)$ reference distribution).

References

Agresti, A. and Pendergast, J. 1986: Comparing mean ranks for repeated measures data. *Communication in Statistics, Theory and Methods* **15**, 1417–34.

Akritas, M. G. 1991: Limitations of the rank transform procedure: a study of repeated measures designs, part I. *Journal of the American Statistical Association* **86**, 457–60.

Akritas, M. G. 1993: Limitations of the rank transform procedure: a study of repeated measures designs, part II. *Statistics and Probability Letters* **17**, 149–56.

Akritas, M. G. and Arnold, S. F. 1994: Fully nonparametric hypotheses for factorial designs, I: multivariate repeated measures designs. *Journal of the American Statistical Association* **89**, 336–43.

Altman, N. S. 1990: Kernel smoothing of data with correlated errors. *Journal of the American Statistical Association* **85**, 749–59.

Ashby, D., Pocock, S. J. and Shaper, A. G. 1986: Ordered polytomous regression: an example relating serum biochemistry and haematology to alcohol consumption. *Applied Statistics* **35**, 289–301.

Benard, A. and van Elteren, P. 1953: A generalization of the method of *m* rankings. *Proceedings Koninklijke Nederlands Akademie van Wetenschappen (A)* **56**, 358–69.

Bhapkar, V. P. 1984: Univariate and multivariate multisample location and scale tests. In Krishnaiah, P. R. and Sen, P. K. (eds), *Handbook of statistics, volume 4: nonparametric methods.* Amsterdam: Elsevier, 31–62.

Birch, M. W. 1965: The detection of partial association, II: the general case. *Journal of the Royal Statistical Society (B)* **27**, 111–24.

Bloch, D. A. and Moses, L. E. 1988: Nonoptimally weighted least squares. *American Statistician* **42**, 50–3.

Brown, G. W. and Mood, A. M. 1951: On median tests for linear hypotheses. *Proceedings of the Second Berkeley Symposium on Mathematical Statistics and Probability.* Berkeley, CA: University of California Press.

Carr, G. J., Hafner, K. B. and Koch, G. G. 1989: Analysis of rank measures of association for ordinal data from longitudinal studies. *Journal of the American Statistical Association* **84**, 797–804.

Cochran, W. G. 1950: The comparison of percentages in matched samples. *Biometrika* **37**, 256–66.

Conover, W. J. and Iman, R. L. 1981: Rank transformations as a bridge between parametric and nonparametric statistics. *American Statistician* **35**, 124–33.

Crowder, M. J. and Hand, D. J. 1990: *Analysis of repeated measures.* London: Chapman & Hall.

Crowder, M. J. and Hand, D. J. 1996: *Practical longitudinal data analysis.* London: Chapman & Hall.

Davidian, M. and Giltinan, D. M. 1995: *Nonlinear models for repeated measurement data.* London: Chapman & Hall.

Davis, C. S. 1991: Semi-parametric and non-parametric methods for the analysis of repeated measurements with applications to clinical trials. *Statistics in Medicine* **10**, 1959–80.

Davis, C. S. 1994: A computer program for nonparametric analysis of incomplete repeated measures from two samples. *Computer Methods and Programs in Biomedicine* **42**, 39–52.

Davis, C. S. 1996: Non-parametric methods for comparing multiple treatment groups to a control group, based on incomplete non-decreasing repeated measurements. *Statistics in Medicine* **15**, 2509–21.

Davis, C. S. and Wei, L. J. 1988: Nonparametric methods for analyzing incomplete nondecreasing repeated measurements. *Biometrics* **44**, 1005–18.

Dawson, J. D. 1994: Comparing treatment groups on the basis of slopes, areas-under-the-curve, and other summary measures. *Drug Information Journal* **28**, 723–32.

Diggle, P. J., Liang, K. Y. and Zeger, S. L. 1994: *Analysis of longitudinal data.* Oxford: Clarendon Press.

Durbin, J. 1951: Incomplete blocks in ranking experiments. *British Journal of Mathematical and Statistical Psychology* **4**, 85–90.

Friedman, M. 1937: The use of ranks to avoid the assumption of normality implicit in the analysis of variance. *Journal of the American Statistical Association* **32**, 675–701.

Frison, L. and Pocock, S. J. 1992: Repeated measures in clinical trials: analysis using mean summary statistics and its implications for design. *Statistics in Medicine* **11**, 1685–704.

Ghosh, M., Grizzle, J. E. and Sen, P. K. 1973: Nonparametric methods in longitudinal studies. *Journal of the American Statistical Association* **68**, 29–36.

Hart, J. D. and Wehrly, T. E. 1986: Kernel regression estimation using repeated measurements data. *Journal of the American Statistical Association* **81**, 1080–8.

Hettmansperger, T. R. 1984: *Statistical inference based on ranks.* New York: John Wiley.

Hodges, J. L. and Lehmann, E. L. 1962: Rank methods for combination of independent experiments in analysis of variance. *Annals of Mathematical Statistics* **33**, 482–97.

Jones, R. H. 1993: *Longitudinal data with serial correlation: a state-space approach.* London: Chapman & Hall.

Kalbfleisch, J. D. and Prentice, R. L. 1980: *The statistical analysis of failure time data.* New York: John Wiley.

Kenward, M. G. 1997: *Analysis of repeated measurements.* New York: Oxford University Press.

Kepner, J. L. and Robinson, D. H. 1988: Nonparametric methods for detecting treatment effects in repeated-measures designs. *Journal of the American Statistical Association* **83**, 456–61.

Koch, G. G. 1969: Some aspects of the statistical analysis of 'split plot' experiments in completely randomized layouts. *Journal of the American Statistical Association* **64**, 485–505.

Koch, G. G., Amara, I. A., Stokes, M. E. and Gillings, D. B. 1980: Some views on parametric and non-parametric analysis for repeated measurements and selected bibliography. *International Statistical Review* **48**, 249–65.

Koch, G. G. and Sen, P. K. 1968: Some aspects of the statistical analysis of the mixed model. *Biometrics* **24**, 27–48.

Kruskal, W. H. and Wallis, W. A. 1952: Use of ranks in one-criterion variance analysis. *Journal of the American Statistical Association* **47**, 583–621.

Kshirsagar, A. M. and Smith, W. B. 1995: *Growth curves.* New York: Marcel Dekker.

Lachin, J. M. 1992: Some large-sample distribution-free estimators and tests for multivariate partially incomplete data from two populations. *Statistics in Medicine* **11**, 1151–70.

Landis, J. R., Heyman, E. R. and Koch, G. G. 1978: Average partial association in three-way contingency tables: a review and discussion of alternative tests. *International Statistical Review* **46**, 237–54.

Landis, J. R., Miller M. E., Davis, C. S. and Koch, G. G. 1988: Some general methods for the analysis of categorical data in longitudinal studies. *Statistics in Medicine* **7**, 109–37.

Leppik, I. E. *et al.* 1987: A controlled study of progabide in partial seizures: methodology and results. *Neurology* **37**, 963–8.

Lindsey, J. K. 1993: *Models for repeated measurements.* New York: Oxford University Press.

Madansky, A. 1963: Test of homogeneity for correlated samples. *Journal of the American Statistical Association* **58**, 97–119.

Matthews J. N. S., Altman, D. G., Campbell, M. J. and Royston, P. 1990: Analysis of serial measurements in medical research. *British Medical Journal* **300**, 230–5.

McNemar, Q. 1947: Note on the sampling error of the difference between correlated proportions or percentages. *Psychometrika* **12**, 153–7.

Moore, D. S. and McCabe, G. P. 1993: *Introduction to the practice of statistics.* New York: W. H. Freeman.

Müller, H. G. 1988: *Nonparametric regression analysis of longitudinal data.* Berlin: Springer.

O'Brien, P. C. 1984: Procedures for comparing samples with multiple endpoints. *Biometrics* **40**, 1079–87.

Page, E. B. 1963: Ordered hypotheses for multiple treatments: a significance test for linear ranks. *Journal of the American Statistical Association* **58**, 216–30.

Palesch, Y. Y. and Lachin, J. M. 1994: Asymptotically distribution-free multivariate rank tests for multiple samples with partially incomplete observations. *Statistica Sinica* **4**, 373–87.

Pocock, S. J. 1983: *Clinical trials: a practical approach.* New York: John Wiley.

Potthoff, R. and Roy, S. N. 1964: A generalized multivariate analysis of variance model useful especially for growth curve problems. *Biometrika* **41**, 313–26.

Puri, M. L. and Sen, P. K. 1971: *Nonparametric methods in multivariate analysis.* New York: John Wiley.

Raz, J. 1989: Analysis of repeated measurements using nonparametric smoothers and randomization tests. *Biometrics* **45**, 851–71.

Schwertman, N. C. 1982: Algorithm AS 174: multivariate multisample nonparametric tests. *Applied Statistics* **31**, 80–5.

Schwertman, N. C. 1985: Multivariate median and rank sum tests. *Encyclopedia of statistical sciences.* New York: John Wiley.

Sen, P. K. 1984: Nonparametric procedures for some miscellaneous problems. In Krishnaiah, P. R. and Sen, P. K. (eds), *Handbook of statistics, volume 4: nonparametric methods.* Amsterdam: Elsevier, 699–739.

Shapiro, S. S. and Wilk, M. B. 1965: An analysis of variance test for normality (complete samples). *Biometrika* **52**, 591–611.

Simpson, G. M. and Angus, J. W. 1970: A rating scale for extrapyramidal side effects. *Acta Psychiatrica Scandinavica, Supplementum* **212**, 11–19.

Thall, P. F. and Lachin, J. M. 1988: Analysis of recurrent events: nonparametric methods for random-interval count data. *Journal of the American Statistical Association* **83**, 339–47.

Thall, P. F. and Vail, S. C. 1990: Some covariance models for longitudinal count data with overdispersion. *Biometrics* **46**, 657–71.

Thompson, G. L. 1991: A unified approach to rank tests for multivariate and repeated measures designs. *Journal of the American Statistical Association* **86**, 410–19.

Vonesh, E. F. and Chinchilli, V. M. 1996: *Linear and nonlinear models for the analysis of repeated measurements.* New York: Marcel Dekker.

Wei, L. J. and Johnson, W. E. 1985: Combining dependent tests with incomplete repeated measurements. *Biometrika* **72**, 359–64.

Wei, L. J. and Lachin, J. M. 1984: Two-sample asymptotically distribution-free tests for incomplete multivariate observations. *Journal of the American Statistical Association* **79**, 653–61.

Zerbe, G. O. 1979a: Randomization analysis of the completely randomized design extended to growth and response curves. *Journal of the American Statistical Association* **74**, 215–21.

Zerbe, G. O. 1979b: Randomization analysis of randomized blocks extended to growth and response curves. *Communication in Statistics, Theory and Methods* **8**, 191–205.

Zerbe, G. O. and Walker, S. H. 1977: A randomization test for comparison of groups of growth curves with different polynomial design matrices. *Biometrics* **33**, 653–7.

8 Regression models for discrete longitudinal data

Garrett M. Fitzmaurice

8.1 Introduction

Longitudinal studies have become increasingly popular in the health, social and behavioural sciences. In the health sciences, longitudinal studies have proven to be important for understanding the development and persistence of disease and for identifying factors which can alter the course of disease development. For example, in studies such as the Framingham Heart Study (Dawber, 1980) and the Six Cities Study of Air Pollution and Health (Ware *et al.*, 1984, Dockery *et al.*, 1989) investigators have followed populations of different ages over time to study the development of chronic illnesses and to detect risk factors for disease.

The distinguishing feature of a longitudinal study is that the response variable of interest and a set of covariates are measured repeatedly over time. The main objective of a longitudinal study is to characterize change in the response variable over time and to examine covariates which contribute to that change. Because repeated observations are made on the same individual, the repeated measures on the response variable will usually be (positively) correlated. This within-subject association or time dependence must be accounted for in order to make correct inference. The focus of this chapter is on longitudinal studies where the response variable is discrete. For simplicity, this chapter is concerned with the special case where the discrete responses are binary. The generalization to ordinal and nominal categorical variables having more than two levels is, in principle, straightforward since each categorical variable can be replaced by a set of binary indicator variables. In order to focus ideas, consider the following example from the Six Cities Study of Air Pollution and Health (Ware *et al.*, 1984, Dockery *et al.*, 1989), a longitudinal study designed to characterize the adverse health effects of exposure to air pollutants. In this study a binary response, the child's wheeze status (wheeze, no wheeze), as well as information about maternal smoking were recorded annually for a sample of children from each of the participating cities. One of the objectives of this study was to determine the effects of maternal smoking and outside air quality on respiratory illness in children. We return to this example later in order to illustrate and compare a number of different analytic approaches for analysing discrete longitudinal data.

In this chapter we distinguish between longitudinal studies where the *marginal* expectation of the responses is of scientific interest, and studies where the *conditional* expectation of the responses is of main interest. Therefore, it is important at this stage to clarify what we mean by the terms *marginal* and *conditional* in this particular context. In the former, the main focus is on the regression parameters for the marginal expectation of each response separately, while in the latter, the regression parameters modelling the conditional expectation of each response, given either the values of previous responses or a set of random effects, are of primary interest. Thus, models for the marginal expectation or mean response are referred to as marginal regression models, since it is of interest to relate the mean response to covariates. The term *marginal* is used here to emphasize that the mean response being modelled is conditional only on the covariates and not on the values of previous responses or random effects. The model parameters then have familiar interpretations, similar to the parameters in repeated measures ANOVA or growth curve models for continuous outcomes. Models for the conditional expectation of the response are referred to as conditional regression models. The term *conditional* is used to emphasize that the mean response being modelled is conditional not only on the covariates, but also on values of previous responses or on unobserved random effects.

The recent literature on both likelihood-based approaches and non-likelihood approaches to analysing longitudinal binary data is reviewed. The objective is to give a brief survey of the different regression models that have recently been proposed, outlining the main features of each approach with particular emphasis on issues of interpretation. In Section 8.2, some notation is introduced and the example from the Six Cities Study of Air Pollution and Health is described in greater detail. This example is used to make comparisons between the various analytic approaches described throughout the remainder of the chapter. In Section 8.3, marginal regression models for longitudinal binary data are considered. We review and contrast two general approaches for estimating the parameters of marginal regression models: a full likelihood-based approach based on a 'mixed parameter' model, and a non-likelihood generalized estimating equations (GEE) approach. We demonstrate that there is a very close connection between these two approaches, and make some recommendations concerning their application. In Section 8.4, conditional regression models for longitudinal binary data are considered. We distinguish two main classes of models: transitional models and random effects models. All of the methods are illustrated using a subset of data from the Six Cities Study of Air Pollution and Health. Finally, we conclude with some remarks concerning the choice between the various models for any particular application. For the reader interested in studying models for discrete longitudinal data and other related topics in greater detail, we recommend the recent textbooks by Diggle *et al.* (1994), Fahrmeir and Tutz (1994) and Hand and Crowder (1996).

8.2   Notation

In longitudinal studies, there is an implied ordering of the times of the repeated observations. For simplicity, we assume that each of N individuals is observed at T occasions. Letting Y_{it} denote the binary response variable, we can form the $T \times 1$ vector $\mathbf{Y}_i = (Y_{i1}, \ldots, Y_{iT})'$, where $Y_{it} = 1$ if the ith individual has response 1 (say, success) at time t, and 0 otherwise. Each individual also has a $J \times 1$ vector of covariates or explanatory variables, $\mathbf{x}_{it}$, measured at occasion t, and we let $\mathbf{x}_i = (\mathbf{x}_{i1}, \ldots, \mathbf{x}_{iT})'$ represent the $T \times J$ matrix of covariates. Typically, the first element of $\mathbf{x}_{it}$ is unity for all i and t, and thus the corresponding regression coefficient represents the intercept term. Note that in longitudinal studies the covariates can be both time stationary, that is constant across occasions, and time varying. Thus, the data for the ith individual consist of the observation $(\mathbf{Y}_i, \mathbf{x}_i)$, $i = 1, \ldots, N$.

Before considering the different approaches to analysing discrete longitudinal data, we first describe an example which is used throughout this chapter to illustrate the different methods, and to compare and contrast the various analytic approaches.

8.2.1   Example: Ohio children's wheeze data

A single example is used to illustrate the methods that are discussed in the following sections. The example uses a subset of data from the Six Cities Study, a longitudinal study of the health effects of air pollution (Ware *et al.*, 1984). The data set contains complete records on 537 children from Steubenville, Ohio, one of the participating cities. Each child was examined annually at ages 7 through 10, and the repeated binary response is the wheezing status (1 = yes, 0 = no) of a child at each measurement occasion. Information about whether each child's mother smoked was ascertained at the beginning of the study and maternal smoking was categorized as 1 if the mother smoked regularly and 0 otherwise. Although maternal smoking is a time-varying covariate, it was treated as fixed at its value at the first year of study. The data are displayed in Table 8.1 and were first reported by Laird *et al.* (1984). These data have previously been analysed by Laird *et al.* (1984), Zeger *et al.* (1988), Fitzmaurice and Laird (1993) and others.

Table 8.1 Ohio children's wheeze data set

Maternal smoking	Age 7	Age 8	Age 9	Age 10 No	Yes
				Child's wheeze status	
No	No	No	No	237	10
			Yes	15	4
		Yes	No	16	2
			Yes	7	3
	Yes	No	No	24	3
			Yes	3	2
		Yes	No	6	2
			Yes	5	11
Yes	No	No	No	118	6
			Yes	8	2
		Yes	No	11	1
			Yes	6	4
	Yes	No	No	7	3
			Yes	3	1
		Yes	No	4	2
			Yes	4	7

8.3   Marginal regression models

One of the distinguishing features of marginal regression models is that the focus is on population averages or rates. In marginal regression models, the regression parameters for the marginal expectation of each response separately, $E[Y_{it}]$, are of primary interest. The marginal distribution of Y_{it} is Bernoulli, and we assume

$$g(\mu_{it}) = \mathbf{x}_{it}\beta^{(M)} \qquad (8.1)$$

where $\mu_{it} = E[Y_{it}|\mathbf{x}_{it}] = \Pr(Y_{it} = 1|\mathbf{x}_{it})$ is the probability of success at time t, $g(\cdot)$ is a monotone link function relating μ_{it} to the covariates, and $\beta^{(M)}$ is a $J \times 1$ vector of marginal regression parameters. With binary responses, the logit link function is a very natural choice,

$$\text{logit}(\mu_{it}) = \log[\mu_{it}/(1 - \mu_{it})] = \mathbf{x}_{it}\beta^{(M)} \qquad (8.2)$$

and is the link function selected to illustrate the various analytic methods throughout the remainder of this chapter. However, in principle, any link function $g(\cdot)$ could be chosen. The $\mu_{it}(\beta^{(M)})$ can be grouped together to form a vector $\mu_i(\beta^{(M)}) = E[\mathbf{Y}_i|\mathbf{x}_i] = (\mu_{i1}, \ldots, \mu_{iT})'$. Note that in marginal regression models there is an implicit assumption that

$$E[Y_{it}|\mathbf{x}_i] = E[Y_{it}|\mathbf{x}_{it}]$$

That is, it is assumed that $\mathbf{x}_{it}$ are *external* time-varying covariates in the sense described by Kalbfleisch and Prentice (1980); otherwise, commonly used estimators of the parameters of the marginal regression model may be inconsistent (a more detailed discussion of this point can be found in Fitzmaurice *et al.* (1993) and Pepe and Anderson (1994)).

In the above, we have described regression models only for the distribution of each response separately, given the covariates. However, to account for the time dependence or within-subject association among responses, the entire joint distribution of the T binary responses must be considered. This joint distribution of Y_i is multinomial with a 2^T probability vector $\pi_i = \{\pi_{ij_1 j_2 \ldots j_T}\}$, where $j_1, \ldots, j_T = 0, 1$. For example, if $T = 4$

$$\pi_{i_{0000}} = \Pr(Y_{i1} = 0, Y_{i2} = 0, Y_{i3} = 0, Y_{i4} = 0)$$
$$\pi_{i_{0001}} = \Pr(Y_{i1} = 0, Y_{i2} = 0, Y_{i3} = 0, Y_{i4} = 1)$$
$$\pi_{i_{0010}} = \Pr(Y_{i1} = 0, Y_{i2} = 0, Y_{i3} = 1, Y_{i4} = 0)$$
$$\vdots$$
$$\pi_{i_{1111}} = \Pr(Y_{i1} = 1, Y_{i2} = 1, Y_{i3} = 1, Y_{i4} = 1)$$

Note that unlike the multivariate normal distribution for continuous responses, this distribution cannot, in general, be represented by the first two moments of Y_i. The fully parameterized distribution has $2^T - 1$ non-redundant parameters (since there is the single constraint that the 2^T probabilities must sum to unity). Thus as the number of occasions, T, increases, the number of parameters proliferates rapidly and it becomes increasingly necessary to find parsimonious models for the data.

Next, consider the interpretation of $\beta^{(M)}$ in marginal regression models. These parameters address questions concerning the marginal or population-averaged distribution of the Y_{it}, given the covariates. That is, the $\beta^{(M)}$ address scientific questions concerned with prevalence in the population. In particular, each parameter can be interpreted in terms of the changes in the prevalence of a positive response (e.g. disease) in the population, for a unit change in the given covariate (while holding all of the remaining covariates constant). For a marginal regression model with a logit link function, each parameter can be interpreted in terms of the log odds of, or logit of the proportion with, a positive response in the population. Thus, marginal regression models are best suited to longitudinal studies where the question of main interest concerns populations rather than individuals.

Given that we are interested in estimating the marginal regression parameters, $\beta^{(M)}$, there are a number of possible ways to parameterize models for the multinomial probabilities. An important distinction between the various approaches that have been proposed in the statistical literature is how the time dependence or association among responses is modelled – specifically, whether the association is parameterized in terms of *marginal* or *conditional* metrics of within-subject association.

There is an extensive statistical literature on modelling the within-subject association among the binary responses in terms of marginal associations. For example, Bahadur (1961), and more recently Zhao and Prentice (1990), describe maximum likelihood estimation where the association among responses is parameterized in terms of marginal correlations or covariances. Ekholm (1991) parameterizes the association in terms of the higher order marginal probabilities (also, see Ekholm *et al.*, 1995). McCullagh and Nelder (1989), Lipsitz *et al.* (1990), Liang *et al.* (1992), Becker and Balagtas (1993), Molenberghs and Lesaffre (1994), Lang and Agresti (1994), Glonek and McCullagh (1995) and others describe maximum likelihood estimation where the association is parameterized in terms of marginal odds ratios. What all of the above approaches have in common is that they parameterize the joint probabilities, π_i, in terms of (i) a model for the mean, $\mu_i(\beta^{(M)})$, and (ii) a model for the higher order *marginal* probabilities. Therefore all of these approaches can be thought of as fully marginal models. However, there are two potential drawbacks of these fully marginal models. The first, and probably the most important, is that estimation of the marginal regression parameters is not robust to misspecification of the time dependence. That is, if the model for the mean has been correctly specified but the model for the within-subject association is incorrect, the fully marginal estimators of $\beta^{(M)}$ will fail to converge in probability to the true mean parameters. Secondly, as noted by Prentice (1988), with binary responses the marginal association parameters are constrained in a very complicated manner by the mean parameters. For example, the pairwise correlations must satisfy certain linear inequalities determined by the means and, by symmetry, vice versa. Such constraints are generally considered to be an unattractive feature of these models.

An alternative approach is to parameterize the within-subject association among the binary responses in terms of *conditional* associations. For example, Fitzmaurice and Laird (1993) parameterize the association in terms of conditional odds ratios. These conditional odds ratios are exactly the same measures of association used in ordinary log-linear modelling of contingency tables (where, neglecting covariates, each individual's response falls into a cell of the 2^T contingency table formed by cross-classifying the T binary responses). Since the joint probabilities are parameterized in terms of (i) a model for the mean, $\mu_i(\beta^{(M)})$, and (ii) a model for the higher order *conditional* probabilities, this can be thought of as a 'mixed parameter' model. The model is 'mixed' in the sense of combining marginal parameters for the mean with the complementary set of conditional parameters for the within-subject association. In the next section, mixed parameter models for longitudinal binary data are considered in greater detail.

8.3.1   Mixed parameter models

A widely used probability model for multivariate binary data is the log-linear model (Bishop *et al.*, 1975). Following Cox (1972) and Zhao and Prentice (1990), this has led Fitzmaurice and Laird (1993) to assume that the joint distribution of $\mathbf{Y}_i$ has the general exponential form

$$f(\mathbf{y}_i, \mathbf{\Psi}_i, \mathbf{\Omega}_i) = \exp[\mathbf{\Psi}_i' \mathbf{y}_i + \mathbf{\Omega}_i' \mathbf{w}_i - A(\mathbf{\Psi}_i, \mathbf{\Omega}_i)] \tag{8.3}$$

where $\mathbf{W}_i = (Y_{i1} Y_{i2}, \ldots, Y_{iT-1} Y_{iT}, \ldots, Y_{i1} Y_{i2} \cdots Y_{iT})'$ denotes a $K \times 1$ vector of two- and higher way cross-products among the $\mathbf{Y}_i$ (with $K = 2^T - T - 1$), $\mathbf{\Psi}_i = (\psi_{i1}, \ldots, \psi_{iT})'$ and $\mathbf{\Omega}_i = (\omega_{i12}, \ldots, \omega_{iT-1,T}, \ldots, \omega_{i12\cdots T})'$ are vectors of canonical parameters, and $A(\mathbf{\Psi}_i, \mathbf{\Omega}_i)$ is a normalizing constant, $\exp(A(\mathbf{\Psi}_i, \mathbf{\Omega}_i)) = \sum \exp(\mathbf{\Psi}_i' \mathbf{y}_i + \mathbf{\Omega}_i' \mathbf{w}_i)$ where summation is over all 2^T possible values of $\mathbf{Y}_i$. The parameters of $\mathbf{\Psi}_i$ can be interpreted in terms of conditional probabilities,

$$\psi_{ir} = \text{logit}[\Pr(Y_{ir} = 1 | Y_{is} = 0, s \neq r)]$$

while the parameters of $\mathbf{\Omega}_i$ can be interpreted in terms of conditional log odds ratios, for example

$$\exp(\omega_{irs}) = \frac{\Pr(Y_{ir}=1, Y_{is}=1 | Y_{it}=0, t \neq r, s)\Pr(Y_{ir}=0, Y_{is}=0 | Y_{it}=0, t \neq r, s)}{\Pr(Y_{ir}=1, Y_{is}=0 | Y_{it}=0, t \neq r, s)\Pr(Y_{ir}=0, Y_{is}=1 | Y_{it}=0, t \neq r, s)}$$

Similar expressions hold for the three-way and higher way association parameters (see Fitzmaurice and Laird, 1993). Note that μ_i is a function of both $\mathbf{\Psi}_i$ and $\mathbf{\Omega}_i$.

Fitzmaurice and Laird (1993) suggest making a one-to-one transformation from $(\mathbf{\Psi}_i, \mathbf{\Omega}_i)$ to the mixed parameters $(\mu_i, \mathbf{\Omega}_i)$. They assume that $\mathbf{\Omega}_i$ can be expressed as a function of a $Q \times 1$ parameter vector $\alpha = (\alpha_1, \ldots, \alpha_Q)'$. In principle, any dependence link function could be used; a natural one in this setting is the identity link function

$$\mathbf{\Omega}_i = \mathbf{z}_i \alpha \tag{8.4}$$

where $\mathbf{z}_i$ is a $K \times Q$ design matrix. With this formulation the model for the within-subject association can be saturated by including all terms up to the T-way association. However, with moderate sample sizes this may only be practical when T is relatively small. Alternatively, more parsimonious models can be fitted, such as the pairwise model (Bishop *et al.*, 1975) which assumes that all association terms except the $\binom{T}{2}$ pairwise terms are zero, or the first-order Markov chain model which assumes that all association terms are zero except adjacent pairwise terms (also, see Azzalini, 1994). Finally, with the model given by (8.4) the within-subject association can be allowed also to depend on covariates. In the next section we briefly describe the likelihood equations for this mixed parameter model.

8.3.2   Likelihood equations

Assuming that the joint distribution of $\mathbf{Y}_i$ is given by (8.2)–(8.4), the likelihood equations for $(\beta^{(M)}, \alpha)$ can be written,

$$\sum_{i=1}^{N} \begin{pmatrix} \partial l_i / \partial \beta^{(M)} \\ \partial l_i / \partial \alpha \end{pmatrix} = \sum_{i=1}^{N} \left[\begin{array}{c} \mathbf{x}_i' \mathbf{\Delta}_i \mathbf{\Sigma}_{y_i}^{-1} (\mathbf{y}_i - \mu_i) \\ \mathbf{z}_i' [(\mathbf{y}_i - \mu_i) - \mathbf{\Sigma}_{w_i y_i} \mathbf{\Sigma}_{y_i}^{-1} (\mathbf{w}_i = v_i)] \end{array} \right] = 0$$

where $\mu_i = E[Y_i]$, $v_i = E[\mathbf{W}_i]$, $\mathbf{\Sigma}_{y_i} = \text{cov}(\mathbf{Y}_i)$, $\mathbf{\Delta}_i = \text{diag}\{\text{var}(Y_{it})\}$, and $\mathbf{\Sigma}_{w_i y_i} = \text{cov}(\mathbf{W}_i, \mathbf{Y}_i)$. Maximum likelihood estimates, $(\hat{\beta}^{(M)}, \hat{\alpha})$, can be obtained as the solution to these likelihood equations. The covariance of $(\hat{\beta}^{(M)}, \hat{\alpha})$ can be approximated by the inverse of the Fisher information matrix, $I_{(\beta^{(M)}, \alpha)}$,

$$\text{cov}(\hat{\beta}^{(M)}, \hat{\alpha}) \approx I_{(\beta^{(M)}, \alpha)}^{-1} = \left[\begin{array}{cc} \sum_{i=1}^{N} \mathbf{x}_i' \mathbf{\Delta}_i \mathbf{\Sigma}_{y_i}^{-1} \mathbf{\Delta}_i \mathbf{x}_i & 0 \\ 0 & \sum_{i=1}^{N} \mathbf{z}_i' (\mathbf{\Sigma}_{w_i} - \mathbf{\Sigma}_{w_i y_i} \mathbf{\Sigma}_{y_i}^{-1} \mathbf{\Sigma}_{w_i y_i}') \mathbf{z}_i \end{array} \right]^{-1}$$

Note that the $(\beta^{(M)}, \alpha)$ component of the Fisher information matrix is zero, implying that $\beta^{(M)}$ and α are orthogonal.

Finally, assuming that the model for the mean has been correctly specified by (8.2), it can easily be shown that $\hat{\beta}^{(M)}$ is a consistent estimate of $\beta^{(M)}$. This is the case regardless of whether $\mathbf{\Omega}_i$ has been correctly specified. However, when $\mathbf{\Omega}_i$ has been misspecified, the inverse of the Fisher information matrix can give inconsistent estimates of the asymptotic variance of $\hat{\beta}^{(M)}$. To make correct inferences about $\beta^{(M)}$, the so-called 'sandwich' estimate of $\text{cov}(\hat{\beta}^{(M)})$ first suggested by Cox (1961), and later proposed by Huber (1967), White (1982) and Royall (1986), can be used.

In summary, the mixed parameter model makes the one-to-one transformation from $(\mathbf{\Psi}_i, \mathbf{\Omega}_i) \rightarrow (\mu_i, \mathbf{\Omega}_i) \rightarrow (\beta^{(M)}, \alpha)$. This mixed para-meterization for the joint distribution is attractive because: (i) it yields likelihood equations for the marginal regression parameters, $\beta^{(M)}$, that are robust to misspecification of the association among the responses; (ii) as a consequence of $\beta^{(M)}$ and α being orthogonal, in large samples the estimated conditional association parameters are uncorrelated with the regression parameters (implying that the standard errors of the regression coefficients are not inflated by fitting complex association models with many unknown parameters); and (iii) unlike marginal association parameters, the conditional association parameters are not constrained by the regression parameters (Fitzmaurice *et al.*, 1993). Finally, there is a very close connection with the generalized estimating equations approach (Liang and Zeger, 1986) and this is explored further in the next section.

8.3.3 Relation to generalized estimating equations

In companion papers, Liang and Zeger (1986) and Zeger and Liang (1986) introduced a general method for incorporating within-subject correlation in generalized linear models. In their proposed generalized estimating equations (GEE), the within-subject correlation (or the correlation within subunits) is accounted for in terms of a 'working' correlation matrix. In a general sense, GEE can simply be regarded as a multivariate analogue of the quasi-score function introduced by Wedderburn (1974). GEE only require specification of the form of the first two moments, the success probabilities and correlations, of the vector of binary responses. The joint distribution of $\mathbf{Y}_i$ is left completely unspecified. Instead of modelling the association between a pair of binary responses in terms of the marginal correlations, Lipsitz *et al.* (1991), Liang *et al.* (1992), Carey *et al.* (1993) and others have proposed extensions of GEE using the marginal odds ratios. With binary responses, the odds ratio is a natural metric for measuring association and may also be easier to interpret.

The GEE for $\beta^{(M)}$ in the logistic regression model given by (8.2) can be written

$$\sum_{i=1}^{N} \mathbf{x}_i' \mathbf{\Delta}_i \mathbf{V}_i^{-1}(\mathbf{y}_i - \mu_i) = \mathbf{0}$$

where $\mathbf{V}_i$ is a 'working' or approximate covariance matrix. Note that the estimating equations for $\beta^{(M)}$ are identical in form to the corresponding likelihood equations for $\beta^{(M)}$ in the mixed parameter model,

$$\sum_{i=1}^{N} \mathbf{x}_i' \mathbf{\Delta}_i \mathbf{\Sigma}_{y_i}^{-1}(\mathbf{y}_i - \mu_i) = \mathbf{0}$$

The only difference is in the 'weighting' matrix. In the GEE, $\mathbf{V}_i$ is a 'working' or approximate covariance matrix usually obtained by the method of moments or using an additional set of estimating equations. In the mixed parameter model, $\mathbf{\Sigma}_{y_i}$ is the covariance matrix implied by a fully parametric model. In a certain sense, this relationship provides a likelihood rationale or justification for the GEE with binary data.

The notion of a mixed parameterization can be extended to a more general class of models than is considered here. Glonek (1996) describes a wider class of mixed parameter models, where certain subsets of marginal parameters are combined with the complementary subset of conditional parameters. For example, in some applications both the marginal means and marginal pairwise odds ratios may be of scientific interest. In that case, it will be useful to consider a mixed parameter model, where the parameters for the marginal means and pairwise odds ratios are combined with the complementary subset of conditional higher order association parameters. An attractive feature of such a model is that the resulting likelihood equations for the mean and pairwise odds ratio parameters are robust to misspecification of the conditional higher order associations. Furthermore, note that there is a close relation between the resulting likelihood equations for the mean and pairwise odds ratio parameters and the corresponding GEE. That is, when the GEE are extended to estimate the mean and pairwise association parameters simultaneously, often referred to as GEE2 (Zhao and Prentice, 1990, Prentice and Zhao, 1991; and also see Liang *et al.*, 1992, Heagerty and Zeger, 1996, Molenberghs and Ritter, 1996), they have the exact same form as the likelihood equations from the corresponding mixed parameter model and again only differ in terms of the 'weighting' matrix.

Finally, we make some comments concerning the choice between using a full likelihood-based approach or the semi-parametric GEE approach in applications. When T is relatively small, say $T < 7$, a full likelihood-based approach may be preferred and some attempt to model adequately the second- and higher order moments can usually be made. However, for larger T the GEE approach may be somewhat more attractive owing to its computational simplicity. For example, when $T = 10$ a likelihood-based approach would involve a probability vector of length 1024 and the computations could be very prohibitive. On the other hand, this poses no such difficulty for the GEE approach since it would only require inversion of a 10×10 'working' covariance matrix.

8.3.4   Example

To illustrate the methods discussed in the previous section, we present analyses of the Ohio children's wheeze data. Recall that the data set contains complete records on 537 children from Steubenville, Ohio, each of whom was examined annually at ages 7 through 10. The repeated binary response is the wheezing status (1 = yes, 0 = no) of a child at each occasion. Maternal smoking was categorized as 1 if the child's mother smoked regularly and 0 otherwise.

The marginal expectation of the response is modelled as a logistic function of two covariates, linear age and maternal smoking,

$$\text{logit}\{E[Y_{it}]\} = \beta_0^{(M)} + \beta_1^{(M)} A + \beta_2^{(M)} S$$

where $S = 1$ if the child's mother smokes, 0 otherwise, and A is the age in years since the child's ninth birthday. Prior analyses indicated that a linear age $\times$ maternal smoking interaction was not required. We modelled the within-subject association among the binary responses using the following five models:

I   Independence: $\boldsymbol{\Omega}_i = \mathbf{0}$

II   Common pairwise: $\boldsymbol{\Omega}_i = \alpha_{CP}$

III   First-order Markov: $\boldsymbol{\Omega}_i = \alpha_M$

IV   Pairwise: $\boldsymbol{\Omega}_i = \alpha_P$

V   Saturated: $\boldsymbol{\Omega}_i = \alpha_S$

where $\boldsymbol{\Omega}_i = (\omega_{i12}, \ldots, \omega_{i34}, \omega_{i123}, \ldots, \omega_{i234}, \omega_{i1234})'$, $\alpha_{CP} = (\alpha, \alpha, \alpha, \alpha, \alpha, \alpha, 0, \ldots, 0)'$, $\alpha_M = (\alpha_{12}, 0, 0, \alpha_{23}, 0, \alpha_{34}, 0, \ldots, 0)'$, $\alpha_P = (\alpha_{12}, \ldots, \alpha_{34}, 0, \ldots, 0)'$, and $\alpha_S = (\alpha_{12}, \ldots, \alpha_{34}, \alpha_{123}, \ldots, \alpha_{234}, \alpha_{1234})'$.

Table 8.2 Parameter estimates and standard error (SE) for the marginal regression models using the Ohio children's wheeze data

Marginal parameters					Time dependence parameters		
Model		Estimate	Model SE	Robust SE		Estimate	Model SE
I	$\beta_0^{(M)}$	−1.884	0.084	0.114			
	$\beta_1^{(M)}$	−0.113	0.054	0.044			
	$\beta_2^{(M)}$	0.272	0.124	0.178			
	$G^2 = 241.49\,\mathrm{df} = 27$						
II	$\beta_0^{(M)}$	−1.880	0.114	0.114	α	1.265	0.073
	$\beta_1^{(M)}$	−0.112	0.044	0.044			
	$\beta_2^{(M)}$	0.265	0.178	0.178			
	$G^2 = 17.02\,\mathrm{df} = 26$						
III	$\beta_0^{(M)}$	−1.899	0.107	0.115	α_{12}	1.940	0.264
	$\beta_1^{(M)}$	−0.116	0.055	0.045	α_{23}	2.433	0.282
	$\beta_2^{(M)}$	0.240	0.164	0.180	α_{34}	2.228	0.291
	$G^2 = 49.08\,\mathrm{df} = 24$						
IV	$\beta_0^{(M)}$	−1.885	0.114	0.114	α_{12}	1.326	0.305
	$\beta_1^{(M)}$	−0.115	0.045	0.044	α_{13}	0.749	0.332
	$\beta_2^{(M)}$	0.255	0.178	0.178	α_{14}	1.282	0.318
					α_{23}	1.912	0.312
					α_{24}	0.868	0.348
	$G^2 = 10.12\,\mathrm{df} = 21$				α_{34}	1.513	0.338
V	$\beta_0^{(M)}$	−1.885	0.114	0.114	α_{12}	1.429	0.414
	$\beta_1^{(M)}$	−0.115	0.045	0.044	α_{13}	1.078	0.508
	$\beta_2^{(M)}$	0.256	0.178	0.178	α_{14}	1.489	0.449
					α_{23}	2.011	0.440
					α_{24}	0.871	0.640
					α_{34}	1.720	0.522
					α_{123}	−0.467	0.792
					α_{124}	−0.184	0.928
					α_{134}	−0.816	0.942
					α_{234}	−0.172	0.942
	$G^2 = 9.30\,\mathrm{df} = 16$				α_{1234}	0.841	1.411

Note: $\mathrm{df} = 2 \times (2^4 - 1) -$ number of parameters estimated

In Table 8.2 the parameter estimates and both model-based and so-called 'robust' standard errors (i.e. based on the 'sandwich' estimator of variance) for the five models are presented.[1] The results of all of these analyses indicate a decline in the rate of wheeze over time, and a moderate, although not statistically discernible, increase in the rate of wheeze for children of mothers who smoke. Note that the estimates of $\beta^{(M)}$ are very similar in all five models. However, the independence model tends to underestimate the model-based standard errors of the time-stationary effects (intercept, S) and overestimate the model-based standard error of the time-varying effect (A). This observation is entirely consistent with what would be expected in linear models with continuous responses.

Likelihood-ratio goodness-of-fit statistics for the five models indicate that model II, the model with common pairwise associations, provides an adequate fit to the observed data. Model III, the first-order Markov chain association model, does not appear to fit the data. Comparing G^2 with more complex models, we find that neither model IV nor V provides a statistically significant improvement in fit over model II. Note that both the model-based and robust standard errors obtained from models II, IV and V are almost identical. This suggests that the time dependence has been adequately modelled by model II. The estimate of the age effect, $\hat{\beta}_1^{(M)} = -0.112$, indicates that the prevalence of wheeze in children is decreasing as they get older. More specifically, the odds of wheeze decrease annually by a factor of 0.894 ($e^{-0.112}$). The estimate of the maternal smoking effect, $\hat{\beta}_2^{(M)} = 0.265$, indicates that the prevalence of wheeze is higher among children of women who smoke. This result suggests that the odds of wheeze for children whose mothers smoke is 1.30 (or $e^{0.265}$) times that of children whose mothers do not smoke. Note that this marginal regression coefficient contrasts the odds or prevalence of wheeze in the population of children whose mothers smoke with the population of children whose mothers do not smoke, and thus has a 'population-averaged' interpretation.

Next, retaining the logistic model for the marginal expectation,

$$\text{logit}\{E[Y_{it}]\} = \beta_0^{(M)} + \beta_1^{(M)} A + \beta_2^{(M)} S$$

we used the GEE approach to obtain estimates of the logistic regression parameters. However, instead of modelling the association among the binary responses in terms of the marginal correlations, we considered models for the marginal odds ratios. Note that the marginal odds ratios,

$$\eta_{irs} = \frac{\Pr(Y_{ir} = 1, Y_{is} = 1)\Pr(Y_{ir} = 0, Y_{is} = 0)}{\Pr(Y_{ir} = 1, Y_{is} = 0)\Pr(Y_{ir} = 0, Y_{is} = 1)}$$

---

[1] A statistical software tool, MAREG, for obtaining MLEs for the mixed parameter model has been developed by Fieger *et al.* (1996). The latest version of MAREG can be obtained via anonymous ftp from ftp.stat.uni-muenchen.de.

are not the same as the conditional odds ratios, $\exp(\omega_{irs})$, in the mixed parameter models considered in Section 8.3.1.

In general, longitudinal models for the odds ratio, similar to those for the correlation, have not been well developed. Recently, however, Fitzmaurice and Lipsitz (1995) have proposed serial pattern models for the odds ratio analogous to the exponential correlation patterns so commonly assumed for continuous response data. Recall that in terms of the correlation, $\rho_{ist} = \rho_{ist}(\theta) = \text{corr}(Y_{is}, Y_{it}|\theta)$, an exponential pattern is given by

$$\rho_{ist} = \theta^{|t-s|} \tag{8.5}$$

where $0 < \theta < 1$. This model characterizes a geometrically decreasing correlation between measurements taken further apart in time, as occurs, for example, in autoregressive and Markov models. Thus when $t = s$, there is perfect correlation and $\rho_{ist} = \theta^0 = 1$. When observations are far apart in time, then as $|t - s| \to \infty$, $\rho_{ist} \to \theta^\infty = 0$ and the observations are uncorrelated. Fitzmaurice and Lipsitz (1995) proposed an analogous serial pattern model for the odds ratio,

$$\eta_{ist} = \theta^{1/|t-s|} \tag{8.6}$$

where $1 < \theta < \infty$. Note that as $|t - s| \to 0$, $\eta_{ist} \to \theta^\infty$ and there is perfect association. When observations are far apart in time, then as $|t - s| \to \infty$, $\eta_{ist} \to \theta^0 = 1$ and there is no association among the observations. A slightly more general model than (8.6) is

$$\eta_{ist} = \theta^{1/|t-s|^k}$$

for some given $k \geq 0$. Alternatively, k can be treated as a parameter to be estimated from the data, but this introduces non-linearity. However, this problem can be circumvented using the linearization technique described in Box and Tidwell (1962).

For the Ohio children's wheeze data set, we considered the following linear model for the marginal log odds ratios,

$$\log(\eta_{ist}) = \frac{1}{|t - s|} \log(\theta)$$

and used GEE to obtain estimates of $\beta^{(M)}$ and θ. In Table 8.3 the parameter estimates and standard errors are presented.[2] Note that the

---

[2] Statistical software for GEE is available from a number of sources. Davis (1993) has provided a FORTRAN program that can be used on personal computers and workstations. Karim and Zeger (1988) have developed an SAS macro that can be used in conjunction with the IML (SAS Institute Inc., 1985) procedure. A very similar routine for use with the Splus software (Statistical Sciences, 1991) has been developed by Carey (1989) and is available via anonymous ftp from StatLib at the Carnegie Mellon University Statistics Department (lib.stat.cmu.edu). Finally, in release 6.12 (and all later releases) of the SAS System, GEE have been incorporated as an option in the GENMOD procedure.

Table 8.3 Parameter estimates and standard error (SE) for the marginal regression model using the Ohio children's wheeze data

Marginal parameters				Time dependence parameter		
	Estimate	Model SE	Robust SE		Estimate	Model SE
$\beta_0^{(M)}$	−1.896	0.111	0.114	$\log(\theta)$	2.497	0.219
$\beta_1^{(M)}$	−0.113	0.054	0.045			
$\beta_2^{(M)}$	0.241	0.172	0.180			

results of these analyses are remarkably similar to those reported in Table 8.2. That is, the GEE estimates of $\beta^{(M)}$ in Table 8.3 are very similar to those reported for the five models in Table 8.2. This result is not too surprising considering that the GEE only differ from the likelihood equations in terms of the 'weighting' matrix.

The estimate of the time dependence, $\log(\hat{\theta}) \approx 2.5$, indicates that the odds ratio for measurements one year apart is $\hat{\theta} \approx 12.2$, whereas for measurements two years apart, the odds ratio is $\hat{\theta}^{1/2} \approx 3.5$; while for observations three years apart, the odds ratio is $\hat{\theta}^{1/3} \approx 2.3$. Note that $\log(\hat{\theta})$ is substantially larger than any of the conditional log odds ratios for adjacent years given in Table 8.2 (see, for example, the estimates obtained under model IV). However, given that the repeated binary responses are expected to be positively correlated, one might also expect that the conditional odds ratio will be somewhat smaller in magnitude than the corresponding marginal odds ratio, since it is conditional on the other two remaining responses.

8.4   Conditional regression models

In this section we consider conditional regression models where the *conditional* expectation of the responses, either $E[Y_{it}|y_{is}, s < t]$ or $E[Y_{it}|\mathbf{b}_i]$ (where the $\mathbf{b}_i$ are random effects), is of main interest. That is, the focus is on regression parameters modelling the conditional expectation of each response, given the values of previous responses or a set of latent (or unobserved) random variables. First, we consider transitional models where the mean response being modelled is conditional not only on the covariates, but also on values of previous responses.

8.4.1   Transitional models

Recall that one of the distinguishing features of marginal regression models is that the mean is modelled separately from the time dependence or within-subject association. Transitional models differ from marginal regression models in that the mean and time dependence are modelled simultaneously (Ware *et al.*, 1988). In transitional models it is assumed that

$$g\{E[Y_{it}|\mathbf{x}_{it}, Y_{is}, s < t]\} = \mathbf{x}_{it}\beta^{(T)} + \sum_{j=1}^{P} \gamma_j h_j(Y_{i1}, \ldots, Y_{i,t-1}) \qquad (8.7)$$

where $g(\cdot)$ is some suitable link function and the $h_j(\cdot)$ are functions (usually, but not necessarily, linear functions) of previous responses (Zeger *et al.*, 1985). Transitional models are considered to be *conditional* regression models in the sense of modelling the conditional distribution (and moments) of the response at time t given previous responses and the covariates at time t. For example, Bonney (1987) proposed a class of logistic models for longitudinal data which take the autoregressive form

$$\text{logit}\{E[Y_{it}|\mathbf{x}_{it}, y_{is}, s < t]\} = \mathbf{x}_{it}\beta^{(T)} + \gamma_1 y_{i,t-1} + \gamma_2 y_{i,t-2} + \cdots + \gamma_{t-1} y_{i1}$$

(see also Cox, 1972, Korn and Whittemore, 1979, Zeger *et al.*, 1985, Ware *et al.*, 1988).

Markov chain models form an important subclass of transitional models and are most suited to the case where there are equally spaced observation times. Markov chain models of different order are obtained by allowing only a fixed number of previous responses to be included as regressors in (8.7). For example, a first-order Markov chain model is given by

$$g\{E[Y_{it}|\mathbf{x}_{it}, y_{is}, s < t]\} = \mathbf{x}_{it}\beta^{(T)} + \gamma y_{i,t-1}$$

Similarly, a second-order Markov chain model is obtained by allowing dependence on the values of the previous two responses,

$$g\{E[Y_{it}|\mathbf{x}_{it}, y_{is}, s < t]\} = \mathbf{x}_{it}\beta^{(T)} + \gamma_1 y_{i,t-1} + \gamma_2 y_{i,t-2}$$

and so on.

The assumption that $\beta^{(T)}$ is constant across time and across individuals can be relaxed, in principle, in a number of different ways. For example, homogeneity of $\beta^{(T)}$ across individuals might only be assumed for individuals within certain well-defined subgroups. Alternatively, it may be possible to fit a model with separate parameters to each wave of data, Y_{it} (see Stram *et al.*, 1988). The general model given by (8.7) also allows additional interaction terms, such as $y_{i,t-1} \times y_{i,t-2}$, to be incorporated. Furthermore, interactions between the previous response and covariates can easily be included. For example, Muenz and Rubinstein (1985) considered a first-order Markov chain model, where the two transition probabilities, $\Pr(Y_{it} = 1|\mathbf{x}_{it}, Y_{i,t-1} = 0)$ and $\Pr(Y_{it} = 1|\mathbf{x}_{it}, Y_{i,t-1} = 1)$, are modelled using a logit link function,

$$\text{logit}\{E[Y_{it}|\mathbf{x}_{it}, Y_{i,t-1} = 0]\} = \mathbf{x}_{it}\beta_0^{(T)} + \gamma_0 y_{i,t-1}$$
$$\text{logit}\{E[Y_{it}|\mathbf{x}_{it}, Y_{i,t-1} = 1]\} = \mathbf{x}_{it}\beta_1^{(T)} + \gamma_1 y_{i,t-1}$$

However, note that this model can be incorporated within Bonney's (1987) formulation in a straightforward manner by simply including interactions between all of the covariates and the lagged response.

With transitional models, the joint distribution of $\mathbf{Y}_i$ can be factored into the product of T conditional distributions,

$$f(y_{i1}, \ldots, y_{iT}; \beta^{(T)}, \gamma) = \prod_{t=1}^{T} f(y_{it} | y_{i,t-1}, \ldots, y_{i1}; \beta^{(T)}, \gamma)$$

For the case of a pth-order Markov chain model this is, strictly speaking, a conditional likelihood, given a set of p initial or starting values y_{i0}, $y_{i,-1}$, $\ldots$, $y_{i,-p+1}$. In a pth-order Markov chain model, $f(y_{it} | y_{i,t-1}, \ldots, y_{i1}; \beta^{(T)}, \gamma) = f(y_{it} | y_{i,t-1}, \ldots, y_{i,t-p}; \beta^{(T)}, \gamma)$, and the ith individual's contribution to the likelihood is simply

$$f(y_{i1}, \ldots, y_{iT}; \beta^{(T)}, \gamma) = f(y_{i1}, \ldots, y_{ip}; \beta^{(T)}, \gamma) \prod_{t=p+1}^{T} f(y_{it} | y_{i,t-1}, \ldots, y_{i,t-p}; \beta^{(T)}, \gamma)$$

However, since the marginal distribution of $f(y_{i1}, \ldots, y_{ip}; \beta^{(T)}, \gamma)$ cannot usually be determined from the conditional distributions, $f(y_{it} | y_{i,t-1}, \ldots, y_{i,t-p}; \beta^{(T)}, \gamma)$, conditional maximum likelihood estimates are generally obtained by ignoring the contribution of $f(y_{i1}, \ldots, y_{ip};$ $\beta^{(T)}, \gamma)$ to the likelihood. The price that is paid for not making additional assumptions concerning $f(y_{i1}, \ldots, y_{ip}; \beta^{(T)}, \gamma)$ is that there will be some loss of efficiency in estimating $\beta^{(T)}$ and γ.

Note that the distinguishing feature of transitional models is that previous responses are essentially accorded the same status as the main explanatory variables in a single regression equation. As such, previous responses are simply treated as additional covariates. Furthermore, assuming that the conditional distribution of Y_{it}, given Y_{is} and $\mathbf{x}_{it}$, is Bernoulli, the transitional model for the mean completely determines the variance, that is

$$\operatorname{var}(Y_{it} | \mathbf{x}_{it}, Y_{is}, s < t) = E[Y_{it} | \mathbf{x}_{it}, Y_{is}, s < t]\{1 - E[Y_{it} | \mathbf{x}_{it}, Y_{is}, s < t]\}$$

Thus, if the model for the conditional mean has been correctly specified, the repeated transitions for an individual can be regarded as independent observations. This allows straightforward application of standard fitting procedures for generalized linear models. That is, the unknown parameters can be estimated by maximum likelihood methods. For example, by simply treating the previous responses as additional covariates, algorithms developed for generalized linear models with independent observations (e.g. weighted iterative least squares) can be used. Consistent parameter estimation is obtained provided only that the model for the conditional mean has been correctly specified. That is, given only a correctly specified model for the conditional mean, $E[Y_{it} | \mathbf{x}_{it}, Y_{is}, s < t]$, the (quasi-)likelihood equations yield estimates which are consistent and asymptotically normal. However, if the conditional mean has been correctly specified but the conditional variance has not, the inverse of the Fisher information matrix can give inconsistent estimates of the asymptotic covariance matrix of $\hat{\beta}^{(T)}$ and $\hat{\gamma}$. To make correct inferences about $\beta^{(T)}$ and γ, the so-called 'sandwich' estimator of the variance must be used instead.

Next, we consider the interpretation of $\beta^{(T)}$. Each parameter can be interpreted in terms of changes in an individual's response probability, conditional on or adjusted for the values of the previous responses. That is, each regression parameter measures the change in the probability of a positive response associated with a unit change in the particular covariate, holding all other covariates and the individual's response history fixed. Note, however, that the interpretation of $\beta^{(T)}$ depends critically on both P and the functional form of the $h_j(\cdot)$ in (8.7). That is, the interpretation of $\beta^{(T)}$ is somewhat different when $P = 1$ as compared to $P = 2$, and so on. This is in marked contrast to marginal regression models where the interpretation of $\beta^{(M)}$ is completely invariant to the choice of model for the covariance or time dependence structure. In order to highlight some of these aspects of interpretation, we next consider transitional models for the Ohio children's wheeze data set.

8.4.2 Example

We return to the Ohio children's wheeze data set to illustrate the methods discussed in the previous section. The conditional expectation of the response is modelled as a logistic function of the previous response and the two covariates, linear age and maternal smoking,

$$\text{logit}\{E[Y_{it}|y_{i,t-1}]\} = \beta_0^{(T)} + \beta_1^{(T)}A + \beta_2^{(T)}S + \gamma y_{i,t-1} \quad \text{for } t = 2, 3, 4$$

where $S = 1$ if the child's mother smokes, 0 otherwise, and A is the age in years since the child's ninth birthday. In a preliminary analysis, which allowed for additional interaction terms between the lagged response and the covariates, none of the interactions were found to be statistically significant.

The results of the analysis are presented in Table 8.4.[3] The regression parameter for the lagged response, γ, measures the dependence of the response probability at a given time on the previous response. The parameter e^{γ} is the ratio of odds of wheeze among those children who did and did not have wheeze on the previous occasion. The estimated coefficient, $\hat{\gamma} = 2.211$, suggests that there is a strong time dependence or association over time among the responses for the same individual. Next, we consider the interpretation of $\hat{\beta}_2^{(T)}$. This can be interpreted in terms of the conditional log odds of wheeze among children, conditional on their response at the previous occasion. That is, given a child's wheeze status at the previous occasion, the conditional odds of wheeze among children of

---

[3] Note that conditional maximum likelihood estimates and model-based standard errors can be obtained using any existing statistical software for ordinary logistic regression.

Table 8.4 Parameter estimates and standard error (SE) for the transitional model using the Ohio children's wheeze data

Transitional parameters

	Estimate	Model SE	Robust SE
$\beta_0^{(T)}$	−2.478	0.115	0.117
$\beta_1^{(T)}$	−0.243	0.094	0.090
$\beta_2^{(T)}$	0.296	0.156	0.155
γ	2.211	0.158	0.187

mothers who smoke is 1.34 ($e^{0.296}$) times that of children whose mothers do not smoke. Somewhat surprisingly, the estimate of $\beta_2^{(T)}$ is slightly larger than the estimate of $\beta_2^{(M)}$ obtained in Section 8.3.4. We might have expected that adjusting for the previous response would eliminate part of the maternal smoking effect. Indeed, Neuhaus (1992) has suggested that conditioning on lagged responses may remove the effects of time-invariant covariates from the model. However, as was demonstrated by this example, this is not always the case.

Note that the interpretation of $\beta_2^{(T)}$ depends on the first-order Markov assumption. If, instead, a second-order Markov chain model is considered, where

$$\text{logit}\{E[Y_{it}|y_{i,t-1}, y_{i,t-2}]\} = \beta_0^{(T)} + \beta_1^{(T)}A + \beta_2^{(T)}S + \gamma_1 y_{i,t-1} + \gamma_2 y_{i,t-2} \quad \text{for } t = 3, 4$$

the interpretation of $\beta_2^{(T)}$ changes. With a second-order Markov chain model $\hat{\beta}_2^{(T)} = 0.174$, indicating that the conditional odds of wheeze among children of mothers who smoke is 1.20 ($e^{0.174}$) times that of children whose mothers do not smoke. Furthermore, note that the magnitude of the estimated maternal smoking effect is somewhat smaller when conditioning is on the lagged responses from the previous two occasions. This is in marked contrast to the interpretation of $\beta_2^{(M)}$ which is completely invariant to the choice of model for the covariance or time dependence structure.

In the next section we consider a second class of conditional regression models where, instead of conditioning on the values of previous responses, conditioning is on a set of unobserved random effects.

8.4.3   Random effects models

Drawing on direct analogies with linear models for continuous responses (e.g. Laird and Ware, 1982), various authors (e.g. Korn and Whittemore, 1979; Stiratelli *et al.*, 1984; Anderson and Aitkin, 1985; Zeger *et al.*, 1988;

and others) have suggested the use of random effects models for discrete responses. In random effects models it is assumed that

$$g\{E[Y_{it}|\mathbf{x}_{it}, \mathbf{b}_i]\} = \mathbf{x}_{it}\beta^{(R)} + \mathbf{z}_{it}\mathbf{b}_i \tag{8.8}$$

where $g(\cdot)$ is some suitable link function, $\mathbf{z}_{it}$ is a function of covariates whose effects are assumed to vary across individuals (usually, but not necessarily, a subset of $\mathbf{x}_{it}$), and $\mathbf{b}_i$ is a vector of random effects. The $\mathbf{b}_i$ are random regression coefficients, with mean $E[\mathbf{b}_i] = \mathbf{0}$ and unknown covariance matrix $\mathrm{cov}(\mathbf{b}_i) = \mathbf{D}$. The $\mathbf{b}_i$ are often assumed to be distributed as multivariate normal, $N(\mathbf{0}, \mathbf{D})$.

Random effects models can be thought of as two-stage models. In the first stage, the observations, Y_{it}, are typically assumed to be conditionally independent given a vector of underlying latent individual parameters, $\mathbf{b}_i$. This is known as the local independence assumption. A regression model is specified, having a vector of fixed regression coefficients, $\beta^{(R)}$, and a vector of random regression coefficients, $\mathbf{b}_i$. In the second stage, the individual-specific random effects, $\mathbf{b}_i$, are assumed to have a particular multivariate distribution, with probability density function $f(\mathbf{b}_i)$ (often assumed to be multivariate normal). That is, $f(\mathbf{b}_i)$ defines the distribution of the random effects over the population of individuals. Note that since the conditional covariance between any pair of responses on an individual is assumed to be zero, that is $\mathrm{cov}(Y_{ir}, Y_{is}|\mathbf{b}_i) = 0$, any marginal correlation among the Y_{it} is being driven by the shared random effects, $\mathbf{b}_i$. The simplest possible example is the random intercepts model. Consider the logistic regression model

$$\mathrm{logit}\{E[Y_{it}|\mathbf{x}_{it}, b_i]\} = \mathbf{x}_{it}\beta^{(R)} + b_i$$

where $\mathbf{x}_{it}$ is assumed to contain the intercept term, and the b_i are randomly varying intercepts, assumed to be $N(0, d)$. This model can be considered to be the discrete data analogue of the compound symmetry (or exchangeable correlation) model for continuous response data. Discussion of some other closely related models can also be found in Ochi and Prentice (1984), Wong and Mason (1985), Gilmour *et al.* (1985), Conaway (1989) and McCulloch (1994).

In random effects models, the local independence assumption is typically made. Thus, given the vector of latent individual parameters, $\mathbf{b}_i$, the Y_{it} are assumed to be conditionally independent Bernoulli, with $\phi_{it} = \mathrm{Pr}(Y_{it} = 1|\mathbf{x}_{it}, \mathbf{b}_i) = E[Y_{it}|\mathbf{x}_{it}, \mathbf{b}_i] = g^{-1}(\mathbf{x}_{it}\beta^{(R)} + \mathbf{z}_{it}\mathbf{b}_i)$. Given some parametric assumption concerning the distribution of the $\mathbf{b}_i$, the likelihood of the data is given by

$$\prod_{i=1}^{N} \int \prod_{t=1}^{T} \phi_{it}^{y_{it}}(1 - \phi_{it})^{1-y_{it}} f(\mathbf{b}_i)\mathrm{d}\mathbf{b}_i$$

where $f(\mathbf{b}_i)$ is the probability density function of the $\mathbf{b}_i$. This likelihood is often called the marginal or integrated likelihood, since it is averaged over the distribution of the unobserved random effects, $\mathbf{b}_i$.

In the past, a potential limitation of random effects models for discrete response data was their computational burden. The main computational difficulty arises because, in general, there is no simple closed form solution for the above likelihood. This necessitates the use of high dimensional numerical integration techniques. The one exception is when $\mathbf{b}_i$ are scalar, in which case the computations are fairly modest. Indeed, much of the early literature on random effects models for discrete data has been concerned with ways of circumventing part of the computational burden, for example by using various approximations of the likelihood. However, many of the recent advances in Monte Carlo techniques, such as Gibbs sampling (Geman and Geman, 1984, Gelfand and Smith, 1990) have now made the computations feasible for even the most complex of models. For example, Zeger and Karim (1991) have applied Gibbs sampling and showed how to simulate from the required conditional distribution. A detailed discussion of the various computational approaches to random effects models can be found in Fahrmeir and Tutz (1994, ch. 7).

Next, we consider the interpretation of the fixed effects, $\beta^{(R)}$. Each of the parameters can be interpreted in terms of the effects of a particular covariate within the same individual. That is, $\beta^{(R)}$ measures the change in the probability of a positive response, for a unit change in the particular covariate, for a specific individual with underlying propensity to respond positively, $\mathbf{b}_i$. Note that unlike the linear random effects model for continuous data, the $\beta^{(R)}$ and the marginal regression parameters are not, in general, equal. The unconditional or marginal mean of Y_{it} is obtained by integrating over the distribution of the $\mathbf{b}_i$ and, in general,

$$\int \phi_{it} f(\mathbf{b}_i) d\mathbf{b}_i \neq g^{-1}(\mathbf{x}_{it}\beta^{(R)})$$

That is, unless an identity link function is assumed, the fixed effects, $\beta^{(R)}$, do not have a marginal interpretation. Zeger *et al.* (1988), Neuhaus and Jewell (1990) and Neuhaus *et al.* (1991) have studied the relationship between the regression parameters in marginal and random effects models for binary responses. They have shown that, in general, the effects of covariates are greater in absolute magnitude in the random effects models than they are in the marginal regression model. That is, in general, $|\beta^{(M)}| < |\beta^{(R)}|$ and consequently the marginal regression parameters will be closer to zero. Unfortunately there are no similar general analytic results comparing $\beta^{(T)}$ to $\beta^{(R)}$ (or $\beta^{(M)}$). Zeger and Liang (1992) have shown that in certain very special cases $|\beta^{(T)}| \leq |\beta^{(M)}| < |\beta^{(R)}|$. Neuhaus (1992) has also suggested that one might expect that conditioning on previous or lagged responses should remove the effects of time-invariant covariates from the model. However, as was demonstrated earlier, this is not always the case.

8.4.4   Example

We return to the Ohio children's wheeze data set to illustrate the methods discussed in the previous section. The conditional expectation of the

Table 8.5 Parameter estimates and standard error (SE) for the random intercepts model using the Ohio children's wheeze data

Random effects parameters

	Estimate	Model SE
$\beta_0^{(R)}$	−3.101	0.222
$\beta_1^{(R)}$	−0.176	0.067
$\beta_2^{(R)}$	0.399	0.273

Standard deviation of b_i:

d	2.165	0.179

response is modelled using the following random effects logistic regression model, with randomly varying intercepts,

$$\text{logit}\{E[Y_{it}|b_i]\} = \beta_0^{(R)} + \beta_1^{(R)}A + \beta_2^{(R)}S + b_i$$

where $S = 1$ if the child's mother smokes, 0 otherwise, and A is the age in years since the child's ninth birthday. The b_i are assumed to have a normal distribution, with unknown variance, d^2. In a preliminary analysis, a model where children were allowed to vary both in terms of their intercepts and their trend across time (i.e. randomly varying intercepts and slopes) was considered, but this did not improve the overall fit to the data.

Maximum marginal likelihood methods were used to obtain estimates of the model parameters. The estimates given in Table 8.5 were obtained using Gauss–Hermite quadrature to integrate numerically over the distribution of the random effects.[4] The results provide clear evidence that there is significant variation in the individual intercepts. The estimated variance of the b_i can also be interpreted in terms of an intraclass correlation of approximately 0.60. Next, consider the interpretation of $\hat{\beta}_2^{(R)}$. This can be interpreted in terms of the log odds of wheeze for a specific child. That is, the odds ratio of wheeze for a given child who has a mother who smokes, versus

---

[4] Statistical software for random effects models is widely available from both commercial and non-commercial sources. For example, Goldstein (1995) and colleagues have developed a general-purpose multi-level modelling package, MLn (Rasbash and Woodhouse, 1995), that is commercially available and can be used for fitting random effects models to discrete longitudinal data. Based on the article by Hedeker and Gibbons (1994), Hedeker and Gibbons (1996) have provided a DOS and Windows version of a computer program, MIXOR, for random effects models for binary and ordinal responses. MIXOR is available via anonymous ftp from the 'MIXOR homepage', http://www.uic.edu/~hedeker/mix.html. Finally, Bayesian estimation is possible using Markov chain Monte Carlo (MCMC) methods, which have been incorporated in the BUGS software package (Spiegelhalter *et al.*, 1995). BUGS is available via anonymous ftp from ftp.mrc-bsu.cam.ac.uk in directory pub/methodology/bugs.

the same child (or a child with identical latent, underlying risk) who has a mother who does not smoke, is 1.49 ($e^{0.399}$). Note that the value of $\hat{\beta}_2^{(R)}$ depends on the assumed distribution of the random effects. This is in contrast to $\hat{\beta}_2^{(M)}$ which is relatively insensitive to the choice of model for the covariance or time dependence structure.

8.5   Conclusions

In this chapter we have reviewed and contrasted two general classes of models for analysing longitudinal binary responses, marginal regression models and conditional regression models. We have further distinguished two kinds of conditional regression models: transitional models, where the conditioning is on the response history, and random effects models, where the conditioning is on a set of unobserved random coefficients. The distinction between these models is somewhat artificial and was made primarily to emphasize certain aspects of interpretation that arise when analysing discrete longitudinal data. However, it should be mentioned that it is possible to combine certain features of these models, thus blurring some of the distinctions. For example, Conaway (1989, 1990) has suggested extending the random effects model to include lagged responses as additional covariates. By symmetry, Conaway's proposal can also be thought of as an extension of the transitional model to incorporate random effects. The regression parameters in Conaways's model then reflect changes within an individual, adjusted for that individual's response history.

While most longitudinal studies are designed to collect data on every individual in the sample at a planned sequence of observation times, these studies habitually suffer from problems with missing data. For example, attrition is a common problem in most studies; that is, some individuals 'drop out' of the study prematurely and thus have incomplete data records. Attrition gives rise to a monotone missing data pattern, where if Y_{ik} is missing then $Y_{ik+1}, \ldots, Y_{iT}$ are also missing. In contrast, the data can be missing intermittently, giving rise to a considerably larger number of potential missing data patterns. When there are missing data, the key issue is whether those with incomplete data records and those with complete data records differ in any further relevant way. If they do not, then analyses restricted to those with complete data records yield valid (albeit inefficient) inferences. If they do differ, then such analyses are potentially biased. In this chapter we have not considered the difficult, but practically important, problem of handling missing data in the analysis of discrete longitudinal data. The interested reader is referred to the excellent review paper by Laird (1988) for a general overview of this topic. A survey of much of the recent statistical literature on methods for modelling drop-out can be found in Little (1995).

Although the recent advances in statistical methodology described in this chapter provide the data analyst with a wide variety of tools for analysing discrete longitudinal data, the appropriate choice amongst the various models is not always obvious. We conclude with some remarks on the appropriate choice between these classes of models for any particular medical study. In general, we hold the view that the choice of model should be guided by the specific scientific question of primary interest. Where the purpose of a study is to make inferences about changes in the rates of disease in a population, and to compare these changes in the populations with and without certain risk factors, marginal regression models are the appropriate choice. On the other hand, where the purpose of a study is the prediction or understanding of disease within an individual, conditional regression models are required. For example, random effects models are appropriate where the purpose of the study is to describe an individual's rate of change over time, and how that is related to various risk factors. On the other hand, when the goal of the study is prediction of an individual's probability of disease, transitional models are a more suitable choice.

In summary, we find ourselves in substantial agreement with Drum and McCullagh (1993, p. 300) when they express the opinion that 'the megalomaniacal strategy of fitting a grand unified model, supposedly capable of answering any conceivable question that might be posed, is, in our view, dangerous, unnecessary and counterproductive'. The answers to different scientific questions concerning longitudinal change demand that different models have to be applied to the data at hand. In short, one size does not fit all.

Acknowledgements

This work was supported in part by the Economic and Social Research Council award H519255004, as part of the Analysis of Large and Complex Datasets Programme.

References

Anderson, D. A. and Aitkin, M. 1985: Variance component models with binary response: interviewer variability. *Journal of the Royal Statistical Society (B)* **47**, 203–10.

Azzalini, A. 1994: Logistic regression for autocorrelated data with application to repeated measures. *Biometrika* **81**, 767–75.

Bahadur, R. R. 1961: A representation of the joint distribution of responses to n dichotomous items. In Solomon, H. (ed.), *Studies in item analysis and prediction*. Stanford Mathematical Studies in the Social Sciences VI. Stanford, CA: Stanford University Press, 158–68.

Becker, M. P. and Balagtas, C. C. 1993: Marginal modeling of binary cross-over data. *Biometrics* **49**, 997–1009.

Bishop, Y. M. M., Fienberg, S. E. and Holland, P. W. 1975: *Discrete multivariate analysis: theory and practice*. Cambridge, MA: MIT Press.

Bonney, G. E. 1987: Logistic regression for dependent binary observations. *Biometrics* **43**, 951–73.

Box, G. E. P. and Tidwell, P. W. 1962: Transformation of the independent variables. *Technometrics* **4**, 531–50.

Carey, V. 1989: Data objects for matrix computations: an overview. *Proceedings of Computer Science and Statistics: 21st Symposium on the Interface*, vol. 21, 157–61.

Carey, V., Zeger, S. L. and Diggle, P. J. 1993: Modelling multivariate binary data with alternating logistic regressions. *Biometrika* **80**, 517–26.

Conaway, M. R. 1989: Analysis of repeated categorical measurements with conditional likelihood methods. *Journal of the American Statistical Association* **84**, 53–62.

Conaway, M. R. 1990: A random effects model for binary data. *Biometrics* **46**, 317–28.

Cox, D. R. 1961: Tests of separate families of hypotheses. In *Proceedings of the 4th Berkeley Symposium on Mathematics, Probability and Statistics*, vol. 1. Berkeley, CA: University of California Press, 105–23.

Cox, D. R. 1972: The analysis of multivariate binary data. *Applied Statistics* **21**, 113–20.

Davis, C. S. 1993: A computer program for regression of repeated measures using. generalized estimating equations. *Computer Methods and Programs in Biomedicine* **40**, 15–31.

Dawber, T. R. 1980: *The Framingham study: the epidemiology of atherosclerotic disease*. Cambridge, MA: Harvard University Press.

Diggle, P. J., Liang, K. Y. and Zeger, S. L. 1994: *Analysis of longitudinal data*. Oxford: Clarendon Press.

Dockery, D. W., Speizer, F. E., Stram, D. O., Ware, J. H., Spengler, J. D. and Ferris, B. G. 1989: Effects of inhalable particles on respiratory health of children. *American Review of Respiratory Disease* **139**, 587–94.

Drum, M. and McCullagh, P. 1993: Comment on 'Regression models for discrete longitudinal responses'. *Statistical Science* **8**, 300–1.

Ekholm, A. 1991: Fitting regression models to a multivariate binary response. In G. Rosenqvist, K. Juselius, K. Nordström and J. Palmgren (eds), *A spectrum of statistical thought: essays in statistical theory, economics, and population genetics in honour of Johan Fellman*. Helsinki: Swedish School of Economics and Business Administration, 19–32.

Ekholm, A., Smith, P. W. F. and McDonald, J. W. 1995: Marginal regression analysis of a multivariate binary response. *Biometrika* **82**, 847–54.

Fahrmeir, L. and Tutz, G. 1994: *Multivariate statistical modelling based on generalized linear models*. New York: Springer.

Fieger, A., Heumann, C. and Kastner, C. 1996: MAREG and WinMAREG. SFB. *Discussion Paper 45*, Universität München, Germany.

Fitzmaurice, G. M. and Laird, N. M. 1993: A likelihood-based method for analysing longitudinal binary responses. *Biometrika* **80**, 141–51.

Fitzmaurice, G. M., Laird, N. M. and Rotnitzky, A. G. 1993: Regression models for discrete longitudinal responses (with discussion). *Statistical Science* **8**, 248–309.

Fitzmaurice, G. M. and Lipsitz, S. R. 1995: A model for binary time series data with serial odds ratio patterns. *Applied Statistics* **44**, 51–61.

Gelfand, A. E. and Smith, A. F. M. 1990: Sampling based approaches to calculating marginal densities. *Journal of the American Statistical Association* **85**, 398–409.

Geman, S. and Geman, D. 1984: Stochastic relaxation, Gibbs distributions and the Bayesian restoration of images. *IEEE Transactions on Pattern Analysis and Machine Intelligence* **6**, 721–41.

Gilmour, A. R., Anderson, R. D. and Rae, A. L. 1985: The analysis of binomial data by a generalized linear mixed model. *Biometrika* **72**, 593–9.

Glonek, G. F. V. 1996: A class of regression models for multivariate categorical responses. *Biometrika* **83**, 15–28.

Glonek, G. F. V. and McCullagh, P. 1995: Multivariate logistic models. *Journal of the Royal Statistical Society (B)* **57**, 533–46.

Goldstein, H. 1995: *Multilevel statistical models*. London: Edward Arnold.

Hand, D. J. and Crowder, M. 1996: *Practical longitudinal data analysis*. London: Chapman & Hall.

Heagerty, P. J. and Zeger, S. L. 1996: Marginal regression models for clustered ordinal measurements. *Journal of the American Statistical Association* **91**, 1024–36.

Hedeker, D. and Gibbons, R. D. 1994: A random-effects ordinal regression model for multilevel analysis. *Biometrics* **40**, 933–44.

Hedeker, D. and Gibbons, R. D. 1996: MIXOR: a computer program for mixed-effects ordinal regression analysis. *Computer Methods and Programs in Biomedicine* **49**, 157–76.

IIuber, P. J. 1967: The behavior of maximum likelihood estimates under nonstandard conditions. In *Proceedings of the 5th Berkeley Symposium on Mathematical Statistics and Probability*, vol. 1. Berkeley, CA: University of California Press, 221–33.

Kalbfleisch, J. D. and Prentice, R. L. 1980: *The statistical analysis of failure time data*. New York: John Wiley.

Karim, M. R. and Zeger, S. L. 1988: GEE: a SAS macro for longitudinal data analysis. *Technical Report 674*, Department of Biostatistics, The Johns Hopkins University.

Korn, E. L. and Whittemore, A. S. 1979: Methods for analyzing panel studies of acute health effects of air pollution. *Biometrics* **35**, 795–802.

Laird, N. M. 1988: Missing data in longitudinal studies. *Statistics in Medicine* **7**, 305–15.

Laird, N. M., Beck, G. J. and Ware, J. H. 1984: Mixed models for serial categorical response. Unpublished manuscript. Department of Biostatistics, Harvard School of Public Health, Boston, MA.

Laird, N. M. and Ware, J. H. 1982: Random effects models for longitudinal data. *Biometrics* **38**, 963–74.

Lang, J. and Agresti, A. A. 1994: Simultaneously modeling joint and marginal distributions on multivariate categorical responses. *Journal of the American Statistical Association* **89**, 625–32.

Liang, K. Y. and Zeger, S. L. 1986: Longitudinal data analysis using generalized linear models. *Biometrika* **73**, 13–22.

Liang, K. Y., Zeger, S. L. and Qaqish, B. 1992: Multivariate regression analyses for categorical data (with discussion). *Journal of the Royal Statistical Society (B)* **54**, 3–40.

Lipsitz, S. R., Laird, N. M. and Harrington, D. P. 1990: Maximum likelihood regression methods for paired binary data. *Statistics in Medicine* **9**, 1517–25.

Lipsitz, S. R., Laird, N. M. and Harrington, D. P. 1991: Generalized estimating equations for correlated binary data: using the odds ratio as a measure of association. *Biometrika* **78**, 153–60.

Little, R. J. A. 1995: Modelling the drop-out mechanism in repeated-measures studies. *Journal of the American Statistical Association* **90**, 1112–21.

McCullagh, P. and Nelder, J. A. 1989: *Generalized linear models*, 2nd edn. New York: Chapman & Hall.

McCulloch, C. E. 1994: Maximum likelihood variance components estimation for binary data. *Journal of the American Statistical Association* **89**, 330–5.

Molenberghs, G. and Lesaffre, E. 1994: Marginal modelling of correlated ordinal data using an n-way Plackett distribution. *Journal of the American Statistical Association* **89**, 633–44.

Molenberghs, G. and Ritter, L. L. 1996: Methods for analysing multivariate binary data, with the association between outcomes of interest. *Biometrics* **52**, 1121–32.

Muenz, L. R. and Rubinstein, L. V. 1985: Markov models for covariate dependence of binary sequences. *Biometrics* **41**, 91–101.

Neuhaus, J. M. 1992: Statistical methods for longitudinal and clustered designs with binary responses. *Statistical Methods in Medical Research* **1**, 249–73.

Neuhaus, J. M. and Jewell, N. P. 1990: Some comments on Rosner's multiple logistic model for clustered data. *Biometrics* **46**, 523–34.

Neuhaus, J. M., Kalbfleisch, J. D. and Hauck, W. W. 1991: A comparison of cluster-specific and population averaged approaches for analyzing correlated binary data. *International Statistical Review* **59**, 25–36.

Ochi, Y. and Prentice, R. L. 1984: Likelihood inference in a correlated probit regression model. *Biometrika* **71**, 531–43.

Pepe, M. S. and Anderson, G. L. 1994: A cautionary note on inference for marginal regression models with longitudinal data and general correlated response data. *Communications in Statistics* **23**, 939–51.

Prentice, R. L. 1988: Correlated binary regression with covariates specific to each binary observation. *Biometrics* **44**, 1033–48.

Prentice, R. L. and Zhao, L. P. 1991: Estimating equations for parameters in means and covariances of multivariate discrete and continuous responses. *Biometrics* **47**, 825–39.

Rasbash, J. and Woodhouse, G. 1995: *MLn command reference*. London: Institute of Education.

Royall, R. M. 1986: Model robust confidence intervals using maximum likelihood estimators. *International Statistical Review* **54**, 221–6.

SAS Institute Inc. 1985: *SAS/IML user's guide (version 5 edn)*. Cary, NC: SAS Institute Inc.

Spiegelhalter, D. J., Thomas, A., Best, N. G. and Gilks, W. R. 1995: *BUGS manual and examples: version 0.50*. Cambridge: MRC Biostatistics Unit.

Statistical Sciences 1991: *Splus user's manual*. Seattle: Statistical Sciences.

Stiratelli, R., Laird, N. M. and Ware, J. H. 1984: Random effects models for serial observations with binary responses. *Biometrics* **40**, 961–71.

Stram, D. O., Wei, L. J. and Ware, J. H. 1988: Analysis of repeated ordered categorical outcomes with possibly missing observations and time-dependent covariates. *Journal of the American Statistical Association* **83**, 631–7.

Ware, J. H., Dockery, D. W., Spiro, A., Speizer, F. E. and Ferris, B. G. 1984: Passive smoking, gas cooking and respiratory health in children living in six cities. *American Review of Respiratory Disease* **129**, 366–74.

Ware, J. H., Lipsitz, S. R. and Speizer, F. E. 1988: Issues in the analysis of repeated categorical outcomes. *Statistics in Medicine* **7**, 95–107.

Wedderburn, R. W. M. 1974: Quasi-likelihood functions, generalized linear models and the Gaussian method. *Biometrika* **61**, 439–47.

White, H. 1982: Maximum likelihood estimation of misspecified models. *Econometrica* **50**, 1–26.

Wong, G. Y. and Mason, W. M. 1985: The hierarchical logistic regression model for multilevel analysis. *Journal of the American Statistical Association* **80**, 513–24.

Zeger, S. L. and Karim, M. R. 1991: Generalized linear models with random effects: a Gibbs sampling approach. *Journal of the American Statistical Association* **86**, 79–86.

Zeger, S. L. and Liang, K. Y. 1986: Longitudinal data analysis for discrete and continuous outcomes. *Biometrics* **42**, 121–30.

Zeger, S. L. and Liang, K. Y. 1992: An overview of methods for the analysis of longitudinal data. *Statistics in Medicine* **11**, 1825–39.

Zeger, S. L., Liang, K. Y. and Albert, P. S. 1988: Models for longitudinal data: a generalized estimating equation approach. *Biometrics* **44**, 1049–60.

Zeger, S. L., Liang, K. Y. and Self, S. G. 1985: The analysis of binary longitudinal. data with time-independent covariates. *Biometrika* **72**, 31–8.

Zhao, L. P. and Prentice, R. L. 1990: Correlated binary regression using a quadratic exponential model. *Biometrika* **77**, 642–8.

9 Dealing with missing values in longitudinal studies

Peter J. Diggle

9.1 Introduction

The simplest protocol for a longitudinal study is one in which each of m subjects provides a sequence of n measurements at a common set of time points, $t_j : j = 1, \ldots, n$. A convenient notation for the resulting data is $y_{ij} : j = 1, \ldots, n; i = 1, \ldots, m$, in which y_{ij} denotes the jth measurement on the ith subject. In practice, it is often the case that not all subjects provide the intended sequence of measurements. In particular, some subjects may drop out of the study; the ith subject is a *drop-out* at time t_k if y_{ij} is missing for $j = k, k+1, \ldots, n$.

Missing values may also occur at intermittent times during the study. We shall focus on the drop-out problem, with only brief discussion of intermittent missing values. We shall also assume, if only implicitly, that drop-outs are for unspecified reasons. In practice, if it is feasible to record the reason for each drop-out this provides potentially valuable information which ought to be considered when formulating a model for the data.

Drop-outs give rise to difficulties in the analysis at two different levels. On a purely technical level, some methods of analysis require the array of measurements y_{ij} to be complete, although this restriction is becoming less common. More fundamentally, the reason for a subject dropping out may be related to the phenomenon being investigated by the measurements y_{ij}. For example, if y_{ij} is an indication of health status and the subject drops out because of poor health, then stochastic dependence between the measurement and drop-out processes cannot be ruled out, and this complicates the modelling and interpretation of the data.

Throughout this chapter, we shall assume that the response variable y is measured on a continuous scale, as this is a sufficiently general setting in which to discuss issues concerning missing values. The analysis of

Table 9.1 Frequency distribution
of reasons for drop-out

Abnormal lab. result	4
Adverse experience	26
Inadequate response	183
Intercurrent illness	3
Lost to follow-up	3
Other reason	7
Uncooperative	25
Withdrew consent	19

longitudinal studies with a discrete response variable is a major topic in its own right. See, for example, Diggle *et al.* (1994, chs 7 to 10).

As an example of a longitudinal data set with drop-out, we shall consider data from a trial comparing different drug regimes in the treatment of chronic schizophrenia. The trial was a multi-centre, double-blind, parallel group phase III study. Data are available from 523 patients, randomly allocated amongst the following six treatments: placebo, haloperidol 20 mg and risperidone at dose levels 2 mg, 6 mg, 10 mg and 16 mg. Haloperidol is regarded as a standard therapy. Risperidone is described as 'a novel chemical compound with useful pharmacological characteristics, as has been demonstrated in *in vitro* and *in vivo* experiments'. The primary response variable was the total score obtained on the positive and negative symptom rating scale (PANSS), a measure of psychiatric disorder. The study design specified that this score should be taken at weeks -1, 0, 1, 2, 4, 6 and 8, where -1 refers to selection into the trial and 0 to baseline. The week between selection and baseline was used to establish a stable regime of medication for each patient. Eligibility criteria included: age between 18 and 65; good general health; total score at selection between 60 and 120. A reduction of 20% in the mean score was regarded as demonstrating a clinical improvement.

Of the 523 patients, only 253 are listed as completing the study,

Table 9.2 Numbers of drop-outs and completers by treatment group. The treatment codes are: p = placebo, h = haloperidol 20 mg, r2 = risperidone 2 mg, r6 = risperidone 6 mg, r10 = risperidone 10 mg, r16 = risperidone 16 mg

	p	h	r2	r6	r10	r16	Total
Drop-outs	61	51	51	34	39	34	270
Completers	27	36	36	52	48	54	253
Total	88	87	87	86	87	88	523

although a further 16 provided a complete sequence of PANSS scores. Table 9.1 gives the distribution of the stated reasons for drop-out. Table 9.2 gives the numbers of drop-outs and completers in each of the six treatment groups. The most common reason for drop-out is 'inadequate response', which accounts for 183 out of the 270 drop-outs. The highest

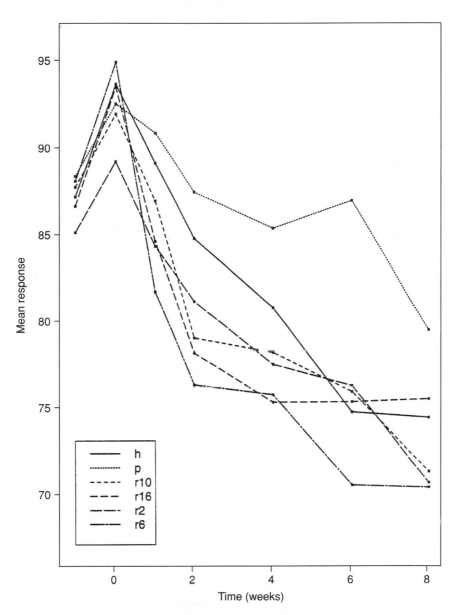

Fig. 9.1 Observed mean response profiles for the schizophrenia trial data. The treatment codes are: p = placebo; h = haloperidol 20 mg; r2 = risperidone 2 mg; r6 = risperidone 6 mg; r10 = risperidone 10 mg; r16 = risperidone 16 mg

drop-out rate occurs in the placebo group, followed by the haloperidol group and the lowest dose risperidone group. One patient provided no data at all after the selection visit, and will not be considered further in the analysis.

Figure 9.1 shows the observed mean response as a function of time

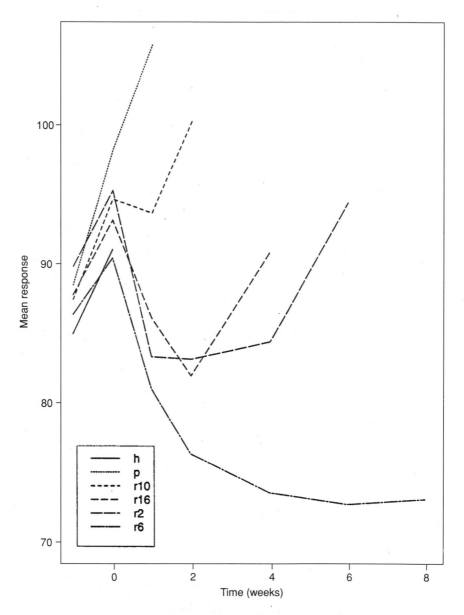

Fig. 9.2 Observed mean response profiles for the schizophrenia trial data within each drop-out cohort, ignoring treatments. Treatment codes as in Fig. 9.1

within each treatment group, that is each average is over those patients who have not yet dropped out. All six groups show a mean response profile with the following features: increasing between selection and baseline; decreasing post-baseline; slower rate of decrease towards the end of the study. The mean response in the placebo group shows a much smaller overall decrease than any of the five active treatment groups. The risperidone treatments all show a faster rate of decrease than haloperidol initially, but the final mean responses for all five active treatment groups are similar. The overall reduction in mean response within each active treatment group is very roughly from 90 to 70, which appears to meet the criterion for clinical improvement. However, at each time point these observed means are, necessarily, calculated only from those subjects who have not yet dropped out of the study, and should therefore be interpreted as conditional means. As we shall see, these conditional means may be substantially different from the means which are estimated in a conventional model-based analysis of the data.

A useful exploratory tool for data of this kind is to divide the subjects retrospectively into cohorts, according to their drop-out times. Figure 9.2 shows the observed mean response as a function of time within each of the resulting drop-out cohorts, ignoring treatments. The mean response profile for the completers is qualitatively similar to all of the profiles shown in Fig. 9.1, albeit with a steeper initial decrease and a levelling out towards the end of the study. Within each of the other drop-out cohorts a quite different picture emerges. In particular, in every case the mean score increases immediately prior to drop-out. This is consistent with the information that most of the drop-outs are due to an inadequate response to treatment. It also underlines the need for a cautious interpretation of the empirical mean response profiles.

We shall return to the analysis of these data in Section 9.4.

In the remainder of this chapter, we first discuss some simple methods which have been proposed for dealing with drop-outs. We would argue that this simplicity is misleading in the sense that it hides, rather than solves, the inherent problems. We then describe approaches to modelling the drop-out process as an integral part of the analysis, and present a model-based analysis of the schizophrenia trial data.

9.2 Simple solutions and their limitations

9.2.1 Last observation carried forward

As the name suggests, this method of dealing with drop-outs consists of extrapolating the last observed measurement for the subject in question to the remainder of his or her intended time sequence. A refinement of this method would be to estimate a time trend, either for an individual subject or for a group of subjects allocated to a particular treatment, and to extrapolate not at a constant level, but relative to this estimated trend; that is, if y_{ij} is the last observed measurement on the ith subject, $\hat{\mu}_i(t)$ is his or her estimated time trend and $r_{ij} = y_{ij} - \hat{\mu}_i(t_j)$, we impute the missing values as $y_{ik} = \hat{\mu}_i(t_k) + r_{ij}$ for all $k > j$.

In its basic form, last observation carried forward has an obvious potential for bias when there are non-zero time trends. The refined version is still subject to bias, albeit of a more subtle kind, if drop-out and measurement processes are related. It also begs the question of exactly how to estimate the time trends or to allow for this estimation in any subsequent inference.

We do not recommend last observation carried forward as a general approach. A very limited argument in its favour is that it allows a randomization-valid test of the null hypothesis of no difference between treatment groups in a randomized parallel group trial.

9.2.2 Complete case analysis

Another very simple way of dealing with drop-outs is to discard all incomplete sequences. This is obviously wasteful of data when the drop-out process is unrelated to the measurement process. Perhaps more seriously, it has the potential to introduce bias if the two processes are related, as the complete cases cannot then be assumed to be a random sample with respect to the distribution of the measurements y_{ij}.

In general, we do not recommend complete case analysis. Perhaps the only exception is when the scientific questions of interest are genuinely confined to the subpopulation of completers, but situations of this kind would seem to be rather specialized. There are many instances in which the questions of interest concern the mean, or other properties, of the measurement process conditional on completion, but this is not quite the same thing. In particular, if we accept that drop-out is a random event, and if we are prepared to make modelling assumptions about the relationship between the measurement process and the drop-out process, then the incomplete data from the subjects *who happened to be drop-outs in this particular realization of the trial* provide additional information about the properties of the underlying measurement *process* conditional on completion. This information would be lost in a complete case analysis.

9.2.3 Unbalanced designs

If we are prepared to assume that the drop-out process is independent of the measurement process then, at least from a likelihood-based perspective, it is legitimate to analyse the incomplete data as if the missing measurements were never intended to be taken.

Modern approaches to longitudinal data analysis can cope quite generally with *unbalanced designs*, in which the observation times are allowed to vary between subjects. In an obvious notation, the data can now be represented as $(y_{ij}, t_{ij}) : j = 1, \ldots, n_i; i = 1, \ldots, m$. Such data can be modelled by assuming that there is an underlying continuous-time stochastic process, $Y_i(t)$ say, for each subject, and that the observed data are sampled from this underlying process so that y_{ij} is the realized value of $Y_i(t_{ij})$. When the response variable is measured on a continuous scale, the usual approach would be to describe the mean response profiles, $\mu_i(t) = E[Y_i(t)]$, by a general linear model, and to describe the stochastic variation about the mean by a Gaussian random process. A reasonably flexible class of models, obtained by combining ideas in Laird and Ware (1982) and Diggle (1988), takes the form

$$Y_i(t_{ij}) = \mu_i(t_{ij}) + d_{ij}'U_i + W_i(t_{ij}) + Z_{ij} \qquad (9.1)$$

The stochastic ingredients of (9.1) have the following interpretations. Firstly, $Z_{ij} \sim N(0, \tau^2)$ are mutually independent and represent measurement errors; in particular, different Z_{ij} and Z_{ik} on the same subject are mutually independent irrespective of the separation between the times t_{ij} and t_{ik}, which might even be coincident if the measurements in question identify duplicate subsamples. Secondly, $W_i(t) : i = 1, \ldots, m$ are independent replicates of a stationary Gaussian process with mean 0, variance σ^2 and correlation function $\rho(u) = \mathrm{corr}(W_i(t), W_i(t-u))$; typically, $\rho(u)$ will be a decreasing function of u, with $\rho(0) = 1$ and $\rho(u)$ approaching zero as u becomes large; this component of the model reflects the fact that pairs of measurements taken close together in time tend to be more strongly correlated, that is more similar, than observations further apart in time. Thirdly, $U_i : i = 1, \ldots, m$ are independent replicates of a zero-mean Gaussian random vector and represent a set of random effects for each subject, with associated explanatory variables d_i; for example, in the bivariate case if $d_{ij}' = (1, t_{ij})$ then the two components of U_i represent a random intercept and slope for a time trend in the response profile specific to the ith subject.

In the setting of unbalanced longitudinal data, it is convenient to describe the covariance structure of the Y process in terms of the *variogram*, defined as follows. Let $Y_i(t)$ and $Y_i(s)$ denote two measurements on the same individual at times t and s, respectively. Then the variogram ordinate, $V(t, s)$, is defined as

$$V(t, s) = \tfrac{1}{2}\mathrm{var}(Y_i(t) - Y_i(s))$$

A useful simplification occurs if we are prepared to replace the term $d_{ij}'U_i$ in (9.1) by a scalar U_i, representing a random intercept for the ith subject. Then, $V(t, s)$ depends only on $u = |t - s|$, and takes the form

$$V(u) = \tau^2 + \sigma^2[1 - \rho(u)] \quad u \geq 0$$

Note that the intercept, $V(0) = \tau^2$, represents the measurement error variance and that $V(u) \to \tau^2 + \sigma^2$ as $u \to \infty$, whereas $\mathrm{var}(Y_i(t)) = \tau^2 + \sigma^2 + v^2$, that is the difference between the variance of $Y_i(t)$ and the asymptote of its variogram is v^2. We can also obtain a non-parametric estimate of the variogram using the *empirical variogram ordinates*, $v_{ijk} = \frac{1}{2}(r_{ij} - r_{ik})^2$, where r_{ij} denotes the residual corresponding to y_{ij} from an ordinary least squares fit to a model specifying a separate mean response for each combination of time and treatment. Then, our non-parametric estimate of $V(u)$ is simply the average of all quantities v_{ijk} corresponding to pairs of measurements on the same subject with time separation u. Similarly, one-half of the average squared difference between pairs of residuals from different subjects estimates the variance of $Y_i(t)$.

Analyses using the model (9.1) or variants of it are now straightforward to implement in a range of software systems, for example SAS PROC MIXED (SAS, 1992), BMDP 5V (available from Statistical Solutions, Cork Technology Park, Model Farm Road, Cork, Ireland) or the Splus-based package Oswald (Smith *et al.*, 1996), for any combination of intermittent missing values and drop-outs. Methodological details are discussed in Diggle *et al.* (1994, chs 4 to 6). The apparent flexibility and ease of implementation of such analyses should not, however, blind us to their implicit assumption that the missing value and measurement processes are independent.

9.3   Modelling the missing value process

The author's opinion is that a proper treatment of drop-outs in longitudinal studies requires the joint modelling of the drop-out and measurement processes. This does not necessarily solve the attendant problems of interpretation but it brings them out into the open and forces the data analyst to make any simplifying assumptions explicit.

9.3.1   Rubin's hierarchy of missing value processes

In general, let Y^* denote an intended complete sequence of measurements on a single subject, and M a vector of binary indicators identifying the observed and unobserved elements of Y^*. A model for the observed data, Y say, can be specified in terms of the joint distribution of Y^* and M. In a fundamental paper, Rubin (1976) gives a careful discussion of the conditions under which valid inferences can be drawn from data with missing values. Little and Rubin (1987) subsequently introduced the following nomenclature for a useful hierarchy of missing value processes. Missingness is defined to be: *completely random* if M and Y^* are independent; *random* if the conditional distribution of M given Y^* depends only on the observed elements of Y^*; and *informative* otherwise. Completely random or random drop-out mechanisms are together called *non-informative*. Within this hierarchy, for likelihood-based inference the crucial distinction is between informative and non-informative missingness. Under the further restriction that there are no parameters in common between the models for Y^* and for M given Y^*, non-informative missingness is called *ignorable* missingness. Note that this classification only refers to the type of *stochastic* dependence between Y^* and M. In practice, there may also be non-stochastic dependence. For example, the models for Y^* and for M may share explanatory variables or parameters, and an investigation of dependencies of this kind may well be of interest in specific applications.

The importance of the distinctions made in Rubin's hierarchy is best demonstrated through specific examples. In doing so, we shall again focus on the drop-out problem, so that the random vector M can be reduced to a scalar drop-out time, D say. Following Diggle and Kenward (1994), we then adopt the notational convention that the complete set of intended measurements, $Y^* = (Y_1^*, \ldots, Y_n^*)$, the observed measurements $Y = (Y_1, \ldots, Y_n)$ and the drop-out time D obey the relationship

$$Y_j = \begin{cases} Y_j^* & j < D \\ 0 & j \geq D \end{cases}$$

We emphasize that in this notation a zero value for Y is simply a code for missingness, not a measured zero. Note also that $2 \leq D \leq n+1$, with $D = n+1$ indicating that the subject in question has not dropped out.

9.3.2 Selection models

In a *selection model*, the joint distribution of Y^* and D is factorized as the marginal distribution of Y^* and the conditional distribution of D given Y^*, thus $P(Y^*, D) = P(Y^*)P(D|Y^*)$. The terminology is due to Heckman (1976), and conveys the notion that drop-outs are *selected* according to their measurement history. Selection models fit naturally into Rubin's hierarchy, as follows: drop-outs are completely random if $P(D|Y^*) = P(D)$, that is D and Y^* are independent; drop-outs are random if $P(D|Y^*) = P(D|Y_1^*, \ldots, Y_{D-1}^*)$; otherwise, drop-outs are informative.

Diggle and Kenward (1994) propose the following specific selection model for informative drop-outs. Firstly, Y^* is specified by a Gaussian linear model of the kind described in Section 9.2.3. Secondly, the drop-out mechanism consists of a sequence of independent Bernoulli trials, with $P(D = d|D \geq d, Y^*) = p_d$, say, and

$$\text{logit}(p_d) = \alpha_d + \sum_{u=0}^{k} \beta_u Y_{d-u}^* \qquad (9.2)$$

for some prespecified integer k. Note that if $k > 1$, then (9.2) does not properly define the drop-out probabilities p_d for $d \leq k$, since the Y_j^* sequence only begins at $j = 1$. The model reduces to completely random drop-out if all β_u are zero, and to random drop-out if only β_0 is zero.

In the Diggle and Kenward model, let θ and ϕ denote the parameters of the submodel for Y^* and of the submodel for D conditional on Y^*, respectively. Then it is easy to show that the log likelihood for (θ, ϕ) can be written as the sum of three components,

$$L(\theta, \phi) = L_1(\theta) + L_2(\phi) + L_3(\theta, \phi) \tag{9.3}$$

in which $L_1(\theta)$ is the log likelihood which would be used in an analysis of the measurement data alone. It follows that the drop-outs can indeed be ignored, *for likelihood-based inference about* θ, provided that $L_3(\theta, \phi) = 0$. The term $L_3(\theta, \phi)$ is derived from the probability of observing a drop-out at time $D = d$, say, conditional on the sequence of observed measurements, $y_1, \ldots, y_{d-1}$. According to the model, the probability of drop-out at time d depends on these observed measurements but also, in general, on the unobserved y_d. Hence, the required probability is

$$P(D = d|y_1, \ldots, y_{d-1}) = \int P(D = d|y_1, \ldots, y_{d-1}, y_d) f(y_d|y_1, \ldots, y_{d-1}) \mathrm{d}y_d.$$

$$\tag{9.4}$$

If $\beta_0 = 0$ in (9.2), then $P(D = d|y_1, \ldots, y_{d-1}, y_d)$ does not depend on y_d. This conditional probability can therefore be taken outside the integral sign in (9.4), the integral reduces to 1 (as the integrand is a pdf) and (9.3) reduces to

$$L(\theta, \phi) = L_1(\theta) + L_2(\phi) \tag{9.5}$$

In (9.5), $L_2(\phi)$ is the log likelihood associated with the logistic regression model (9.2). It follows that the stochastic structure of the measurement process can be ignored *for likelihood-based inference about* ϕ. Note that for each subject the sequence of binary responses in this logistic regression model consists of a sequence of negatives terminated by a single positive, and that these can be treated as if they were mutually independent for purposes of constructing the log likelihood, because of the conditioning within the definition of the drop-out probabilities p_d.

In summary, under random drop-out, the log likelihood separates into two components, one for the parameters of the measurement submodel, the other for the parameters of the drop-out submodel, and it is in this sense that the drop-out process is ignorable for inferences about the measurement process, and vice versa. Equally, it is clear that this would not hold if there were parameters in common between the two submodels, or a more general functional relationship between θ and ϕ.

The separation of the log likelihood under the assumption of random drop-outs and separate parameterizations of the measurement and drop-out submodels is not specific to the Diggle and Kenward model, but holds quite generally, and is the basis for the widely held belief that random drop-outs are ignorable. The author's point of view is that unqualified use of the term 'ignorable' is potentially misleading, as it assumes that the relevant scientific questions are addressed by inference about the Y^* process. This may not be a reasonable assumption in particular applications. For example, if drop-outs occur primarily because subjects with a poor response are withdrawn from the study on ethical grounds, it might be relevant to ask what the trial would have shown if these subjects had not been removed, and this is precisely what is addressed by an analysis of the Y^* process. On the other hand, if drop-outs occur because some subjects experience an adverse reaction to treatment (as distinct from a poor clinical response), then inferences about Y^* relate to a fictitious population of subjects for whom such adverse reactions do not occur, and it might be of more practical relevance to analyse both the incidence of adverse reactions and the pattern of responses amongst the subpopulation of subjects with no adverse reaction. This leads on to the idea of pattern mixture models, which we discuss in Section 9.3.3.

When the drop-out process is informative, in Rubin's sense, the log likelihood for θ and ϕ does not separate and the statistical analysis becomes more complex. Furthermore, in practice the analysis then rests on modelling assumptions which are difficult, or even impossible, to validate from the observed data. A related difficulty with models for informative drop-out is that they may not be identifiable; see, for example, Fitzmaurice *et al.* (1996). We return to this point in Section 9.3.3.

The Diggle and Kenward model, as described here, is implemented within the Oswald software (Smith *et al.*, 1996).

9.3.3   Pattern mixture models

Pattern mixture models, introduced by Little (1993), work with the factorization of the joint distribution of Y^* and D into the marginal distribution of D and the conditional distribution of Y^* given D; thus $P(Y^*, D) = P(D)P(Y^*|D)$. From a theoretical point of view, it is always possible to express a selection model as a pattern mixture model and vice versa, as they are simply alternative factorizations of the same joint distribution. In practice, the two approaches lead to different kinds of simplifying assumptions, and hence to different analyses.

From a modelling point of view, a possible rationale for pattern mixture models is that each subject's drop-out time is somehow predestined, and that the measurement process varies between drop-out cohorts. This literal interpretation would seem unlikely to apply very often, although an ironic exception is one of the examples analysed by Diggle and Kenward (1994) using a selection model. This example concerned the protein content of weekly milk samples taken from cows for between 15 and 19 weeks after calving. In the discussion of Diggle and Kenward's paper, Verbyla (1994) revealed that time in the experiment was measured relative to calving date and that the experiment terminated at a fixed calendar date. Thus, the different 'drop-out times' correspond precisely to different cohorts and the literal interpretation of a pattern mixture model would be exactly right for these data.

More usually, the arguments in favour of pattern mixture modelling are of the following more pragmatic kind.

Firstly, classification of subjects in a longitudinal trial according to their drop-out time provides an obvious way of dividing the subjects into subgroups after the event, and it is eminently sensible to ask whether the response characteristics which are of primary interest do or do not vary between these subgroups; indeed, separate inspection of subgroups defined in this way is a very natural piece of exploratory analysis which many a statistician would carry out without formal reference to pattern mixture models. See, for example, Grieve (1994).

Secondly, writing the joint distribution for Y^* and D in its pattern mixture factorization brings out very clearly those aspects of the model which are assumption driven rather than data driven. As a simple example, consider a trial in which it is intended to take two measurements on each subject, $Y^* = (Y_1^*, Y_2^*)$, but that some subjects drop out after providing the first measurement. Let $f(y|d)$ denote the conditional distribution of Y^* given $D = d$, for $d = 2$ (drop-outs) and $d = 3$ (non-drop-outs). Quite generally, $f(y|d) = f(y_1|d)f(y_2|y_1, d)$ but the data can provide no information about $f(y_2|y_1, 2)$ since, by definition, $D = 2$ means that Y_2^* is not observed.

Extensions of the kind of example given above demonstrate that pattern mixture models cannot be identified without placing restrictions on the conditional distributions $f(y|d)$. For example, Little (1993) discusses the use of *complete case missing variable* restrictions, which correspond to assuming that for each $d < n + 1$ and $t \geq d$,

$$f(y_t|y_1, \ldots, y_{t-1}, d) = f(y_d|y_1, \ldots, y_{t-1}, n + 1)$$

At first sight, pattern mixture models do not fit naturally into Rubin's hierarchy. However, Molenberghs *et al.* (1998) show that random drop-out corresponds precisely to the following set of restrictions, which they call *available case missing value* restrictions:

$$f(y_t|y_1, \ldots, y_{t-1}, d) = f(y_t|y_1, \ldots, y_{t-1}, D > t)$$

This result, henceforth referred to as the MMKD result, implies that the hypothesis of random drop-out cannot be tested without making additional assumptions to restrict the class of alternatives under consideration.

The identifiability problems associated with informative drop-out models, and the impossibility of validating a random drop-out assumption on empirical evidence alone, serve as clear warnings that the analysis of a longitudinal data set with drop-outs needs to be undertaken with extreme caution. However, in the author's opinion this is no reason to adopt the superficially simpler strategy of automatically assuming that drop-outs are ignorable.

9.3.4   Random effects models

Random effects models are extremely useful to the longitudinal data analyst. They formalize the sensible idea that a subject's pattern of responses in a study is likely to depend on many characteristics of that subject, including some which are unobservable. These unobservable characteristics are then included in the model as random variables, that is as random effects.

It is therefore natural to formulate models in which a subject's propensity to drop out also depends on unobserved variables, that is on random effects, as in Wu and Carroll (1988). In the present context, a simple formulation of a model of this kind would be to postulate a bivariate random effect, $U = (U_1, U_2)$, and to model the joint distribution of Y^*, D and U as

$$f(y, d, u) = f_1(y|u_1)f_2(d|u_2)f_3(u). \tag{9.6}$$

In (9.6), the dependence between Y^* and D is a by-product of the dependence between U_1 and U_2, or to put it another way, Y^* and D are conditionally independent given U. In terms of Rubin's hierarchy, the drop-outs in (9.6) are completely random if U_1 and U_2 are independent, whereas if U_1 and U_2 are dependent then in general the drop-outs are informative. Strictly, the truth of this last statement depends on the precise formulation of $f_1(y|u_1)$ and $f_2(d|u_2)$. For example, it would be within the letter, but clearly not the spirit, of (9.6) to set either $f_1(y|u_1) = f_1(y)$ or $f_2(d|u_2) = f_2(d)$, in which case the model would reduce trivially to one of completely random drop-outs whatever the distribution of U.

9.3.5 A synthesis

In the author's opinion, the MMKD result implies that debates about the relative merits of selection and pattern mixture models *per se* are unhelpful; models for drop-out in longitudinal studies should be considered on their merits in the context of particular applications. In this spirit, Fig. 9.3 shows a schematic view of selection, pattern mixture and random effects models which takes the point of view that random effects are almost always with us (whether or not we recognize them in our models), and that one consideration in formulating a model for a longitudinal trial with drop-outs would be to think about what kinds of causal relationship might plausibly exist amongst *three* sets of random variables: measurements Y, drop-out times D and random effects U. Each diagram in Fig. 9.3 is a conditional independence graph for these three random variables, in which the absence of an edge between two vertices indicates that the two random variables in question are conditionally independent given the third (Whittaker, 1990). The most general kind of model is represented by the complete graph in the top-left panel, whilst the remaining graphs, each of which has a single edge deleted, correspond to random effects, selection and pattern mixture models.

Figure 9.3 is intended as an aid to the kind of thought experiment that the data analyst must conduct in deciding how to deal with drop-outs. Figure 9.3(a) represents a denial that any simplifying assumptions are possible. Under this scenario, we would be more or less compelled to

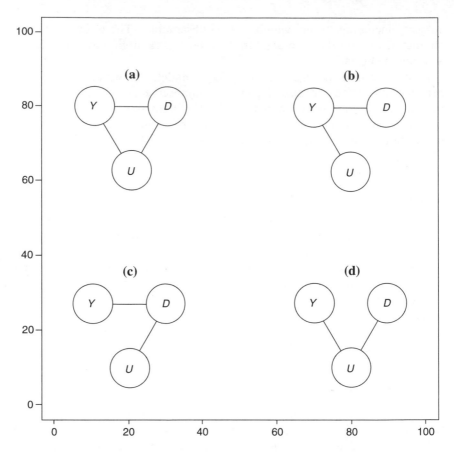

Fig. 9.3 Graphical representation of (a) saturated, (b) selection, (c) pattern mixture and (d) random effects drop-out models

express a model for the data as a collection of joint distributions for Y and U conditional on each of the possible discrete values of D. Figure 9.3(b) invites interpretation as a causal chain in which random effects or latent subject-specific characteristics, U, influence the properties of the measurement process, Y, for the subject in question, with propensity to drop out subsequently determined by the realization of the measurement process. In contrast, Fig. 9.3(c) invites the interpretation that the subject-specific characteristics initially determine propensity to drop out, with a consequential variation in the measurement process between different, predestined drop-out cohorts. Finally, Fig. 9.3(d) suggests that measurement and drop-out processes are a joint response to subject-specific characteristics; we could think of these characteristics as unidentified explanatory variables, discovery of which would convert the model to one in which Y and D were independent, that is completely random drop-out.

9.4   Case study

We now present an analysis of the schizophrenia trial data described briefly in Section 9.1. All computations were carried out using the Oswald package.

For the schizophrenia trial data, Fig. 9.2 provides strong empirical evidence of a relationship between the measurement and drop-out processes. Nevertheless, we shall initially analyse the measurement data ignoring the drop-outs, to provide a basis for comparison with an integrated analysis of measurements and drop-outs. From now on, we ignore the pre-baseline measurements because these preceded the establishment of a stable drug regime for each subject.

As a first step in fitting a model to the measurement data, we convert the responses to residuals from an ordinary least squares fit to a model which specifies a separate mean value for each combination of time and treatment. We then estimate the variogram of this residual process, as described in Section 9.2.3, under the assumption that the variogram depends only on the time separation u. The resulting variogram estimate is shown in Fig. 9.4. Its salient features are: a substantial intercept; a relatively smooth increase with u; a maximum value substantially less than the process variance. These features suggest fitting a model of the form (9.1) with a scalar random effect. Thus

$$Y_i(t_{ij}) = \mu_i(t_{ij}) + U_i + W_i(t_{ij}) + Z_{ij} \tag{9.7}$$

where $U_i \sim N(0, v^2)$, $W_i(t)$ is a zero-mean, stationary Gaussian process with

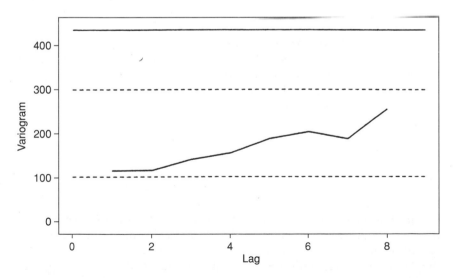

Fig. 9.4 The estimated variogram for the schizophrenia trial data. The horizontal solid line is an estimate of the variance of the measurement process. The dashed horizontal lines are rough initial estimates of the intercept and asymptote of the variogram

covariance function $\sigma^2 \exp(-\phi u^2)$ and $Z_{ij} \sim N(0, \tau^2)$. Initial estimates of the three variance components are obtained by dividing the range of $V(u)$ roughly into three pieces, defined by the intercept (τ^2), the asymptote $(\tau^2 + \sigma^2)$ and the process variance $(\tau^2 + \sigma^2 + v^2)$. This gives the values $\tilde{\tau}^2 = 100$, $\tilde{v}^2 = 140$ and $\tilde{\sigma}^2 = 200$. The assumed form of the correlation function of $W_i(t)$ reflects the ogive shape of the estimated variogram, and a crude initial estimate of ϕ is $\tilde{\phi} = 0.05$, based on the observation that the variogram might be close to its asymptote by about $u = 10$.

With regard to the mean response profiles $\mu_i(t)$, Fig. 9.1 suggests a collection of convex, non-parallel curves in the six treatment groups. The simplest model consistent with this behaviour is

$$\mu_i(t) = \mu + \delta_k + \theta_k t + \gamma_k t^2 \quad k = 1, \ldots, 6 \tag{9.8}$$

where $k = k(i)$ denotes the treatment group to which the ith subject is allocated. A more sophisticated non-linear model, perhaps incorporating a constraint that the mean response should be monotone and approach a horizontal asymptote as time increases, might be preferable on biological grounds. But for an empirical description of the data we feel that a low order polynomial should be adequate.

The focus of scientific interest is the set of estimated mean response curves. In particular, we wish to investigate possible simplifications of the assumed mean response model by testing whether the corresponding sets of contrasts are significantly different from zero. If μ denotes the generic vector of mean response parameters, $\hat{\mu}$ the estimate of μ and V the estimated variance matrix of $\hat{\mu}$, then a test statistic for the hypothesis $Q\mu = 0$, where Q has rank r, is the quadratic form $(Q\hat{\mu})'(QVQ')^{-1}(Q\hat{\mu})$, whose approximate null sampling distribution is chi-square on r degrees of freedom.

In the present context, two different kinds of simplification are of interest. Firstly, we can ask whether the quadratic terms are necessary, that is whether or not the six quadratic parameters γ_k in (9.8) are all zero. The chi-square statistic is 16.97 on six degrees of freedom, corresponding to a P value of 0.009, so we retain the quadratic terms in the model. Secondly, in Fig. 9.1 the differences amongst the mean response curves for the four risperidone treatments were relatively small, and the estimated values of the risperidone parameters are not related in any consistent way to the corresponding dose levels. This suggests a possible simplification to a three-group model, in which all four risperidone doses are considered as a single group. Within the overall model (9.8) the reduction to three groups is a linear hypothesis on nine degrees of freedom (three each for the constant, linear and quadratic effects). The chi-square statistic is 16.38, corresponding to a P value of 0.059. We therefore arrive at a model of the form (9.8), but with $k = 1, 2$ and 3 corresponding to haloperidol, placebo and risperidone, respectively.

How well does the model fit the data? Figure 9.5 shows the correspondence between non-parametric and parametric maximum likelihood

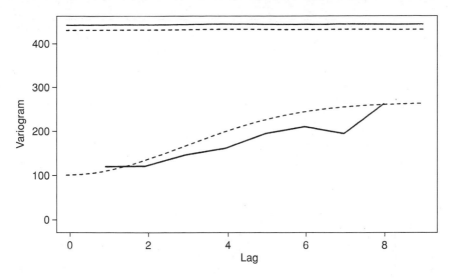

Fig. 9.5 The estimated variogram for the schizophrenia trial data (solid lines), together with a fitted parametric model (dashed lines)

estimates of the variogram. The fit is reasonably good, in that the values of $V(u)$ are closely modelled throughout the observed range of time lags in the data. Notice, however, that the estimate of τ^2 involves an extrapolation to zero time lag which is heavily influenced by the assumed parametric form of the correlation function. Figure 9.6 shows the observed and fitted mean responses in the haloperidol, placebo and risperidone groups. On the face of it, the fit is qualitatively wrong, but the diagram is not comparing like with like. As noted earlier, the observed means are estimating the mean response at each observation time conditional on not having yet dropped out, whereas the fitted means are actually estimating what the mean response would have been had there been no drop-outs – note that this is *not* the same as the mean response for completers only.

Setting aside possible quibbles about the precise specification of the parametric model, the fitted mean and covariance structures illustrated in Figs 9.5 and 9.6 are what would be produced by many widely used packages. They result from a likelihood-based fit to a model which recognizes the likely correlation between repeated measurements on the same subject and treats missing values as ignorable. But the qualitative discrepancy between the observed and fitted means surely deserves further investigation.

We therefore proceed to a joint analysis of measurements and drop-outs. The empirical behaviour of Fig. 9.2, in which the mean response within each drop-out cohort shows a sharp increase immediately before drop-out, coupled with the overwhelming preponderance of 'inadequate response' as the reason for drop-out, suggests modelling the probability of drop-out as a function of the measured response, that is a selection model.

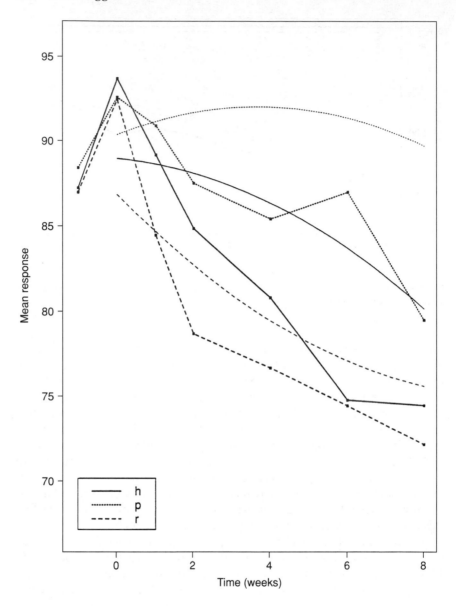

Fig. 9.6 Observed and means in the placebo (heavy dotted line), haloperidol (heavy solid line) and risperidone (heavy dashed line) treatment groups, compared with fitted means (dotted, solid and dashed lines, respectively) from an analysis ignoring drop-outs

In the first instance, we fit a simple logistic regression model for dropout, with the most recent measurement as an explanatory variable. Thus, if p_{ij} denotes the probability that patient i drops out at the jth time point (so that the jth and all subsequent measurements are missing), then

$$\text{logit}(p_{ij}) = \alpha + \beta_1 y_{i,j-1} \tag{9.9}$$

The standard output from the fitting of this model using the Oswald software is shown below:

```
Longitudinal Data Analysis Model
assuming random drop-out based on 1 previous observations
Call:
pcmid(formula = reduce.bal ~ group + group:time + group:time^2, vparms = c(150,
    100, 0.05), drop.parms = c(0, 1), drop-out.est = T, maxfn = 2000)

Analysis Method: Maximum Likelihood (ML)
Correlation structure: exp(- phi * |u| ^ 2 )

Maximised likelihood:
[ 1] -20743.85

Mean Parameters:
          (Intercept)      group1       group2 group1time group2time  group3time
PARAMETER  88.586001   0.7149764   -0.9456852   -0.206645  0.9268766  -2.2666378
STD.ERROR   0.956137   1.3516221    0.5524827    0.563144  0.5889424   0.2751296
          group1I(time^2)  group2I(time^2)  group3I(time^2)
PARAMETER     -0.11295433      -0.12909728       0.10560498
STD.ERROR      0.08120405       0.08795066       0.03890633

Variance Parameters:
   nu.sq  sigma.sq    tau.sq         phi
 161.8178   170.091  95.31707  0.05553844

Drop-out parameters:
 (Intercept) y.d        y.d-1
  -4.816878    0  0.03101689

Iteration converged after 157 iterations.
```

The Oswald function which performs the fit is called pcmid. This function offers a long list of optional arguments whose omission results in their being assigned sensible default values. The non-default arguments specified in this example are as follows:

- formula – a *model formula* expressed in the Splus style to include a main effect for the treatment group (recognized by Oswald as a reserved name, and treated as a factor) together with linear and quadratic interactions between time (again recognized by Oswald as a reserved name, but treated as a measured variable) and treatment; note that treatments are here identified by the alphanumeric order of their codified names, so that 1 = haloperidol, 2 = placebo; 3 = risperidone;

- vparms – initial estimates of the parameters v^2, τ^2 and ϕ which specify the covariance structure, in this case using the correlation function $\rho(u) = \exp(-\phi u^2)$ by default;

- drop.parms – the zero instructs the function to fit a random drop-out model (by specifying a zero coefficient for the regression on the unobservable measurement that would have been taken had the subject not dropped out), the one is an initial estimate of the parameter β in the drop-out model (9.9).

The output also lists:

- the value of the maximized log likelihood;

- a table of estimates of the parameters in the mean response model, and their standard errors – this particular analysis uses the GLIM parameterization, corresponding to the constraint $\delta_1 = 0$ in (9.8);

- point estimates of the parameters defining the covariance structure;

- point estimates of the parameters defining the drop-out model;

- the number of iterations to convergence.

Within the formulation (9.9), the generalized likelihood ratio statistic to test the submodel with $\beta_1 = 0$ is $D = 103.3$ on one degree of freedom, which is overwhelmingly significant. We therefore reject completely random drop-out (MCAR) in favour of random drop-out (MAR). At this stage, results obtained by ignoring the drop-out process would remain valid, as they rely only on the drop-out process being either completely random or random.

Within the random drop-out framework, we have considered two possible extensions to the model: including a dependence on the previous measurement but one; and including a dependence on the treatment allocation. Thus, we replace (9.9) by

$$\text{logit}(p_{ij}) = \alpha_k + \beta_1 y_{i,j-1} + \beta_2 y_{i,j-2} \qquad (9.10)$$

where $k = k(i)$ denotes the treatment allocation for the ith subject. Both extensions yield a significant improvement in the log likelihood, as indicated in Table 9.3. Finally, we test the random drop-out assumption by embedding (9.10) within the informative drop-out model

$$\text{logit}(p_{ij}) = \alpha_k + \beta_0 y_{ij} + \beta_1 y_{i,j-1} + \beta_2 y_{i,j-2} \qquad (9.11)$$

The generalized likelihood ratio statistic to test the submodel of (9.11) with $\beta_0 = 0$ is $D = 7.4$ on one degree of freedom. This corresponds to a P value of 0.007, leading us to reject the random drop-out assumption in favour of informative drop-out.

We emphasize at this point that rejection of random drop-out is necessarily preconditioned by the particular modelling framework

Table 9.3 Maximized log likelihoods under different drop-out models

$\text{logit}(p_{ij})$	Log likelihood
$\alpha + \beta_1 y_{i,j-1}$	$-20\,743.85$
$\alpha + \beta_1 y_{i,j-1} + \beta_2 y_{i,j-2}$	$-20\,728.51$
$\alpha_k + \beta_1 y_{i,j-1} + \beta_2 y_{i,j-2}$	$-20\,724.73$
$\alpha_k + \beta_0 y_{ij} + \beta_1 y_{i,j-1} + \beta_2 y_{i,j-2}$	$-20\,721.03$

Table 9.4 Maximum likelihood estimates of covariance parameters under random drop-out and informative drop-out models

Drop-out	Parameter			
	v^2	σ^2	τ^2	ϕ
Random	161.8	170.1	95.3	0.0555
Informative	175.4	137.4	103.8	0.0704

adopted, as a consequence of the MMKD result. Nevertheless, the unequivocal rejection of random drop-out within this modelling framework suggests that we should establish whether the conclusions regarding the measurement process are materially affected by whether or not we assume random drop-out. One aspect of the fitted model which does change substantially is the covariance structure of the measurement process. Table 9.4 shows the maximum likelihood estimates of the covariance parameters under the random and informative drop-out models. Some of the numerical changes are substantial, but the values of the fitted variogram within the range of time lags encompassed by the data are almost identical, as is demonstrated in Fig. 9.7.

Of more direct practical importance is the inference concerning the set of mean response profiles. Under the random drop-out assumption, a linear hypothesis concerning the mean response profiles can be tested using either a generalized likelihood ratio statistic, comparing the maximized log likelihoods for the two models in question, or a quadratic form based

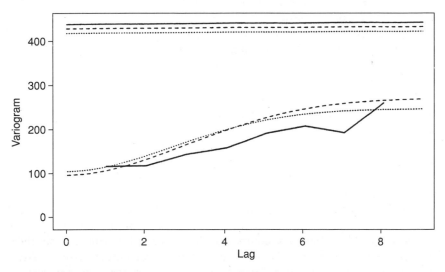

Fig. 9.7 The estimated variogram for the schizophrenia trial data (solid lines), together with fitted parametric models assuming random drop-outs (dashed lines) and informative drop-outs (dotted lines)

Table 9.5 Maximum likelihood estimates of mean value parameters under random drop-out (with standard errors in parentheses) and informative drop-out models

	Parameter								
Drop-out	μ	δ_2	δ_3	θ_1	θ_2	θ_3	γ_1	γ_2	γ_3
Random	88.83	1.43	−2.13	−0.21	0.93	−2.27	−0.11	−0.13	0.11
	(1.92)	(2.70)	(2.14)	(0.56)	(0.59)	(0.28)	(0.08)	(0.09)	(0.04)
Informative	88.79	0.74	−2.29	−0.55	0.33	−2.62	−0.15	−0.16	0.09

on the approximate multivariate normal sampling distribution of the estimated mean parameters in the full model. Under the informative drop-out assumption, only the first of these methods is available, because the current methodology does not provide standard errors for the estimated treatment effects within the informative drop-out model.

Under the random drop-out model (9.10), the generalized likelihood ratio statistic to test the hypothesis of no difference between the three mean response profiles is $D = 42.32$ on six degrees of freedom, whereas under the informative drop-out model (9.11), the corresponding statistic is $D = 35.02$. The conclusion that the mean response profiles differ significantly between treatment groups is therefore unchanged. As shown in Table 9.5, the estimated treatment effects also do not change substantially, relative to their estimated standard errors, when we move from the random drop-out model to the informative drop-out model.

The evidence for curvature in the mean response profiles is less strong. Under the random drop-out model, the generalized likelihood ratio test of the hypothesis that the quadratic terms are all zero is $D = 8.72$ on three degrees of freedom, corresponding to a P value of 0.033. Under the informative drop-out model, this changes only slightly, to $D = 8.34$ ($P = 0.039$).

We can also formally test the assumption that the drop-out probabilities depend on the treatment allocation. Within the framework of the informative drop-out model (9.11), the generalized likelihood ratio statistic is $D = 14.72$ on two degrees of freedom, corresponding to $P = 0.0006$. The estimated drop-out probabilities are highest in the placebo group, second highest in the haloperidol group and lowest in the risperidone group.

Finally, to emphasize how the dependence between the measurement and drop-out processes affects the interpretation of the observed mean response profiles, Fig. 9.8 compares the observed means in the three groups with their simulated counterparts calculated from 10 000 simulations of the fitted informative drop-out model. In contrast to Fig. 9.6, these fitted means *should* correspond to the observed means if the model fits the data well. The correspondence is reasonably close. The

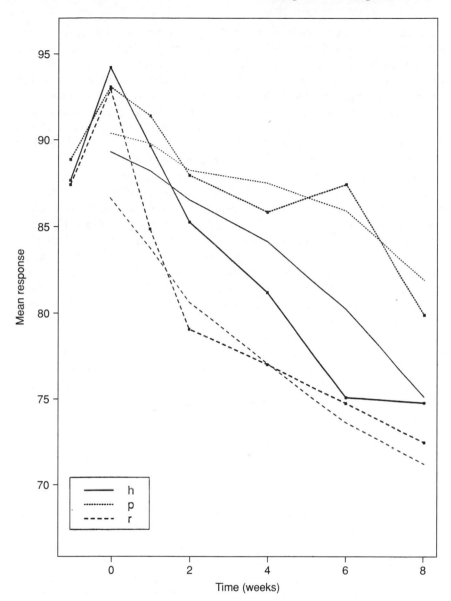

Fig. 9.8 Observed means in the placebo (heavy dotted line), haloperidol (heavy solid line) and risperidone (heavy dashed line) treatment groups, compared with simulated means conditional on not yet having dropped out (dotted, solid and dashed lines, respectively), from an informative drop-out model

contrast between Fig. 9.6 and Fig. 9.8 encapsulates the important practical difference between an analysis which ignores the drop-outs and one which takes account of them. By comparison, the distinction between the random drop-out model (9.10) and the informative drop-out model (9.11) is much less important.

In summary, our conclusions for the schizophrenia trial data are the following. Figure 9.8 demonstrates that all three treatment groups show a downward trend in the mean PANSS score conditional on not having dropped out of the study; the reduction in the mean PANSS score between baseline and eight weeks is from 86.1 to 70.8. If we want to adjust for the selection effect of the drop-outs, the relevant fitted means are those shown in Fig. 9.6. In this case, the fitted mean PANSS score is almost constant in the placebo group but still shows a downward trend in each of the two active treatment groups. The 'on-average' change between baseline and eight weeks in the risperidone group is now from 86.5 to 71.4. In view of the fact that the majority of drop-outs are the result of an inadequate response, and that this artificially deflates the observed average PANSS score, it could be argued that the fitted curves in Fig. 9.6 are the more appropriate indicators of the clinical effectiveness of the treatments than those in Fig. 9.8. From either point of view, risperidone achieves a lower mean PANSS score than haloperidol throughout the trial, and the estimated mean reduction between baseline and eight weeks comes close to the 20% criterion which is regarded as demonstrating a clinical improvement. With regard to the drop-out process, there is significant variation in the drop-out rates between the three treatment groups, with the highest rates in the placebo group and the lowest in the risperidone group. There is also significant evidence that, *within the selection modelling framework represented by equation (9.11)*, the drop-out mechanism is informative. However, this does not materially affect the conclusions regarding the mean PANSS scores by comparison with the analysis under a random drop-out assumption.

9.5   Discussion

This chapter has concentrated on the challenges of formulating and fitting models for longitudinal data in the presence of possibly complex drop-out mechanisms. This topic presents fascinating problems for the methodological research statistician, although an emerging consensus is that analyses of such data must rely on assumptions which are difficult, or even impossible, to justify on purely empirical grounds. A similar conclusion is reached by Copas and Li (1997) in their discussion of inference based on non-random samples.

In the author's opinion, this should certainly act as a warning against uncritical reliance on inferences based on particular modelling assumptions, but should not be taken as an excuse to avoid the issue of how to deal with drop-outs. An important conclusion is that the combination of drop-outs and correlated measurements makes the interpretation of a fitted regression model less than obvious. In any particular investigation, we therefore need to be clear precisely about what inferences are clinically relevant, and to investigate the extent to which these inferences are sensitive to different assumptions about the drop-out process. The models and methods described in this chapter are intended to help this process but should not be taken as definitive.

Acknowledgements

The schizophrenia trial data were provided by Dr Peter Ouyang, Janssen Research Foundation. This work was supported by the ESRC's programme in the Analysis of Large and Complex Datasets.

References

Copas, J. B. and Li, H. G. 1997: Inference for non-random samples (with discussion). *Journal of the Royal Statistical Society, (B)* **59**, 55–95.

Diggle, P. J. 1988: An approach to the analysis of repeated measurements. *Biometrics* **44**, 959–71.

Diggle, P. J. and Kenward, M. G. 1994: Informative dropout in longitudinal data analysis (with discussion). *Applied Statistics* **43**, 49–93.

Diggle, P. J., Liang K. Y. and Zeger, S. L. 1994: *Analysis of longitudinal data.* Oxford: Oxford University Press.

Fitzmaurice, G. M., Heath, A. F. and Clifford, P. 1996: Logistic regression models for binary panel data with attrition. *Journal of the Royal Statistical Society (A)* **159**, 249–63.

Grieve, A. P. 1994: Contribution to the discussion of the paper by Diggle and Kenward. *Applied Statistics* **43**, 74–6.

Heckman, J. 1976: The common structure of statistical models of truncation, sample selection and limited dependent variables, and a simple estimator for such models. *Annals of Economic and Social Measurement* **5**, 475–92.

Laird, N. M. and Ware, J. H. 1982: Random-effects models for longitudinal data. *Biometrics* **38**, 963–74.

Little, R. J. A. 1993: Pattern-mixture models for multivariate incomplete data. *Journal of the American Statistical Association* **88**, 125–34.

Little, R. J. and Rubin, D. B. 1987: *Statistical analysis with missing data.* New York: John Wiley.

Molenberghs, G., Michiels, B., Kenward, M. G. and Diggle, P. J. 1998: Missing data mechanisms and pattern-mixture models. *Statistica Neerlandica* (in press).

Rubin, D. B. 1976: Inference and missing data. *Biometrika* **63**, 581–92.

SAS 1992: The MIXED procedure. *SAS/STAT software: changes and enhancements, release 6.07.* SAS Institute Inc., Cary, NC.

Smith, D. M., Robertson, W. H. and Diggle, P. J. 1996: Oswald: object-oriented software for the analysis of longitudinal data in S. *Technical Report MA96/192,* Lancaster University Department of Mathematics and Statistics.

Verbyla, A. P. 1994: Contribution to the discussion of the paper by Diggle and Kenward. *Applied Statistics* **43**, 87–8.

Whittaker, J. C. 1990: *Graphical models in applied multivariate statistics.* Chichester: John Wiley.

Wu, M. C. and Carroll, R. J. 1988: Estimation and comparison of changes in the presence of informative right censoring by modelling the censoring process. *Biometrics* **44**, 175–88.

10 Comparing institutional performance using Markov chain Monte Carlo methods

E. Clare Marshall and
David J. Spiegelhalter

10.1 Introduction

There has been a growing interest over recent years in the use of performance indicators in healthcare, which may measure aspects of the process of care, clinical outcomes or the incidence of disease (NHS Executive, 1995, Scottish Office, 1995, New York State Department of Health, 1996). In response a sizeable literature has emerged questioning the very use of such indicators as a measure of 'quality of care', as well as stating more specific criticisms of the statistical methods used to obtain estimates adjusted for patient case-mix (DuBois *et al.*, 1987, Jencks *et al.*, 1988, Epstein, 1995, Schneider and Epstein, 1996). We do not attempt to further this general discussion of performance indicators and risk adjustment – see, for example, Goldstein and Spiegelhalter (1996). Rather, the purpose of this chapter is to highlight how recent developments in computer-intensive methods can be used to explore a wide range of plausible statistical models for the variability between institutions.

Several authors have highlighted methodological concerns with the traditional *fixed effects* approach to performance assessment (Thomas *et al.*, 1994, Normand *et al.*, 1997), and have advocated the use of *hierarchical, multi-level* or *random effects* models in which it is assumed that the true underlying institutional effects are drawn from some common distribution: we shall use these terms interchangeably in our context, since we only consider random intercept models. Specifically, the use of such models is intended to (i) overcome *small sample* problems by appropriately pooling information across institutions, introducing some bias or *shrinkage*; (ii) provide a statistical framework that allows one to quantify and explain variability in outcomes through the investigation of institutional-level covariates; and (iii) provide more reliable estimates of performance.

The theoretical advantages of such models have been known for a long time (Efron and Morris, 1977), and they have been widely used in geographical epidemiology (Clayton and Kaldor, 1987, Bernardinelli and Montomoli, 1992) and educational research (Bryk and Raudenbush, 1992, Aitkin and Longford, 1986, Goldstein *et al.*, 1993) but only recently have applications in medical comparisons been promoted (Thomas *et al.*, 1994, Normand *et al.*, 1995, Morris and Christiansen, 1996, Goldstein and Spiegelhalter, 1996, Rice and Leyland, 1996).

A wide variety of statistical software is now available to fit such models, including SAS PROC MIXED (Littell *et al.*, 1996), MLn (Rasbash *et al.*, 1995) and others discussed by Kreft *et al.* (1994). Such software has encouraged the use of multi-level models and allowed attention to focus on vital issues of model choice, diagnostics, influence and so on. However, the methods generally used rely on an explicit or implicit (through the use of a form of least squares) assumption that the institutional effects are drawn from a normal distribution. We shall show in this chapter that a Markov chain Monte Carlo (MCMC) approach not only allows full flexibility in the choice of random effects distribution, but extends in a straightforward manner to institutional covariates with or without measurement error.

Another advantage of using MCMC is that we can easily quantify the uncertainty associated with the rank of an institution and obtain intervals around this rank. This latter point is of interest since the public release of medical outcome data almost inevitably leads to the explicit ranking of institutions. Although this is generally avoided by those responsible for the assessment exercise the media tend to produce 'league tables' of performance. As with any statistical measure, an institution's rank has associated uncertainty – uncertainty which should be taken into account before inferences regarding relative performance can be made.

The remainder of the chapter is organized as follows. Section 10.2 gives a brief introduction to MCMC and its application to practical Bayesian inference. This section merely aims to introduce the ideas behind MCMC, with little rigorous mathematics (for a more detailed description see Gilks *et al.*, 1995). Section 10.3 introduces a data set on one-year survival rates following a kidney transplant in 29 centres within the UK. Section 10.4 contrasts the results of fitting both fixed and normal random effects models, both in terms of estimates and ranks. In Sections 10.5 and 10.6 we then consider a series of realistic elaborations of this model; in particular, we assess the impact on posterior inferences of assuming different forms for the random effects distribution and including institutional-level covariates with or without measurement error. All analyses are carried out using the BUGS program (Spiegelhalter *et al.*, 1995), and computational issues are discussed in Section 10.7. Finally, Section 10.8 summarizes our findings and discusses their implications for routine performance assessment, emphasizing both the possible advantages and disadvantages of an MCMC approach.

10.2   Bayesian statistics and MCMC

10.2.1   Bayesian analysis

A fully Bayesian approach treats both observables (data) and model parameters (unknowns which may include latent variables, missing data and so on) as random quantities and requires the specification of a probability model $p(D|\theta)$ for the data (D), together with a *prior* distribution $p(\theta)$ for the model parameters $\theta = (\theta_1, \theta_2, \ldots, \theta_K)$. Inferences regarding the model parameters, or functions of these parameters, are then based on the *posterior* distribution $p(\theta|D)$, determined by Bayes's theorem:

$$p(\theta|D) = \frac{p(\theta)p(D|\theta)}{\int p(\theta)p(D|\theta)\mathrm{d}\theta} \qquad (10.1)$$

Any features of the posterior distribution of interest can be expressed in terms of the posterior expectation of a function $f(\theta)$:

$$E[f(\theta)|D] = \int f(\theta)p(\theta|D)\mathrm{d}\theta \qquad (10.2)$$

For example, in the simplest of cases where $f(\theta) = \theta$ then equation (10.2) gives the posterior mean of θ.

The appropriate, and often high dimensional, integration needed to evaluate $E[f(\theta)|D]$ has until recently posed most difficulties for the practical application of Bayesian inference. In all but the most simple of situations $E[f(\theta)|D]$ cannot be evaluated analytically. Alternative approaches include numerical quadrature (Smith *et al.*, 1987); analytic approximations such as the Laplace approximation (Tierney and Kadane, 1986); or Monte Carlo integration and specifically MCMC. Below we give a very brief introduction to MCMC methods; see Gelfand and Smith (1990), Casella and George (1992) or Gilks *et al.* (1995) for a more detailed explanation of this rapidly expanding field.

10.2.2   Monte Carlo integration

Suppose we had a sample $\{\theta^{(t)}, t = 1, \ldots, N\}$ from the posterior, $p(\theta|D)$; then the posterior expectation of $f(\theta)$ could be approximated by

$$E[f(\theta)|D] \approx \frac{1}{N}\sum_{t=1}^{N} f(\theta^{(t)}) \qquad (10.3)$$

Thus the integral (10.2) is estimated by a mean of a simulated sample of plausible values of $f(\theta)$. This constitutes a simple yet powerful approach.

Its practical application, however, is dependent on the efficient generation of a sample from the posterior distribution $p(\theta|D)$. Since the posterior distribution will typically be non-standard, drawing independent samples is not feasible. For equation (10.3) to hold, however, the $\theta^{(t)}$ need not be independent and so one way of drawing samples is through a Markov chain having $p(\theta|D)$ as its stationary distribution.

10.2.3   Markov chains

A Markov chain is a sequence of random variables $\{\theta^0, \theta^1, \ldots\}$ such that given θ^t, the next state θ^{t+1} does not depend on the history of the chain $\{\theta^0, \theta^1, \ldots, \theta^{t-1}\}$. Subject to general regularity conditions the chain will gradually 'forget' its starting point θ^0 and will eventually converge to a unique stationary distribution, which we will denote by $\pi(.)$. After a sufficiently long *burn-in* of, say, m iterations, therefore, $\{\theta^{(t)}, t = m+1, \ldots, N\}$ form a sample from $\pi(.)$. The output from the Markov chain can then be used to estimate the expectation of any function $f(\theta)$, where $\theta \sim \pi(.)$. Burn-in samples are discarded giving an estimator,

$$E[f(\theta)|D] \approx \frac{1}{N-m} \sum_{t=m+1}^{N} f(\theta^t) \tag{10.4}$$

The combined approach – of using a sample comprising realizations of a Markov chain to produce Monte Carlo estimates – is referred to as MCMC.

All that is needed now is a Markov chain whose stationary distribution $\pi(.)$ is precisely our posterior of interest, $p(.|D)$. Constructing such a chain is surprisingly easy. We briefly describe one method – the Gibbs sampler.

10.2.4   The Gibbs sampler

The Gibbs sampler is a special case of the single-component Metropolis–Hastings algorithm (Metropolis *et al.*, 1953, Hastings, 1970). Let $p(\theta_i|\theta_{\setminus i}, D), i = 1, \ldots, K$, denote what is known as the 'full conditional density' for each unknown θ_i, which is the conditional distribution of θ_i given the data and known values of all the remaining parameters $\theta_{\setminus i}$.

Then the Gibbs sampler proceeds as follows. Given an arbitrary set of starting values $\theta^{(0)}$ successive random drawings are made from the full conditionals:

$\theta_1^{(1)}$ is drawn from $p(\theta_1|\theta_2^{(0)}, \theta_3^{(0)}, \ldots, \theta_K^{(0)}, D)$

$\theta_2^{(1)}$ is drawn from $p(\theta_2|\theta_1^{(1)}, \theta_3^{(0)}, \ldots, \theta_K^{(0)}, D)$

$$\vdots$$

$\theta_K^{(1)}$ is drawn from $p(\theta_K|\theta_1^{(1)}, \theta_2^{(1)}, \ldots, \theta_{K-1}^{(1)}, D)$

Iteration of the scheme produces a sequence $\{\theta^{(0)}, \theta^{(1)}, \theta^{(2)}, \ldots\}$ which is a realization of a Markov chain. Geman and Geman (1984) show that under mild regularity conditions $\theta^{(t)} \to \theta \sim p(\theta|D)$ as $t \to \infty$. That is, if the chain is run for long enough $\{\theta^{(t)}; t = m + 1, \ldots, N\}$ form a sample from the posterior $p(\theta|D)$, as required. For a discussion of the problems in judging what is a sufficient burn-in and how long to run the 'converged' sampler, see Cowles and Carlin (1996).

10.3   Kidney transplant data

In 1995 the United Kingdom Transplant Support Service Authority (UKTSSA) published its second audit of renal transplantation (UKTSSA, 1995), focusing on the 10 years 1984–93. UKTSSA presents results based on data held in the national transplant database which contains follow-up information on approximately 86% of all transplants carried out in the UK and Republic of Ireland for the period of audit. As well as publishing outcome data at a national level UKTSSA gives transplant survival rates by centre for two epochs, 1984–88 and 1989–93 (table 11.1 of their publication). One-year transplant survival rates are given in both epochs for 29 of the 38 centres audited – these data form the basis for our analysis and are reproduced in Table 10.1. (No adjustment for patient case-mix has been made.) We note that hierarchical models have already been used in the context of kidney transplant survival by Gilks (1987), Van Houlwelingen and Thorogood (1995) and Morris and Christiansen (1996).

Since at least a year of follow-up is available we can assume that there is little allowance for censoring in these survival estimates, and hence it is reasonable to assume they are based on binomial data with the observed denominators shown in Table 10.1. For the most recent epoch, 1989–93, centre 33 has the lowest rate of 61%, although it is also the joint smallest centre. In contrast, centres 2, 4, 35 and 36 all have survival rates of 89%, and they vary considerably in size.

10.4   Basic cross-sectional analyses

In this section we contrast the simplest fixed and random effects analyses for outcomes during 1989–93, and also show how MCMC methods can also provide inferences on the ranks of the institutions.

Let n_{ij} be the number at risk in centre i, epoch j, and let r_{ij} be the observed number of one-year transplant survivals, obtained by multiplying n_{ij} by the quoted survival rate in UKTSSA (1995). The observed number of transplant survivals in each epoch are assumed to be independently binomially distributed with parameters n_{ij} and p_{ij}, where p_{ij} represents the 'true' transplant survival rate in centre i, epoch j. The logit transplant

Table 10.1 One-year transplant survival estimates after first cadaveric kidney transplant in the UK and Republic of Ireland, 1 January 1984 to 31 December 1993, by centre

Centre code	No. at risk		Survival (%)		Centre code	No. at risk		Survival (%)	
	1984–8	1989–93	1984–8	1989–93		1984–8	1989–93	1984–8	1989–93
1	269	334	81	81	21	157	106	83	86
2	266	438	82	89	22	158	146	77	85
3	117	54	67	77	23	98	62	71	78
4	142	133	82	89	24	141	130	68	84
5	74	94	78	78	28	357	389	83	87
6	195	194	79	87	29	77	84	75	82
7	200	270	73	79	30	246	263	83	88
10	114	55	71	78	31	162	176	73	81
11	100	91	84	76	32	284	224	73	79
12	144	142	78	86	33	92	54	68	61
13	364	276	78	86	34	172	164	79	83
15	101	59	83	81	35	114	94	86	89
17	119	130	78	81	36	304	361	80	89
18	308	429	78	84	38	249	245	76	87
19	89	114	69	78					

survival rates $\{b_{ij} : j = 1, 2; i = 1, \ldots, 29\}$ represent the *centre effects* in each epoch. We therefore have a model

$$r_{ij} \sim Bin(n_{ij}, p_{ij}) \tag{10.5}$$

$$\log\left(\frac{p_{ij}}{1 - p_{ij}}\right) = b_{ij} \tag{10.6}$$

10.4.1 Fixed effects model

We first consider the traditional fixed effects analysis, which mirrors that presented in UKTSSA's renal transplantation audit and assumes the independence of centres. Since we are adopting a Bayesian approach we need to select a 'minimally informative' independent prior for each b_{ij}, which we choose to be

$$b_{ij} \sim N(0, 1 \times 10^6) \tag{10.7}$$

This proper normal prior has a standard deviation of 1000, and since the observed empirical logits

$$l_{ij} = \log \frac{r_{ij} + \frac{1}{2}}{n_{ij} - r_{ij} + \frac{1}{2}} \tag{10.8}$$

only vary from 0.45 to 2.1 it seems reasonable that relative to the information in the data this prior provides minimal information. Adopting a normal prior for the centre effects has the advantage that the model falls naturally into a hierarchical structure allowing one easily to impose more complex forms of prior 'similarity'.

10.4.2 Random effects models – assuming normality

Section 10.1 briefly highlighted some of the problems inherent in the use of this fixed effects model and the need for an alternative approach which in some sense pools information across centres to obtain more reliable estimates of performance. By structuring the inevitable heterogeneity between institutions, the aim is to elucidate the underlying distribution of outcome rates, and so help identify institutions with 'genuine' high or low outcomes, compensating for the fact that smaller centres are more likely to be outlying by chance alone. The joint modelling should also help to overcome the classical problem of multiple comparisons when comparing many institutions with some standard.

We begin by considering the common assumption of a normal distribution for the centre effects:

$$b_{ij} \sim N(\mu_j, \sigma_j^2) \tag{10.9}$$

Here μ_j represents the mean survival rate on the logit scale and σ_j^2 the between-centre variability in the jth epoch. Vague but proper priors are specified for these parameters:

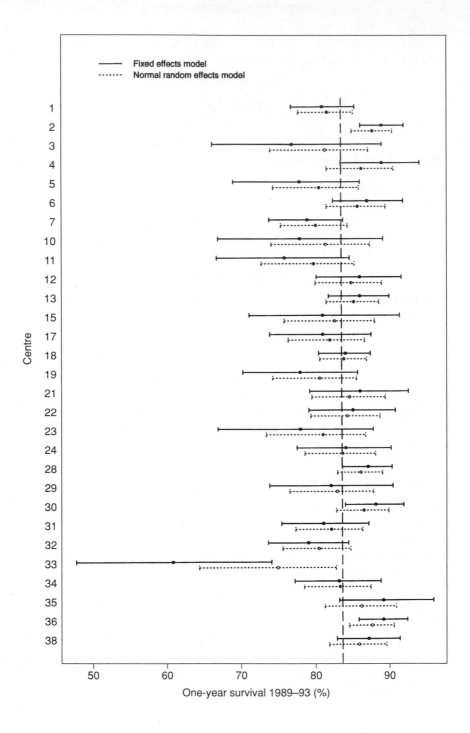

Fig. 10.1 Mean and 95% interval for the one-year survival (%) at each of the centres under both a fixed effects model and that assuming normal random effects. The dashed vertical line represents the mean transplant survival of 83.5%

$$\mu_j \sim N(0, 1 \times 10^6) \tag{10.10}$$

$$\sigma_j^{-2} \sim \Gamma(0.001, 0.001) \tag{10.11}$$

where the gamma distribution for the precision (inverse of the variance) has a mean of 1 and variance of 1000: this 'just proper' prior essentially puts a locally uniform distribution on the logarithm of the variance.

Figure 10.1 shows the mean and associated 95% intervals for one-year transplant survival in the second epoch (1989–93) under both a fixed effects model and one assuming normal random effects. The graph clearly shows *shrinkage* of the random effects estimates towards the overall level, with those centres performing few transplants being shrunk more than those performing a large number. This seems reasonable as estimates based on large populations are preserved yet those based on unreliable data are shrunk – the shrunk estimates have the appealing property of falling between those obtained under the two extremes of independence and the complete pooling of centres. Centre 33, being rather small, is pulled in considerably but still is 'significantly' below average. Centre 4 is pulled more than the larger centre 2, indicating that its good performance is more likely to be due to chance.

Computational details of iterations and burn-in are given in Section 10.7.

10.4.3   Ranks

Using an MCMC approach it is possible at each iteration of the sampler not only to sample from the posterior distribution of each centre's transplant survival rate but to rank this set of parameter realizations. Suppose, for example, that the Gibbs sampler were run for 5000 iterations; discarding an initial *burn-in* of 1000, we are left with 4000 values of each centre's transplant survival rate along with 4000 values of each centre's rank. Point and interval estimates of the ranks can then be reported alongside the estimates of performance. Details are provided in Section 10.7.

Figure 10.2 shows the 95% intervals associated with each centre's rank under the fixed effects and normal random effects models (the higher the rank the better). The intervals around the ranks are wide under both models, particularly the random effects. Thus, assuming the hierarchical model, centre 33 can only be confidently placed in the bottom half of institutions, while no centre can be confidently placed in the top quarter either by the fixed or random effects analysis.

10.5   Alternative forms of random effects distribution

Figure 10.3(a) shows the empirical survival estimates plotted on a logit scale, which suggest the normal assumption may well be inappropriate. There is evidence of a multimodal distribution, possibly with outliers, perhaps indicating there is some important institutional covariate that is

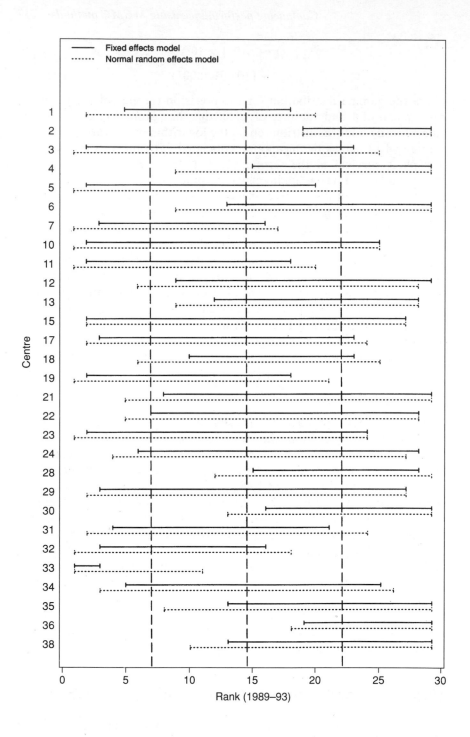

Fig. 10.2 Mean and 95% interval for the rank of each centre under both a fixed effects model and that assuming normal random effects. The dashed vertical lines divide the centres into quarters according to their rank

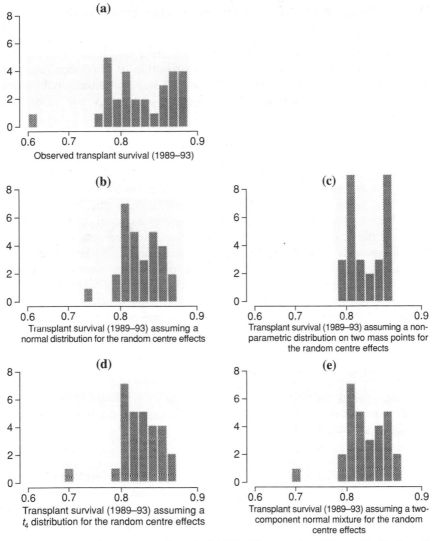

Fig. 10.3 Empirical histograms of survival (1989–93), assuming different distributions for the random centre effects

not being taken into account. Inappropriate use of a normality assumption for the underlying population distribution may well result in 'overshrinkage' of the centre effects: Fig. 10.3(b) shows that the estimated centre effects (using the posterior means as estimates) may be being unjustifiably forced towards a normal distribution. In this section we illustrate some alternative models that could be fitted; there is also a general issue of diagnostics of distributional shape (Lange and Ryan, 1989), outliers and influence in such models, but we shall not consider this important topic here.

10.5.1   Non-parametric distribution on two mass points

A non-parametric model is intended to 'let the data decide' the shape of the population distribution, and a simple example that is straightforward to fit within MCMC is to constrain the distribution to be concentrated on a small number of unknown points. Figure 10.3(c) shows the fitted values resulting from an assumption of a two-point non-parametric prior: the model is

$$b_{ij} = \theta_{T_{ij}} \tag{10.12}$$

$$T_{ij} \sim Categorical(P) \tag{10.13}$$

where T_{ij} can take on the values 1 or 2 with probabilities P and $1 - P$, and P is given a prior distribution which is uniform on 0–1. Any smoothing in Fig. 10.3(c) is due to uncertainty as to in which of these groups a particular centre belongs. Here the estimated centre effects are shrunk towards a local rather than global point. Although a non-parametric distribution on only two mass points may not be a sensible choice for these data, gradually increasing the number of mass points may help to shed some light on the form of the population distribution. However, the assumption that each centre is one of a limited number of exactly identical types does not seem particularly realistic.

10.5.2   Student's *t* distribution

A heavier-tailed distribution, such as a Student's t distribution on four degrees of freedom, should lead to less shrinkage in extremes and hence accommodate outliers. Assuming the model

$$b_{ij} \sim t_4(\mu_j, \delta_j) \tag{10.14}$$

leads to the fitted centre effects shown in Fig. 10.3(d), the major consequence is that the outlying centre is not shrunk in as much, although the fact that a t_4 distribution is also quite strongly peaked leads to increased shrinkage for the more typical centres, masking any possible bimodality.

10.5.3   Normal mixture with *K* components

The essential idea of a normal mixture model is to expand the non-parametric prior assumption to allow for variability within groups, and hence automatically to identify clusters of institutions. However, fitting mixtures is a notoriously tricky problem in MCMC because components can become empty at some iteration: the sampler may then 'wander off' and that component never receives another member. This problem can be overcome (to a certain extent) through clever parameterization and the assumption of strong prior information for the component parameters, and is claimed to be entirely overcome by recent developments in reversible jump MCMC which handles a mixture of unknown number of components by allowing the 'birth' and 'death' of components (Richardson and Green, 1997).

The model is

$$b_{ij} \sim N(\theta_{T_{ij}}, \sigma^2_{T_{ij}}) \qquad (10.15)$$

$$T_{ij} \sim Categorical(P) \qquad (10.16)$$

Vague priors are put on the θ_k, where $k = 1, \ldots, K$, but they are constrained so that $a < \theta_1 < \theta_2 < \ldots < \theta_K < b$, with appropriate choices of a and b. The following prior is put on the component variances:

$$\sigma_k^{-2} \sim \Gamma(\gamma, \phi), \qquad k = 1, \ldots, K \qquad (10.17)$$

with *hyperprior* for ϕ given by

$$\phi \sim \Gamma(c, d) \qquad (10.18)$$

Following Richardson and Green (1997), d is chosen to be a small multiple of $1/R^2$, where R is the range of the observed centre effects (on a logit scale), and γ and c such that $\gamma > 1 > c$. This prior reflects the belief that the σ_k^2 are similar, but is not informative about their size. We have taken $\gamma = 3$, $c = 0.5$ and $d = 0.5$.

Figure 10.3(e) shows the fitted centre effects assuming a two-component normal mixture prior. There has been some shrinkage but the shape of the fitted distribution seems to reflect the data rather well. Estimates for the component means (and associated 95% intervals) are 78% (57.4, 84.5) and 86.1% (82.4, 96.7). Note that the main bulk of the fitted values lies above the mean of the first component. The posterior distribution of θ_1 (not presented here) appears almost bimodal, with a large peak at $\simeq 1.5$ and a second much smaller mode at $\simeq 0.45$ – which translate to 82% and 61%, respectively, on the probability scale. The outlying centre is having a strong influence, but the sampler cannot decide whether to put it into a component on its own or shrink it towards the main body. Another note of interest is that the 95% interval for the proportion of centres in group 1 spans almost the whole range 0–1. The results provide no evidence, therefore, of the presence of two clear clusters of institutions; nevertheless assuming a normal mixture prior for the b_{ij} has allowed for greater flexibility in the shape of the fitted population distribution. In particular, the small 'lump' of mass at $\simeq 0.45$ ($\equiv 61\%$ on the probability scale) is allowing for the possibility that centre 33 is *genuinely* outlying. Finally, the main body of the fitted population distribution has tails reminiscent of the t_4 distribution but it has a far flatter peak and so typical centres are not 'overshrunk'.

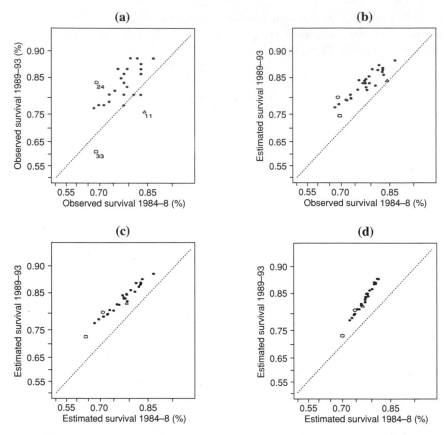

Fig. 10.4 Scatter of estimated transplant survival rates in two epochs under four different models described in Sections 11.6.1 to 11.6.4: (a) the observed rates; (b) the estimated rates when using as a covariate the 1984–8 observed rates; (c) the estimated rates when using as a covariate the 1984–8 'true' rates, estimated as fixed effects; (d) the estimated rates when using as a covariate the 1984–8 'true' rates, estimated as random effects assuming a normal population distribution

10.6   Models using survival rates from previous epoch as a predictor

10.6.1   Comparing observed rates in 1984–8 and 1989–93

Figure 10.4(a) suggests that survival rates in 1984–8 may be predictive of the survival rate in the period 1989–93, and hence instead of analysing each epoch separately, the data for 1984–8 might be used as an institutional-level covariate. A number of means of introducing this covariate are possible and we consider three possibilities in this section. The consequences for three specific institutions are examined in detail: centre 11 which had a low success rate in the recent epoch, centre 24 which had a low success rate in the earlier epoch, and centre 33 which was low in both epochs, but particularly recently. These centres are identified in Fig. 10.4.

10.6.2 Observed rate in 1984–8 as a predictor

First, we consider the empirical logit l_{i1} as a predictor, leading to a regression model for b_{i2}:

$$b_{i2} \sim N(\mu_{i2}, \sigma_2^2) \tag{10.19}$$

$$\mu_{i2} = \beta_0 + \beta_1(l_{i1} - \bar{l}_1) \tag{10.20}$$

where $\bar{l}_1 = (1/n)\sum_i l_i$, and we assume essentially 'non-informative' priors on β_0 and β_1.

The fitted values from this model are shown in Fig. 10.4(b), and it is clear that the estimated 1989–93 rates are pulled towards an estimated regression line, with the greatest effect on cases lying off the line. Figure 10.4(b) and Table 10.2 show that this produces a dramatic influence on centre 11, whose recent decline in performance is largely ignored, while centre 24 is influenced by the low performance in the last epoch.

10.6.3 'True' rate (1984–8) as predictor: estimated as fixed effect

It is perhaps more natural to think of the recent true centre effect b_{i2} depending on the past effect b_{i2}, rather than the observed rate. This

Table 10.2 Impact on estimated one-year survival of assuming different forms for the random effects distribution and of including the survival rate (1984–8) as a covariate

	β	Estimated one-year survival 1989–93 (SE)		
		Centre 11	Centre 24	Centre 33
Without covariate				
Fixed effects model		76 (4.5)	84 (3.2)	61 (6.6)
Random effects models:				
Normal		79.9 (3.2)	83.6 (2.4)	75.0 (4.7)
Non-parametric (two mass points)		80.4 (1.9)	83.6 (3.2)	80.1 (1.4)
Two-component normal mixture		78.2 (3.7)	83.8 (2.8)	71.2 (6.7)
t_4		80.1 (3.3)	83.7 (2.2)	70.5 (6.9)
With covariate				
Observed baseline rate	0.74 (0.18)	85.4 (2.7)	80.2 (2.4)	74.5 (3.9)
True rate; fixed effect	0.78 (0.19)	82.8 (2.9)	80.3 (2.5)	72.7 (4.3)
True rate; random effect	1.27 (0.38)	82.0 (2.8)	80.8 (2.6)	73.0 (4.7)

essentially leads to a regression model with measurement error on the covariate.

$$b_{i2} \sim N(\mu_{i2}, \sigma_2^2) \tag{10.21}$$

$$\mu_{i2} = \beta_0 + \beta_1(b_{i1} - \bar{l}_1) \tag{10.22}$$

Two models have been considered for the prior distribution for the baseline effects b_{i1}.

First, we could allow b_{i1} to have a 'non-informative' distribution, as used in the fixed effect analysis:

$$b_{i1} \sim N(0, 10^6) \tag{10.23}$$

The fitted values are plotted in Fig. 10.4(c). There is little difference between these fitted values and those obtained from fitting the model which makes no allowance for measurement error, except that there is increased tendency towards the regression line.

10.6.4   'True' rate (1984–8) as predictor: estimated as random effect

The second model we consider is a random effects model for the baseline rates, so that

$$b_{i1} \sim N(\mu_1, \sigma_1^2) \tag{10.24}$$

This can be easily shown to be equivalent to assuming a bivariate normal for b_{ij}, with mean $(\mu_1, \beta_0 + \beta_1(\mu - \bar{l}_1))$, variances σ_1^2, $\sigma_2^2 + \beta_1^2 \sigma_1^2$, and correlation $\beta_1 \sigma_1 / (\sigma_2^2 + \beta_1^2 \sigma_1^2)^{1/2}$. The fitted values are shown in Fig. 10.4(d), showing that there is considerable shrinkage of the baseline estimates but very little effect on the estimated values for 1989–93. Table 10.2 shows that the estimated regression coefficient is greatly increased, as is typical when allowing for measurement error and a random effects distribution.

10.7   Computation

The essential idea of the BUGS program is to generate automatically the code to carry out the Gibbs sampling using the minimal specification possible. The simplest method for specifying a full joint distribution over a large number of quantities is to exploit the conditional independence assumptions implicit in the model specification. As explained by Best *et al.* (1996), this graphical representation then directly translates into the expressions that have to be given in order for the full joint distribution to be uniquely specified; these expressions comprise the conditional distribution of each quantity given its 'parents' in the graph. Figure 10.5 shows the graphical representation of the model described in Section 10.6.4.

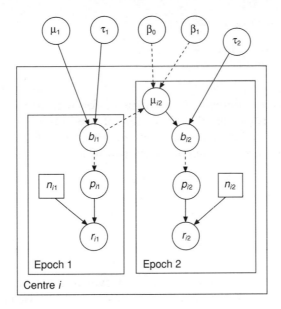

Fig. 10.5 Graphical model for transplant data

The BUGS code for this model is shown below, and should be self-explanatory. The crucial idea is that each node in the graph is represented once and once only on the left-hand side of the description. Thus the code exactly specifies the graph, and the program can build an internal representation of the graph in memory and generate the code to carry out the required sampling operations.

```
{
   for (i in 1:N) {
      r2[i]          ~ dbin(p2[i],n2[i]);
      r1[i]          ~ dbin(p1[i],n1[i]);
      logit(p1[i]) <- b1[i];
      logit(p2[i]) <- b2[i];

      b2[i]      ~ dnorm(mu2[i],tau2);
      mu2[i]     <- beta0 + beta1 * (b1[i] - mean(l1[]));

      b1[i] ~ dnorm(mu1,tau1);
   }
   # priors
   tau1 ~ dgamma(1.0E-3,1.0E-3);
   tau2 ~ dgamma(1.0E-3,1.0E-3);
   sigma1 <- 1/sqrt(tau1);
   sigma2 <- 1/sqrt(tau2);

   beta0 ~ dnorm(0.0,1.0E-6);
```

```
    beta1 ~ dnorm(0.0,1.0E-6);

    mu1 ~ dnorm(0.0,1.0E-6);
    mu2 ~ dnorm(0.0,1.0E-6);
 }
```

The BUGS code to compute the ranks is as follows: at each iteration a matrix `greater` is calculated with a value of one in the (i, j)th position if the current value for p_i is greater than p_j. The rank of centre I at that iteration is then simply the sum of the ith row of `greater`.

```
 for (i in 1:N) {
   for (j in 1:N) {
        greater[ i,j] <- step(p2[i]  - p2[j]);
   }
   rank[i] <-sum(greater[i,]);
 }
```

A burn-in of 5000 iterations was adopted, which is rather cautious but ensured convergence. Estimates and intervals were then based on a further 2000 iterations.

10.8   Discussion

We do not recommend one particular random effects distribution for these particular data, but rather show that one can explore the population heterogeneity with the tools now available. One crucial issue is the sensitivity of the inferences concerning performance change to different model assumptions, and we have only shown informal graphical procedures, although more formal analyses are possible. The other important aspect is the relative fit of these alternative models: again both informal and formal procedures are possible but are not explored here.

   With regard to our exploration of previous performance as a predictor of recent performance, we have tried to illustrate the wide range of models that can be easily fitted using MCMC techniques. It could be questioned whether this is a 'fair' analysis, in that a centre may claim to have improved more than the model predicts. In reality a longer series would be desirable, in which one can allow for heterogeneity of slope (time effects) by fitting a full random coefficient model. This would be straightforward within this framework.

   In conclusion, while making no claim to have performed a definitive analysis on these data, we have tried to illustrate the wide range of models that can be easily fitted using MCMC techniques, and the ability to make inferences on analytically infeasible quantities such as ranks.

Acknowledgements

This work was partly supported by a grant from the UK Economic and Social Science Research Council's initiative for the Analysis of Large and Complex Datasets, award number H519 25 5023.

References

Aitkin, M. and Longford, N. 1986: Statistical modelling issues in school effectiveness studies (with discussion). *Journal of the Royal Statistical Society (A)* **149**, 1–43.

Bernardinelli, L. and Montomoli, C. 1992: Empirical Bayes versus fully Bayesian analysis of geographical variation in disease risk. *Statistics in Medicine* **11**, 983–1007.

Best, N. G., Spiegelhalter, D. J., Thomas, A. and Brayne, C. E. G. 1996: Bayesian analysis of realistically complex models. *Journal of the Royal Statistical Society (A)* **159**, 323–42.

Bryk, A. S. and Raudenbush, S. W. 1992: *Hierarchical linear models.* Newbury Park, CA: Sage.

Casella, G. and George, E. I. 1992: Explaining the Gibbs sampler. *American Statistician* **46**, 167–74.

Clayton, D. and Kaldor, J. 1987: Empirical Bayes estimates of age-standardised relative risks for use in disease mapping. *Biometrics* **43**, 671–81.

Cowles, M. K. and Carlin, B. P. 1996: Markov chain Monte Carlo convergence diagnostics – a comparative review. *Journal of the American Statistical Association* **91**, 883–904.

DuBois, R. W., Brook, R. H. and Rogers, W. H. 1987: Adjusted hospital death rates: a potential screen for quality of medical care. *American Journal of Public Health* **77**, 1162–7.

Efron, B. and Morris, C. 1977: Stein's paradox in statistics. *Scientific American* **236**, 119–227.

Epstein, A. 1995: Performance reports on quality-prototypes, problems and prospects. *New England Journal of Medicine* **333**, 57–61.

Gelfand, A. E. and Smith, A. F. M. 1990: Sampling-based approaches to calculating marginal densities. *Journal of the American Statistical Society* **85**, 398–409.

Geman, S. and Geman, D. 1984: Stochastic relaxation, Gibbs distributions and the Bayesian restoration of images. *IEEE Transactions on Pattern Analysis and Machine Intelligence* **6**, 721–41.

Gilks, W. R. 1987: Some applications of hierarchical models in kidney transplantation. *The Statistician* **36**, 127–36.

Gilks, W. R., Richardson, S. and Spiegelhalter, D. J. 1995: *Markov chain Monte Carlo methods in practice.* New York: Chapman & Hall.

Goldstein, H., Rasbash, J., Yang, M., Woodhouse, G., Pan, H. and Nuttal, D. 1993: A multilevel analysis of school examination results. *Oxford Review of Education* **19**, 425–33.

Goldstein, H. and Spiegelhalter, D. J. 1996: League tables and their limitations: statistical issues in comparisons of institutional performance. *Journal of the Royal Statistical Society (A)* **159**, 385–443.

Hastings, W. K. 1970: Monte Carlo sampling methods using Markov chains and their applications. *Biometrika* **57**, 97–109.

Jencks, S. F., Daley, J., Draper, D., Thomas, N., Lenhart, G. and Walker, J. 1988: Interpreting hospital mortality data. The role of clinical risk adjustment. *Journal of the American Medical Association* **260**, 3611–16.

Kreft, I. G., de Leeuw, J. and van der Leeden, R. 1994: Comparing five statistical packages for hierarchical linear regression: BMDP-5V, GENMOD, HLM, ML3 and VARCL. *American Statistician* **48**, 324–35.

Lange, N. and Ryan, L. 1989: Assessing normality in random effects models. *Annals of Statistics* **17**, 624–42.

Littell, R. C., Milliken, G. A., Stroup, W. W. and Wolfinger, R. D. 1996: *SAS system for mixed models*. Cary, NC: SAS Institute Inc.

Metropolis, N., Rosenbluth, A. W., Teller, M. N. and Tellet, A. H. 1953: Equations of state calculations by fast computing machine. *Journal of Chemical Physics* **21**, 1087–91.

Morris, C. N. and Christiansen, C. L. 1996: Hierarchical models for ranking and for identifying extremes, with applications. In Bernardo, J. O., Berger, J. O., Dawid, A. P. and Smith, A. F. M. (eds), *Bayesian statistics 5*. Oxford: Oxford University Press, 277–97.

New York State Department of Health 1996: *Coronary artery bypass surgery in New York State, 1992–94*. Albany, NY: New York State Department of Health.

NHS Executive 1995: *The NHS performance guide 1994–1995*. Leeds: NHS Executive.

Normand, S.-L. T., Glickman, M. E. and Gatsonis, C. A. 1997: Statistical methods for profiling providers of medical care: issues and applications. *Journal of the American Statistical Association* **92**, 803–41.

Normand, S.-L. T., Glickman, M. E. and Ryan, T. J. 1995: Modelling mortality rates for elderly heart attack patients: profiling hospitals in the cooperative cardiovascular project. In Gatsonis, C., Hodges, J., Kass, R. and Singpurwalla, N. (eds), *Case studies in Bayesian statistics*, pp. 731–58. New York: Springer.

Rasbash, J., Yang, M., Woodhouse, G. and Goldstein, H. 1995: *MLn: command reference guide*. London: Institute of Education.

Rice, N. and Leyland, A. 1996: Multilevel models: applications to health data. *Journal of Health Services Research and Policy* **1**, 154–64.

Richardson, S. and Green, P. J. 1997: On Bayesian analysis of mixtures with an unknown number of components (with discussion). *Journal of the Royal Statistical Society (B)* **59**, 731–92.

Schneider, E. C. and Epstein, A. M. 1996: Influence of cardiac-surgery performance reports on referral practices and access to care. *New England Journal of Medicine* **335**, 251–6.

Scottish Office 1995: *Clinical outcome indicators – 1994*. Edinburgh: Clinical Resource and Audit Group.

Smith, A. F. M., Skene, A. M., Shaw, J. E. H. and Naylor, J. C. 1987: Progress with numerical and graphical methods for practical Bayesian statistics. *The Statistician* **36**, 75–82.

Spiegelhalter, D. J., Thomas, A., Best, N. G. and Gilks, W. R. 1995: *BUGS: Bayesian inference using Gibbs Sampling, version 0.50*. Cambridge: MRC Biostatistics Unit.

Thomas, N., Longford, N. T. and Rolph, J. E. 1994: Empirical Bayes methods for estimating hospital specific mortality rates. *Statistics in Medicine* **13**, 889–903.

Tierney, L. and Kadane, J. B. 1986: Accurate approximations for posterior moments and marginal densities. *Journal of the American Statistical Association* **81**, 82–6.

UKTSSA 1995: *Renal transplant audit 1984–1993*. Bristol: United Kingdom Transplant Support Service Authority.

Van Houlwelingen, H. C. and Thorogood, J. 1995: Construction, validation and updating of a prognostic model for kidney graft survival. *Statistics in Medicine* **14**, 1999–2008.

11 Bayesian meta-analysis

Larry V. Hedges

11.1 Introduction

The use of statistical methods for combining information from different clinical trials or epidemiological studies (an enterprise which is often called meta-analysis) has become widespread in the biomedical sciences. It has been used extensively in various medical specialties such as perinatal medicine (Chalmers, 1988), public health (Louis *et al.*, 1985), and the development of practice policies (McCormick *et al.*, 1994). Given the increasing size of the research literature, in medicine and other empirical sciences, it appears that meta-analysis in some form will be an important part of biostatistical research for some time.

Meta-analysis usually involves representing the result of each study by a numerical index (estimate) of effect size, and then combining these estimates across studies according to some model. The combination model is always implicitly a two-level hierarchical model, recognizing two sources of variation affecting each effect size estimate: a within-study sampling error and a between-study effect. The within-study sampling error reflects the variation which arises because the estimate obtained from a given sample is not identical to the underlying effect parameter of which it is an estimate. The between-study effect is a consequence of the fact that the effect parameters associated with every study may not be identical.

There are two competing classes of models for meta-analysis, usually called fixed and random effects models. Both classes of models conceive within-study sampling error as random. However, they differ in how the between-study effects are conceived. Fixed effects models treat between-study effects as fixed, but unknown, constants. The simplest fixed effects model treats these constants as all zero; that is, such models incorporate the assumption that all of the effect parameters are identical. In this case the object of the analysis is to estimate the common effect parameter across studies.

Random effects models conceive some or all of the between-study effect as a consequence of a random process. For example, one might conceive that differences in experimental, measurement and sampling conditions cause studies to obtain different effect parameters. There is a universe of studies (or more precisely, effect parameters) one might wish to generalize about, which is defined by experimental, measurement and sampling conditions. Any particular study (and its effect parameter) might be seen as having been sampled from the universe. This class of models would suggest that the object of combination is to describe the distribution of effect parameters associated with the universe of studies about which we wish to generalize. This is usually done by estimating the mean and variance (the between-study variance component) of the effect parameters.

Many statisticians believe that random effects models are more appropriate than fixed effects models for meta-analysis because between-study variation is an important source of uncertainty that should not be ignored in assigning uncertainty to pooled results. For example, a report on combining information sponsored by the National Research Council's Committee on Applied and Theoretical Statistics (National Research Council, 1992) concluded that meta-analytic 'modeling would be improved by an increase in the use of **random effects** models in preference to the current default of **fixed effects** models' (p. 3).

Random effects models are typically implemented by obtaining an estimate of the variance component from the data and then treating this estimate as if it were known, a priori (e.g. Hedges and Olkin, 1985, DerSimonian and Laird, 1986).

For example, one might invoke the idea of maximum likelihood estimation of the variance component to obtain the single value that is most likely given the observed study results. Such a procedure is equivalent to plotting the likelihood given the data as a function of variance component and determining which value has the highest likelihood. This value is used whether or not there is a range of other values that are nearly as consistent with the data. If the most likely single value is zero, this is seen as evidence supporting the use of the fixed effects model.

One widely used application of this principle is the use of a preliminary test of the significance of the variance component prior to adopting the fixed effects model. Many authors (e.g. DerSimonian and Laird, 1986) have suggested conducting a test of homogeneity (which is a test of the hypothesis that the between-study variance component is zero) and using fixed effects models if the variance component is not statistically significant. Since the fixed effects model is essentially a random effects model with zero variance component, this procedure is equivalent to substituting an estimated value (zero) as the variance component as if this were a known a priori.

The problem with this approach to random effects analysis is that information about the variance component comes from variation between studies and when the number of studies is small, any estimate of the variance component must be rather uncertain. Therefore an analysis (such as the conventional random effects analysis) that treats an estimated value of the variance component as if it were known with certainty is problematic.

Bayesian analyses address this problem by recognizing that there is a family of random effects analyses, one for each value of the variance component. The Bayesian analyses can be seen as essentially averaging over the family of results, giving each one the weight that is appropriate given the posterior probability of each variance component value conditional on the observed data. In this way the uncertainty of the variance component given the data is incorporated into the analysis in a manner that can make its role transparent to the data analyst.

This chapter describes the basics of Bayesian meta-analysis. Section 11.2 is a discussion of effect size measures and the hierarchical models used. Section 11.3 describes methods for an important special case of Bayesian meta-analysis where the studies are completely exchangeable. Section 11.4 describes methods for meta-analysis in the general case when not all effect sizes are exchangeable. Section 11.5 describes prior distributions that might be used in Bayesian meta-analysis.

11.2   Models for effect sizes

Much of the methodological work on meta-analysis has addressed problems of combining specific estimators under specific models. For example, Hedges (1982) discussed the problem of combining estimates of the standardized differences between group means, Hedges and Olkin (1983) discussed combining estimates of correlation coefficients, and Fleiss (1973) discussed odds ratios, risk differences and risk ratios.

While much of the literature has concentrated on methods for combining specific estimators, the methods used have actually been more general, and the same procedures for fixed and random effects combinations have been rediscovered in new contexts (see Hedges, 1983). These methods depend on the fact that most effect size measures that have been used in meta-analysis are approximately normally distributed with a known variance (or at least a standard error that can be consistently estimated). The accuracy of the standard meta-analytic methods is essentially determined by the accuracy of the normal approximation to the distribution of the individual effect size estimates. A discussion of effect size measures that have been used in meta-analysis can be found in Fleiss (1994) and Shadish and Haddock (1994).

In this chapter we follow the convention of using a general measure of effect size. Suppose that there are k independent studies. Let θ_i and T_i be the effect size parameter and estimate, respectively, in the ith study, and assume that T_i has negligible bias as an estimator of θ_i and that the standard error S_i can be estimated consistently from information observed in the study. In addition, let $\mathbf{x}_i = (x_{i1}, \ldots, x_{ip})'$ be a vector of $p < k$ study-level covariates indicating characteristics of the studies that may be related to effect size.

Form the $(k \times 1)$ vectors of effect size estimates $\mathbf{T} = (T_1, \ldots, T_k)'$, effect size parameters, $\boldsymbol{\theta} = (\theta_1, \ldots, \theta_k)'$, the $(p \times 1)$ vector of covariate effects $\boldsymbol{\beta} = (\beta_1, \ldots, \beta_p)'$, and the $k \times p$ design matrix $\mathbf{X} = (\mathbf{x}'_1, \ldots, \mathbf{x}'_p)'$, which is assumed to be of full rank. Specify the $k \times 1$ vectors of sampling errors $\boldsymbol{\epsilon} = \mathbf{T} - \boldsymbol{\theta}$ and between-study effects as $\boldsymbol{\delta} = \boldsymbol{\theta} - \mathbf{X}\boldsymbol{\beta}$. The hierarchical model is that

$$
\begin{aligned}
\mathbf{T} &= \mathbf{X}\boldsymbol{\beta} + \boldsymbol{\delta} + \boldsymbol{\epsilon}, & \boldsymbol{\epsilon} &\sim N(\mathbf{0}, \mathbf{S}) \\
\boldsymbol{\theta} &= \mathbf{X}\boldsymbol{\beta} + \boldsymbol{\delta}, & \boldsymbol{\delta} &\sim N(\mathbf{0}, \tau^2 \mathbf{I})
\end{aligned}
\tag{11.1}
$$

where $\mathbf{S}$ is a $k \times k$ matrix of known sampling error variances and covariances of $\boldsymbol{\epsilon}$ and $\mathbf{I}$ is a $k \times k$ identity matrix.

The Bayesian formulation of this model places a prior distribution on the unknown parameters $\boldsymbol{\beta}$ and τ. It makes sense to start with the prior distribution for τ, which as shown below need not be specified in detail at this point. Therefore let $\pi(\tau)$ be a prior distribution on τ and let $\boldsymbol{\beta}|\tau$ be p-variate normally distributed with p-dimensional mean vector $\boldsymbol{\mu} = (\mu_1, \ldots, \mu_p)'$ and $p \times p$ covariance matrix $\boldsymbol{\Sigma}$ which are assumed to be known. Thus the hierarchical model becomes

$$
\begin{aligned}
\tau &\sim \pi(\tau) \\
\boldsymbol{\beta}|\tau &\sim N(\boldsymbol{\mu}, \boldsymbol{\Sigma}) \\
\boldsymbol{\theta}|\boldsymbol{\beta}, \tau &\sim N(\mathbf{X}\boldsymbol{\beta}, \tau^2 \mathbf{I}) \\
\mathbf{T}|\boldsymbol{\theta}, \boldsymbol{\beta}, \tau &\sim N(\boldsymbol{\theta}, \mathbf{S})
\end{aligned}
\tag{11.2}
$$

This hierarchical model is essentially identical to the one considered by Rubin (1981), DuMouchel and Harris (1983), Carlin (1992) and chapter 5 of Gelman *et al.* (1995), but it is not the only possibility. Alternatives are given by Box and Tiao (1973), Efron and Morris (1973), Smith (1973), Harville (1977), Laird and Ware (1982) and DuMouchel (1990). One major class of variants includes models where the distribution of $\boldsymbol{\theta}|\boldsymbol{\beta}, \tau$ is not normal, but a heavier-tailed distribution such as a Student's t or gamma distribution (see Seltzer, 1993, Smith *et al.*, 1995, Seltzer *et al.*, 1996). Estimation in such models usually requires the use of Markov chain Monte Carlo methods which are slightly more complex than those discussed in this chapter.

11.3   All effect sizes exchangeable

The analysis that arises most frequently and is the simplest is when all studies and their corresponding effect sizes are exchangeable. It arises, for example, when there are no study-level covariates and all of the effect size estimates are conditionally independent given θ. In this case there is no reason to assign a different prior distribution to any particular study. This case is considered first because it not only is the simplest case, but also gives some insight about the calculations in more complex situations.

11.3.1 Model and notation

Suppose that there are k independent studies and let θ_i and T_i denote the effect size parameter and estimate, respectively, from the ith study. Define the linear model for T_i and θ_i as follows:

$$
\begin{aligned}
T_i &= \theta_i + \epsilon_i, & \epsilon_i &\sim N(0, S_i^2) \\
\theta_i &= \beta + \delta_i, & \delta_i &\sim N(0, \tau^2)
\end{aligned}
\tag{11.3}
$$

where the ϵ_i and the δ_i are distributed independently of one another. The parameter β is the mean of the distribution of effect size parameters. The random effect ϵ_i is a sampling error of the observed effect size (estimate) about the effect size parameter in the ith study and the random effect δ_i is a between-study effect. The standard error of the effect size estimate S_i is treated as known since it can usually be estimated with reasonable precision for each study. The between-studies variance component τ^2 is an index of the heterogeneity of effect size parameters across studies. This linear model is often called the simple random effects model in meta-analysis (see, for example, Hedges, 1983, DerSimonian and Laird, 1986, Raudenbush, 1994).

The Bayesian formulation of this model requires placing prior distributions on the unknown parameters β and τ. It makes sense to start with the prior distribution for τ, which as shown below need not be specified in detail at this point. Therefore let $\pi(\tau)$ be a prior distribution on τ and let $\beta|\tau$ be normally distributed with mean μ and variance σ^2, which are assumed to be known. Thus the hierarchical model becomes

$$
\begin{aligned}
\tau &\sim \pi(\tau) \\
\beta|\tau &\sim N(\mu, \sigma^2) \\
\theta_i|\beta, \tau &\sim N(\beta, \tau^2) \\
T_i|\theta, \beta, \tau &\sim N(\theta_i, S_i^2)
\end{aligned}
\tag{11.4}
$$

Specifying μ with a finite value of σ^2 is equivalent to expressing prior knowledge of β; that is, using an informative prior distribution. If, as in many analyses, the investigator does not wish to include prior information in the analysis, it is possible to let σ^2 tend to infinity, so that β has essentially a uniform prior, which is taken to be uninformative for μ. Analyses using the uninformative prior for β are discussed first and those for informative priors follow afterwards.

11.3.2   Analyses with an uninformative prior on β

The analysis of the hierarchical model involves computing the posterior distribution of β, τ^2 and sometimes the individual effect parameters $\theta_1, \ldots, \theta_k$. These analyses are simplified by recognizing that, conditional on τ, the effect size estimates $T_1, \ldots, T_k$ are normally distributed about β with known variances $\tau^2 + S_1^2, \ldots, \tau^2 + S_k^2$, respectively. Since β itself is normally distributed, the posterior distribution of β and that of any θ_i, given the data vector $\mathbf{T} = (T_1, \ldots, T_k)'$, are normal with a simple form. Specifically, the conditional distribution of β given $\mathbf{T}$ and τ, $f(\beta|\mathbf{T}, \tau)$, is normal with variance

$$\tilde{\sigma}^2(\tau) = \left(\sum_{i=1}^{k} \frac{1}{S_i^2 + \tau^2} \right)^{-1} \tag{11.5}$$

and mean

$$\tilde{\mu}(\tau) = \left(\sum_{i=1}^{k} \frac{T_i}{S_i^2 + \tau^2} \right) \tilde{\sigma}^2(\tau) \tag{11.6}$$

Note that $\tilde{\mu}(\tau)$ is just the weighted mean of the observed effect sizes $T_1, \ldots, T_k$, where the weights are the reciprocals of the variances of the T_i conditional on τ. This is the estimate of β that would be computed in a classical random effects meta-analysis, where the entire analysis would be conditioned on the empirical estimate of τ obtained from the data.

The posterior distribution of τ given $\mathbf{T}$ is only slightly more complicated. A direct computation shows that the posterior distribution of τ given $\mathbf{T}$, $f(\tau|\mathbf{T})$, is proportional to

$$\pi(\tau) \exp\left(\frac{-Q(\tau)}{2} \right) \Bigg/ \sqrt{\prod_{i-1}^{k} (S_i^2 + \tau^2) \left(\sum_{i=1}^{k} \frac{1}{S_i^2 + \tau^2} \right)} \tag{11.7}$$

where $Q(\tau)$ is given by

$$Q(\tau) = \sum_{i=1}^{k} \frac{[T_i - \tilde{\mu}(\tau)]^2}{\tau^2 + S_i^2}$$

and $\tilde{\mu}(\tau)$ is just the posterior mean conditional on τ given above.

To obtain the normalizing constant necessary to make (11.7) a legitimate probability density, it is necessary to integrate the above expression numerically, but this usually poses no particular difficulties with a computational environment such as Splus, Maple, or Gauss. One simple strategy is to search for the maximum of (11.7), then find the point $\tau = c$ where (11.7) is only $1/100$ as large as the maximum, and evaluate the integral as the sum of evaluations of (11.7) over 100 equally spaced points between 0 and c.

Note that $Q(\tau)$ is just the weighted sum of squares about the weighted mean effect size, weighted by the reciprocal of $S_i^2 + \tau^2$ (the total variance of

T_i). It is interesting to note that $Q(0)$ is often used as a test statistic for testing the hypothesis that $\tau = 0$ in classical meta-analysis.

The posterior density of $\beta, f(\beta|\mathbf{T})$, is a mixture of normal densities $f(\beta|\mathbf{T}, \tau)$ indexed by τ with the mixing probabilities given by $f(\tau|\mathbf{T})$, that is

$$f(\beta|\mathbf{T}) = \int_0^\infty f(\beta|\mathbf{T}, \tau) f(\tau|\mathbf{T}) \mathrm{d}\tau$$

$$= \int_0^\infty \phi\left(\frac{\beta - \tilde{\mu}(\tau)}{\tilde{\sigma}(\tau)}\right) f(\tau|\mathbf{T}) \mathrm{d}\tau \tag{11.8}$$

where $\phi(x)$ is the standard normal probability density function. This density is useful for expressing graphically the uncertainty of β given the observed data $\mathbf{T}$, generating a confidence profile for the mean effect (see Eddy *et al.*, 1992). The posterior density (11.8) is relatively easy to evaluate by numerical integration.

Alternatively, $f(\beta|\mathbf{T})$ can be computed by Monte Carlo integration. To do so, compute the integral in (11.8) by first sampling values of τ from $f(\tau|\mathbf{T})$, and then sampling a value of $\beta|\tau, \mathbf{T}$ from $f(\beta|\mathbf{T}, \tau)$ for each value of τ. A thousand values is usually sufficient. To sample from $f(\tau|\mathbf{T})$, compute the inverse of the cumulative distribution of $\tau|\mathbf{T}$ numerically. A crude, but effective, technique for sampling from $\tau|\mathbf{T}$ is to estimate the cumulative distribution by calculating $f(\tau|\mathbf{T})$ for 100 equally spaced values in the region of highest density of $\tau|\mathbf{T}$ to obtain the cumulative distribution function $F(\tau) = F(\tau|\mathbf{T})$. Sampling from $f(\tau|\mathbf{T})$ is then accomplished by sampling uniform deviate U from $[0, 1]$ and obtaining the value of τ as $F^{-1}(U)$. Since $f(\beta|\mathbf{T}, \tau)$ is a normal density, the second stage of the sampling is trivial.

The mean and standard deviation of the posterior distribution are often of great interest in summarizing the meta-analysis. The posterior mean and variance can be obtained by integrating $f(\beta|\mathbf{T})$ given in (11.8) numerically. However, since the mean and variance conditional on τ have a simple closed form expression, the computations are more transparent (and often easier) if the summary statistics are computed conditionally given τ, and then averaged across values of τ weighted by $f(\tau|\mathbf{T})$. Specifically the mean and variance are

$$\tilde{\mu} = \int_0^\infty \tilde{\mu}(\tau) f(\tau|\mathbf{T}) \mathrm{d}\tau$$

$$\tilde{\sigma}^2 = \int_0^\infty \tilde{\sigma}^2(\tau) + [\tilde{\mu}(\tau) - \tilde{\mu}]^2 \mathrm{d}\tau \tag{11.9}$$

One other summary statistic that is often of interest is the posterior probability that the mean effect size is positive. This too can be computed directly from the posterior density $f(\beta|\mathbf{T})$, but is also generally easier to compute conditionally, and then average over the $f(\tau|\mathbf{T})$. Specifically

$$P(\beta > 0) = \int_0^\infty \Phi\left(\frac{\tilde{\mu}(\tau)}{\tilde{\sigma}(\tau)}\right) f(\tau|\mathbf{T})d\tau \tag{11.10}$$

where $\Phi(x)$ is the standard normal cumulative distribution function.

The integrals involved in (11.8)–(11.10) can usually be computed to sufficient accuracy by evaluating the posterior distribution of τ for a small (20–100) ensemble of points covering the range of non-negligible values of $f(\tau|\mathbf{T})$, approximating the function as a step function and then computing the integral as a sum.

The posterior distribution of θ_i, conditional on τ, $f(\theta_i|\mathbf{T}, \tau)$, is also normal with mean $\tilde{\theta}_i(\tau)$ and variance $\tilde{S}_i^2(\tau)$, where

$$\tilde{\theta}_i(\tau) = \tilde{\mu}(\tau) + [T_i - \tilde{\mu}(\tau)]\frac{\tau^2}{\tau^2 + S_i^2}$$

$$\tilde{S}_i^2(\tau) = \frac{\tau^2}{\tau^2 + S_i^2}S_i^2 + \frac{S_i^4}{(S_i^2 + \tau^2)^2}\left(\sum_{i=1}^k \frac{1}{S_i^2 + \tau^2}\right)^{-1} \tag{11.11}$$

As in the case of β, the posterior distribution of θ_i, $f(\theta_i|\mathbf{T})$, is a mixture of normal densities $f(\theta_i|\mathbf{T}, \tau)$ indexed by τ with the mixing probabilities given by $f(\tau|\mathbf{T})$, that is

$$\tilde{\theta}_i = \int_0^\infty \tilde{\theta}_i(\tau) f(\tau|\mathbf{T})d\tau$$

$$\tilde{S}_i^2 = \int_0^\infty \{\tilde{S}_i^2(\tau) + [\tilde{\theta}_i(\tau) - \tilde{\theta}_i]^2\} f(\tau|\mathbf{T})d\tau \tag{11.12}$$

The integrals in the expression for $\tilde{\theta}_i$ and $\tilde{S}_i^2$ can be either computed numerically or evaluated by Monte Carlo methods as in the case of β. That is, evaluate the joint posterior distribution of θ_i by sampling first values of $\tau|\mathbf{T}$, and then for each value of $\tau|\mathbf{T}$, sampling values of $\theta_1, \ldots, \theta_k$ from normal distributions with means $\tilde{\theta}_1(\tau), \ldots, \tilde{\theta}_k(\tau)$ and variances $\tilde{S}_1^2(\tau), \ldots, \tilde{S}_k^2(\tau)$, respectively. A sample of 1000 suites of $\theta_1, \ldots, \theta_k$, values is usually sufficient for most purposes. The posterior means and variances of any θ_i can then be computed as the (sample) mean and variance of the sampled values or the individual posterior distributions can be estimated as the distribution of the sampled values. One advantage of this approach is that the data set of sampled values can easily be used to estimate any other descriptive index (such as quantiles of the proportion of the time that $\theta_1 > \tilde{\theta}$) that might be desired based on the posterior distribution.

Table 11.1 Data from the 11 studies in the USEPA report on the relation between environmental tobacco smoke and lung cancer, and the posterior means and standard deviations of the effect sizes when all studies are exchangeable

Study	T_i	S_i	Flat prior		DuMouchel prior	
			$\tilde{\theta}_i$	$\tilde{S}_i$	$\tilde{\theta}_i$	$\tilde{S}_i$
Brownson *et al.* (1987)	0.405	0.695	0.180	0.188	0.174	0.145
Buffler *et al.* (1984)	−0.386	0.451	0.097	0.170	0.129	0.134
Butler (1988)	0.698	0.730	0.196	0.190	0.182	0.146
Correa *et al.* (1983)	0.637	0.481	0.218	0.173	0.195	0.136
Fontham *et al.* (1991)	0.247	0.134	0.202	0.096	0.191	0.086
Garfinkel *et al.* (1985)	0.239	0.206	0.189	0.123	0.181	0.105
Garfinkel (1981)	0.148	0.163	0.159	0.108	0.162	0.094
Humble *et al.* (1987)	0.693	0.544	0.214	0.178	0.192	0.139
Janerich *et al.* (1990)	−0.236	0.246	0.060	0.135	0.102	0.112
Kabat and Wynder (1984)	−0.315	0.591	0.126	0.182	0.145	0.141
Wu *et al.* (1985)	0.278	0.487	0.178	0.173	0.173	0.136

11.3.2.1 Example

In 1992 the United States Environmental Protection Agency (USEPA) published a meta-analysis of studies of the effects of environmental tobacco smoke on lung cancer. The analysis included epidemiological studies conducted worldwide, but the analyses were conducted separately for each country. The studies were typically case–control studies, but some were cohort studies. The measure of effect size in the case–control studies was the log risk ratio and the effect size for the cohort studies was the log odds ratio. Because of the low prevalence of lung cancer, the log odds ratio used in the cohort studies was regarded as estimating essentially the same parameter as the log risk ratio.

We analyse here the 11 studies from the United States. Table 11.1 is a list of the studies, their effect size estimates (T_i values) and standard errors (S_i values). USEPA used a fixed effects analysis, which is equivalent to assuming that $\tau = 0$ a priori. In that analysis, the average effect was found to be 0.17 with a 95% confidence interval of 0.01 to 0.33, indicating that the mean effect was just statistically significant at the 0.05 level. One obvious question is whether the data are consistent with such a strong assumption about the consistency of the effect size studies. The assumption that $\tau = 0$ is equivalent to assuming that all of the studies estimate exactly the same effect size parameter β.

Figure 11.1 shows plots of three posterior distributions of τ given the data **T** from the 11 studies, each assuming a different prior distribution of τ. These three prior distributions correspond to different prior assumptions about τ, ranging from strong belief that τ is near zero (the prior $\pi(\tau) \propto 1/\tau^2$), relatively diffuse belief that τ was about 0.265, the harmonic

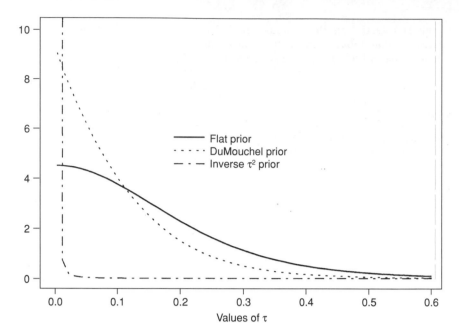

Fig. 11.1 Posterior distributions of τ

mean of the standard errors (the prior suggested by DuMouchel, $\pi(\tau) \propto S_{.}/(S_{.}+\tau)^2$), to diffuse belief favouring large values of τ (the prior $\pi(\tau) \propto 1$). The figure suggests that the likely values of τ depend on the prior distribution chosen, but all suggest that the most likely single value is $\tau = 0$, the single value used in the USEPA analyses. The posterior distributions of τ associated with these three priors differ substantially in their concentration around zero, however. The posterior mean of τ is greater than zero regardless of the prior used, since it is the average of non-negative values over a positive density. The posterior mean is 0.15 with the flat prior, 0.10 with the DuMouchel prior and 0.00 (positive but zero to two decimal places) under the prior proportional to $1/\tau^2$. Thus the first two of the priors lead to a posterior distribution for which there is a substantial chance that τ is larger than zero, and values of τ larger than 0.1 are more likely than values of τ less than 0.1. The third prior, the one proportional to $1/\tau^2$, is so concentrated at zero that analyses based on this prior give essentially the same results as the fixed effects model used in the USEPA analysis (which assumed that $\tau = 0$, a priori).

If one does not have strong prior belief that τ is near zero, this suggests that a fixed effects analysis like that conducted by USEPA may have understated the uncertainty of the average effect size since it did not include the larger uncertainty associated with non-zero values of τ. Alternatively, one might say that belief in the fixed effects analysis corresponds to a prior belief that τ is near zero that is at least as extreme as assuming that it has a density function $\pi(\tau) \propto 1/\tau^2$.

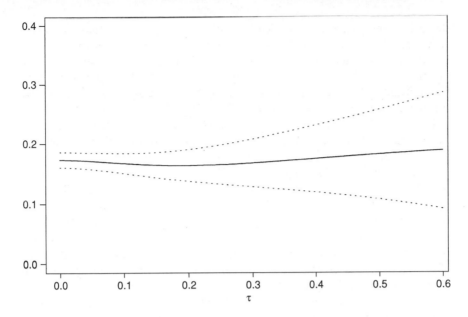

Fig. 11.2 Conditional mean and confidence intervals

Figure 11.2, however, shows the conditional posterior mean $\tilde{\mu}(\tau)$ and two (conditional) standard error intervals $\tilde{\mu}(\tau) - 2\tilde{\sigma}(\tau)$ to $\tilde{\mu}(\tau) + 2\tilde{\sigma}(\tau)$. The plot shows that the conditional mean is little changed by changes in τ, but the uncertainty of the mean as expressed by the posterior standard

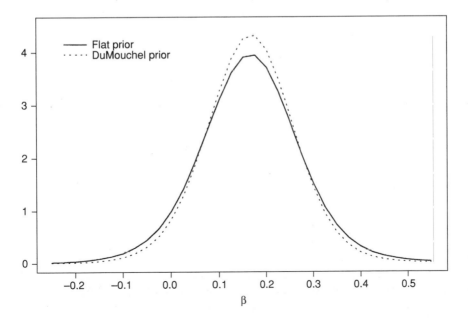

Fig. 11.3 Posterior distributions of β

deviation increases monotonically with τ. The conditional posterior standard deviation increases from about 0.08 for $\tau = 0$ to 0.13 for $\tau = 0.25$, a change of 62% over the range of values of τ that are plausible given the data. Consequently, although understating the value of τ would not substantially affect the mean, it might have a substantial effect on the uncertainty of the mean effect size.

Figure 11.3 shows the posterior density of β given the three prior distributions above. The figure shows that the posterior distributions are slightly skewed and, as expected, the means are only slightly affected by the choice of prior distribution of τ. The posterior means and standard deviations using the flat, DuMouchel and $1/\tau^2$ prior distributions, respectively, are $\tilde{\mu} = 0.165$, 0.166 and 0.170 and $\tilde{\sigma} = 0.110$, 0.095 and 0.081. The posterior probabilities that $\tilde{\mu} > 0$ are 0.94, 0.96 and 0.098 under the three priors, showing the effect of the choice of prior on this summary of the posterior distribution. Indeed, the posterior probability that the effect is positive is greater than 0.95 for two of the priors, but is less than 0.95 for the prior on τ proportional to a constant.

Figure 11.4 shows the conditional Bayes estimates $\tilde{\theta}_i(\tau)$ of the study-specific effect size parameters (the θ_i) for several of the studies. Note that if $\tau = 0$, the Bayes estimates equal the posterior mean of β (i.e. $\tilde{\theta}_i(0) = \tilde{\mu}$), corresponding to the idea that when there is no variation among effect parameters, the best estimate of the effect in any study is the posterior mean. When τ is very large (at least in proportion to the S_i) the Bayes estimates of study-specific effects approach the observed effect sizes

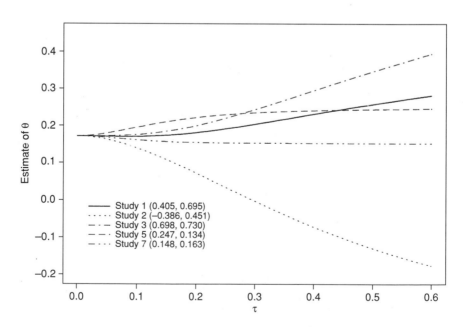

Fig. 11.4 Estimates of θ as a function of τ for selected studies

(i.e. $\tilde{\theta}_i(\tau) \to T_i$ as τ becomes large). When the value of τ is inter-mediate, each $\tilde{\theta}_i(\tau)$ shrinks towards $\tilde{\mu}$ by an amount that depends on the relative size of τ^2 and S_i^2. Therefore the studies with the most uncertain effect size estimates (those with the biggest S_i) shrink more towards the posterior mean than those with more certain estimates. Table 11.1 gives the (unconditional) posterior means and variances for all of the studies given the flat and DuMouchel prior distributions discussed above. The prior proportional to $1/\tau^2$ leads to essentially com-plete shrinkage to $\tilde{\mu}$.

11.3.3 Analyses with an informative prior on β

The analysis with an informative prior is no more complex than that discussed above. As in the case of the uninformative priors on β, the analysis of the hierarchical model involves computing the posterior distribution of β, τ^2 and sometimes the individual effect parameters $\theta_1, \ldots, \theta_k$. Conditional on τ, the effect size estimates $T_1, \ldots, T_k$ are normally distributed about β with known variances $\tau^2 + S_1^2, \ldots, \tau^2 + S_k^2$, respectively. Since β itself is normally distributed, the posterior distribution of β and that of any θ_i, given the data vector $\mathbf{T} = (T_1, \ldots, T_k)'$, are normal. The conditional distribution of β given $\mathbf{T}$ and τ, $f(\beta|\mathbf{T}, \tau)$, is normal with variance

$$\tilde{\sigma}^2(\tau) = \left(\sum_{i=1}^{k} \frac{1}{S_i^2 + \tau^2} + \frac{1}{\sigma^2} \right)^{-1} \tag{11.13}$$

and mean

$$\tilde{\mu}(\tau) = \left(\sum_{i=1}^{k} \frac{T_i}{S_i^2 + \tau^2} + \frac{\mu}{\sigma^2} \right) \tilde{\sigma}^2(\tau) \tag{11.14}$$

Comparing (11.5) and (11.6) with (11.13) and (11.14), the effect of prior information on $\tilde{\mu}(\tau)$ and $\tilde{\sigma}^2(\tau)$ is apparent. Conditional on τ, setting the prior mean at μ with variance σ^2 is the equivalent of adding an observation (an effect size estimate) with value μ and standard error $\sqrt{(\sigma^2 - \tau^2)}$. This provides a way to think about eliciting prior information to set the prior distribution on β. If the prior were determined by the effect size estimate from an empirical study, it could be incorporated either as part of the data or as part of the prior. The principle that either method of incorporating the prior data should give the same result would suggest using a prior mean equal to the estimate and a prior variance of S^2 + the typical value of τ^2. Thus, when a prior study is not available but there is subjective or other information about β, the prior mean and variance should be set by eliciting prior belief in a way that could be expressed as equivalent to the outcome of a study possessing equivalent prior information.

The posterior distribution of τ given $\mathbf{T}$ is only slightly more complicated. A direct computation lead shows that the posterior distribution of τ given $\mathbf{T}, f(\tau|\mathbf{T})$, is proportional to

$$\pi(\tau)\exp\left(-\frac{[Q(\tau)+D(\tau)]}{2}\right)\Big/ \sqrt{\prod_{i=1}^{k}\sigma^2(\tau^2+S_i^2)\left(\frac{1}{\sigma^2}+\sum_{i=1}^{k}\frac{1}{\tau^2+S_i^2}\right)} \quad (11.15)$$

where the two terms $Q(\tau)$ and $D(\tau)$ are given by

$$Q(\tau)=\sum_{i=1}^{k}\frac{[T_i-\overline{T}(\tau)]^2}{\tau^2+S_i^2}$$

and

$$D(\tau)=\frac{[\overline{T}(\tau)-\mu]^2}{\sigma^2+\left(\sum_{i=1}^{k}1/(\tau^2+S_i^2)\right)^{-1}}$$

where $\overline{T}(\tau)$ is the weighted mean of the observed effect sizes $T_1, \ldots, T_k$ conditional on τ given by

$$\overline{T}(\tau)=\sum_{i=1}^{k}\frac{T_i}{\tau^2+S_i^2}\Big/\sum_{i=1}^{k}\frac{1}{\tau^2+S_i^2}$$

Note that there are two components to the exponential in this posterior distribution. The first term, $Q(\tau)$, occurred in the posterior distribution of τ in the non-informative case, so the effect of the prior information is contained in the second term, $D(\tau)$. The first term is a consequence of variation of the observed effect sizes T_i about their mean. The second term, $D(\tau)$, is a consequence of the deviation of the average T_i from μ and represents the degree to which the data agree with the prior mean.

To obtain the normalizing constant necessary to make (11.15) a probability density, it is necessary to integrate the last expression above numerically (which is straightforward) or to use Monte Carlo integration as described in the case of the uninformative prior on β.

The posterior distribution of β, $f(\beta|\mathbf{T})$, is a mixture of normal densities $f(\beta|\mathbf{T}, \tau)$ indexed by τ with the mixing probabilities given by $f(\tau|\mathbf{T})$, that is

$$f(\beta|\mathbf{T})=\int_0^{\infty} f(\beta|\mathbf{T}, \tau)f(\tau|\mathbf{T})d\tau$$

$$=\int_0^{\infty}\Phi\left(\frac{\beta-\tilde{\mu}(\tau)}{\tilde{\sigma}(\tau)}\right)f(\tau|\mathbf{T})d\tau \quad (11.16)$$

This density can be used to express the uncertainty of β given the observed data $\mathbf{T}$, in a confidence profile for the mean effect (see Eddy et al., 1992).

However, the mean and standard deviation of the posterior distribution are often of great interest in summarizing the meta-analysis. As in the case of an uninformative prior distribution on β, it is generally preferable to compute summary statistics conditionally given τ, and then average across values of τ weighted by $f(\tau|\mathbf{T})$. Specifically the mean and variance are

$$\tilde{\mu} = \int_0^\infty \tilde{\mu}(\tau) f(\tau|\mathbf{T}) d\tau$$

$$\tilde{\sigma}^2 = \int_0^\infty \{\tilde{\sigma}^2(\tau) + [\tilde{\mu}(\tau) - \tilde{\mu}]^2\} f(\tau|\mathbf{T}) d\tau \qquad (11.17)$$

Both integrals are easy to compute numerically or by Monte Carlo methods, which provides the full joint distribution of the θ_i.

11.4 The general case

The analyses discussed in previous sections assumed that the prior distribution of β was the same for all effect sizes and that all effect size estimates were conditionally independent (given θ and τ). These assumptions are too restrictive for some problems. In some situations a single experiment may measure the outcome at several points in time or may measure the same outcome by several different methods. Alternatively, a study may have several treatment groups but only a single control group, so that effect size estimates computed from different treatment groups involve the same control group. In such cases, the effect size estimates from the experiment would not be conditionally independent (the S matrix would not be diagonal).

In other situations, study design, study procedures or patient populations may differ so that it is unreasonable to believe that the mean effect size is the same for all studies. Thus, the mean effect size may differ across studies and the estimates may not be conditionally independent. For example, studies may use different dosages of a drug, have different schedules for its administration, or administer it in conjunction with other therapies. If there is no strong model to link these differences (e.g. a model implying that they should be proportional), the differences among studies in their mean effects may be expressed by letting each group of similar studies depend on different components of β.

11.4.1 Informative prior on β

The analysis using an informative prior on β proceeds by finding the posterior distribution given a multivariate normal prior distribution with mean μ and covariance matrix Σ. As in the case of exchangeability among all effect sizes, it proves easier to obtain the posterior density of β

conditional on τ, then the posterior density of τ, and to integrate over τ to obtain the unconditional posterior and its moments.

The conditional distribution of β given τ, $f(\beta|\mathbf{T}, \tau)$, using the informative prior on β is multivariate normal with mean

$$\tilde{\mu}(\tau) = \tilde{\Sigma}(\tau)[\mathbf{X}'\mathbf{W}(\tau)\mathbf{T} + \Sigma^{-1}\mathbf{T}] \tag{11.18}$$

and variance

$$\tilde{\Sigma}(\tau) = [\mathbf{X}'\mathbf{W}(\tau)\mathbf{X} + \Sigma^{-1}]^{-1} \tag{11.19}$$

where $\mathbf{W}(\tau) = (\mathbf{S} + \tau^2\mathbf{I})^{-1}$ is the covariance matrix of $\mathbf{T}$ given β and τ. The form of the posterior distribution is the same as in the case of completely exchangeable effect sizes. The posterior mean $\tilde{\mu}(\tau)$ is just the weighted mean of the least squares estimate of β, $(\mathbf{X}'\mathbf{W}(\tau)\mathbf{X})^{-1}\mathbf{X}'\mathbf{W}(\tau)\mathbf{T}$, and the prior mean of θ, $\mathbf{X}\mu$, weighting each by the inverse of its variance. The variance of the conditional posterior distribution is the inverse of the sum of the weights.

The posterior distribution of τ, $f(\tau|\mathbf{T})$, is proportional to

$$\pi(\tau)|\mathbf{S} + \tau^2\mathbf{I} + \mathbf{X}\Sigma\mathbf{X}'|^{-1/2}\exp\{-(\mathbf{T} - \mathbf{X}\mu)'[\mathbf{S} + \tau^2\mathbf{I} + \mathbf{X}\Sigma\mathbf{X}'](\mathbf{T} - \mathbf{X}\mu)/2\} \tag{11.20}$$

As in the case of completely exchangeable effect sizes, summaries of the posterior distribution of β, such as the mean and variance, are most easily obtained by computing them conditionally and then integrating over τ, weighting according to $f(\tau|\mathbf{T})$. The unconditional mean and variance, $\tilde{\mu}$ and $\tilde{\Sigma}$, are therefore given by

$$\tilde{\mu} = \int_0^\infty \tilde{\mu}(\tau)f(\tau|\mathbf{T})\mathrm{d}\tau \tag{11.21}$$

and

$$\tilde{\Sigma} = \int_0^\infty \{\tilde{\Sigma}(\tau) + [\tilde{\mu}(\tau) - \tilde{\mu}][\tilde{\mu}(\tau) - \tilde{\mu}]'\}f(\tau|\mathbf{T})\mathrm{d}\tau \tag{11.22}$$

As in the case of completely exchangeable effect sizes, the mean is just the expected value of $\tilde{\mu}(\tau)$ over τ and the (co)variance is the expected value of the (co)variance plus the (co)variance of the average.

The posterior density of θ is also a mixture of multivariate normals, each of which is the conditional distribution $f(\theta|\mathbf{T}, \tau)$ of θ on $\mathbf{T}$ and τ. The mean and variance of these conditional distributions are

$$\tilde{\theta}(\tau) = \tilde{\mathbf{S}}(\tau)[\mathbf{S}^{-1}\mathbf{T} + (\mathbf{X}\Sigma\mathbf{X}' + \tau^2\mathbf{I})^{-1}\mathbf{X}\mu] \tag{11.23}$$

and

$$\tilde{\mathbf{S}}(\tau) = [\mathbf{S}^{-1} + (\tau^{-2}\mathbf{I} + \mathbf{X}\Sigma^{-1}\mathbf{X}')^{-1}]^{-1} \tag{11.24}$$

The posterior mean $\tilde{\theta}(\tau)$ is just the weighted sum of the data $\mathbf{T}$ and the prior mean μ, weighted by the inverse of the variance of each, and the variance is the inverse of the sum of the variances.

The posterior mean, $\tilde{\mu}$, and variance, $\tilde{S}$, of θ therefore are given by

$$\tilde{\theta} = \int_0^\infty \theta(\tau) f(\tau|\mathbf{T}) d\tau$$

$$\tilde{S} = \int_0^\infty \{\tilde{S}(\tau) + [\tilde{\theta}(\tau) - \tilde{\theta}][\tilde{\theta}(\tau) - \tilde{\theta}]'\} f(\tau|\mathbf{T}) d\tau$$

(11.25)

11.4.2 Uninformative prior on β

The analysis using the uninformative prior on β proceeds by using the posterior distribution given an informative prior, with arbitrary mean μ and covariance matrix $t\Sigma$, and then finding the limiting distribution as $t \to \infty$. This limit, which does not depend on μ or Σ, is taken as the posterior distribution with an uninformative prior on β. As in the case of exchangeability among all effect sizes, it proves easier to obtain the posterior density of β conditional on τ and the posterior of τ and then integrate over τ to obtain the unconditional posterior and its moments. The conditional distribution of β given τ, $f(\beta|\mathbf{T}, \tau)$, using the uninformative prior on β is multivariate normal with mean

$$\tilde{\mu}(\tau) = \tilde{\Sigma}(\tau) \mathbf{X}' \mathbf{W}(\tau) \mathbf{T} \tag{11.26}$$

and variance

$$\tilde{\Sigma}(\tau) = (\mathbf{X}' \mathbf{W}(\tau) \mathbf{X})^{-1}, \tag{11.27}$$

where $\mathbf{W}(\tau) = (\mathbf{S} + \tau^2 \mathbf{I})^{-1}$ is the covariance matrix of $\mathbf{T}$ given β and τ. Both the conditional mean and covariance are easily computed using just matrix arithmetic.

The posterior distribution of τ, $f(\tau|\mathbf{T})$, is proportional to

$$\pi(\tau) |\mathbf{W}(\tau)|^{1/2} |\mathbf{X}' \mathbf{W}(\tau) \mathbf{X}|^{-1/2} \exp(-\mathbf{T}' \mathbf{V}(\tau) \mathbf{T}/2) \tag{11.28}$$

where $\mathbf{V}(\tau) = \mathbf{W}(\tau) - \mathbf{W}(\tau) \mathbf{X} (\mathbf{X}' \mathbf{W}(\tau) \mathbf{X})^{-1} \mathbf{X}' \mathbf{W}(\tau)$.

As in the case of completely exchangeable effect sizes, summaries of the posterior distribution of β, such as the mean and variance, are most easily obtained by computing them conditionally and then integrating over τ, weighting according to $f(\tau|\mathbf{T})$. The unconditional mean and variance, $\tilde{\mu}$ and $\tilde{\Sigma}$, are therefore given by

$$\tilde{\mu} = \int_0^\infty \tilde{\mu}(\tau) f(\tau|\mathbf{T}) d\tau \tag{11.29}$$

and

$$\tilde{\Sigma} = \int_0^\infty \{\tilde{\Sigma}(\tau) + [\tilde{\mu}(\tau) - \tilde{\mu}][\tilde{\mu}(\tau) - \tilde{\mu}]'\} f(\tau|\mathbf{T}) d\tau \qquad (11.30)$$

As in the case of completely exchangeable effect sizes, the mean is just the expected value over τ and the variance is the expected value of the (co)variance plus the (co)variance of the average.

The posterior density of $\boldsymbol{\theta}$ is a mixture of multivariate normals, each of which is the conditional distribution $f(\boldsymbol{\theta}|\mathbf{T}, \tau)$ of $\boldsymbol{\theta}$ on $\mathbf{T}$ and τ. The mean and variance of these conditional distributions are

$$\tilde{\theta}(\tau) = \tilde{\mathbf{S}}(\tau)\mathbf{S}^{-1}\mathbf{T} \qquad (11.31)$$

and

$$\tilde{\mathbf{S}}(\tau) = \{\mathbf{S}^{-1} + \tau^{-2}[\mathbf{I} - \mathbf{X}(\mathbf{X}'\mathbf{X})^{-1}\mathbf{X}']\}^{-1} \qquad (11.32)$$

The posterior mean, $\tilde{\mu}$, and variance, $\tilde{\mathbf{S}}$, of $\boldsymbol{\theta}$ therefore are given by

$$\tilde{\theta} = \int_0^\infty \theta(\tau) f(\tau|\mathbf{T}) d\tau$$

$$\tilde{\mathbf{S}} = \int_0^\infty \{\tilde{\mathbf{S}}(\tau) + [\tilde{\theta}(\tau) - \tilde{\theta}][\tilde{\theta}(\tau) - \tilde{\theta}]'\} f(\tau|\mathbf{T}) d\tau \qquad (11.33)$$

11.4.3   Example

Continuing with the example of the USEPA meta-analysis of studies of the effects of environmental tobacco smoke on lung cancer, we note that nine of the studies were case–control studies and two of the studies were cohort studies. It seems plausible that studies with these different designs (and subject to different kinds of biases) might not produce the same effect sizes. To explore this idea, specify a two-dimensional distribution for $\boldsymbol{\beta}$, so that $\boldsymbol{\beta} = (\beta_1, \beta_2)'$ and $\mathbf{X} = (\mathbf{x}_1', \ldots, \mathbf{x}_{11}')'$, where $\mathbf{x}_i' = (1\ 0)$ if study i is a case–control study and $\mathbf{x}_i' = (0\ 1)$ if study i is a cohort study. Thus β_1 is the mean of the distribution of effect sizes from case–control studies and β_2 is the mean of the effect sizes of the cohort studies. As before, we assume an uninformative prior on $\boldsymbol{\beta}$, namely a prior density that is proportional to a constant.

Figure 11.5 shows plots of two posterior distributions of τ given the data $\mathbf{T}$ from the 11 studies, assuming two of the prior distributions of τ used earlier. Comparing these posterior distributions with those in Fig. 11.1, when all studies were assumed to be exchangeable, we see that they are not substantially different.

Figure 11.6 shows the marginal posterior densities of β_1 and β_2 given the prior distribution $\pi(\tau) \propto S_\cdot/(S_\cdot + \tau)^2$. The figure shows that the posterior distribution of β_1 is much less dispersed than that of β_2,

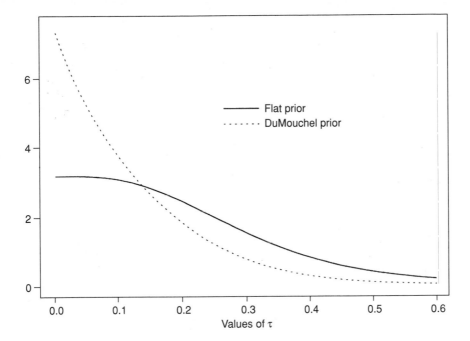

Fig. 11.5 Posterior distributions of τ

indicating the greater amount of information about the mean of the effect sizes of the case–control studies. The posterior means and covariance matrices using the three prior distributions, respectively, are given in Table 11.2. The posterior means and variances given the prior proportional to $1/\tau^2$ are again essentially identical to those in the fixed effects model assuming that $\tau = 0$, a priori.

As in the case when all of the effect sizes were considered exchangeable, the posterior means are not much affected by the choice of prior distribution, but the posterior standard deviation and the posterior probability that the effect is positive are more greatly affected. These analyses suggest that there is some reason to believe that effects are slightly larger for the cohort studies, but there is weak evidence that the mean effects are positive for both types of studies. The posterior probability that

Table 11.2 Posterior means of effect sizes from the USEPA data using the bivariate model (separate effects for case–control and cohort studies) for three prior distributions

Prior	$\tilde{\mu}_1$	$\tilde{\mu}_2$	$\tilde{\sigma}_{11}$	$\tilde{\sigma}_{22}$	$\tilde{\sigma}_{12}$	$P(\tilde{\mu}_1 > 0)$	$P(\tilde{\mu}_2 > 0)$
$\pi(\tau) \propto 1$	0.159	0.270	0.048	0.187	0.000	0.780	0.745
$\pi(\tau) \propto S_{.}/(S_{.}+\tau)^2$	0.159	0.258	0.041	0.155	0.000	0.844	0.800
$\pi(\tau) \propto 1/\tau^2$	0.160	0.248	0.036	0.133	0.000	0.800	0.752

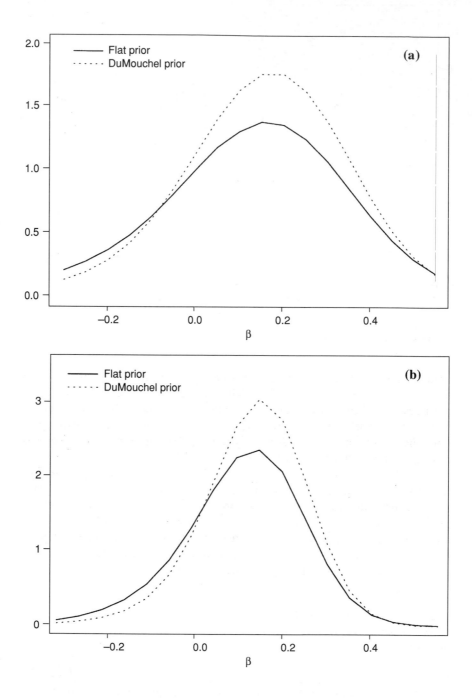

Fig. 11.6 Posterior distribution of (a) β_1 and (b) β_2

Table 11.3 Effect size estimates and posterior means of effect sizes from the USEPA data using the bivariate model (separate effects for case–control and cohort studies)

Study	T_i	S_i	Flat prior $\tilde{\theta}_i$	$\tilde{S}_i$	DuMouchel prior $\tilde{\theta}_i$	$\tilde{S}_i$
Brownson *et al.* (1987)	0.405	0.695	0.187	0.322	0.255	0.333
Buffler *et al.* (1984)	−0.386	0.451	0.091	0.315	0.190	0.323
Butler (1988)	0.698	0.730	0.315	0.467	0.414	0.535
Correa *et al.* (1983)	0.637	0.481	0.225	0.315	0.281	0.333
Fontham *et al.* (1991)	0.247	0.134	0.188	0.249	0.259	0.292
Garfinkel *et al.* (1985)	0.239	0.206	0.181	0.270	0.252	0.304
Garfinkel (1981)	0.148	0.163	0.241	0.374	0.364	0.474
Humble *et al.* (1987)	0.693	0.544	0.226	0.321	0.281	0.336
Janerich *et al.* (1990)	−0.236	0.246	0.085	0.288	0.182	0.307
Kabat and Wynder (1984)	−0.315	0.591	0.111	0.321	0.204	0.327
Wu *et al.* (1985)	0.278	0.487	0.179	0.309	0.249	0.325

the effect is positive is less than 0.85 for all of the priors. Table 11.3 gives the (unconditional) posterior means and variances of the $\tilde{\theta}_i$ given the flat and DuMouchel prior distributions. The individual estimates are essentially equal to the fixed effects estimates of β_1 or β_2 for the prior proportional to $1/\tau^2$.

11.5 Prior distributions

For many statisticians and researchers, the use of prior distributions in Bayesian inference is problematic because it introduces a troubling source of arbitrariness in the analysis. Consequently, many statisticians feel it is desirable to select a prior distribution according to rules that remove the arbitrariness. When the researcher has no real prior information the notion of choosing an 'uninformative' prior which represents complete ignorance has great appeal, but is hard to characterize precisely. A cogent review of principles for choosing uninformative prior distributions is given by Kass and Wasserman (1996), who argue that no one principle is necessarily adequate in all situations. They note, however, that most principles lead to similar choices for uninformative priors in many situations.

In the linear models such as those considered in this chapter, the uninformative prior of choice for β is proportional to a constant, which is used here by assuming a normal distribution whose variance tends to infinity. In the case of τ, a prior proportional to a constant cannot be justified by a principle of uninformativeness, but the choice of $\pi(\tau) \propto 1$

(the flat prior) is often suggested for convenience. For example, Gelman *et al.* (1995) suggest the flat prior as a starting point for analyses, which should include analysis of sensitivity of results to other plausible choices of prior distributions for τ.

The justification of a prior for τ using principles of uninformativeness is more difficult, although most principles, such as Jeffrey's rule or Box and Tiao's (1973) method based on data-translated likelihoods, suggest a prior proportional to $1/\tau$. Unfortunately, this prior does not yield an integrable posterior distribution in the current problem and thus it cannot be used. One might look for alternative distributions that share some of the qualitative properties of $\pi(\tau) \propto 1/\tau$, namely distributions that concentrate mass at zero, but which are highly dispersed. A simple alternative that does give a proper posterior distribution is to make the prior proportional to $1/\tau^2$, but this choice of prior is much more concentrated at $\tau = 0$.

Another approach to specifying a prior distribution is to draw on the substantive meaning of the parameters in the problem. Since τ represents between-study variation in effects, it is reasonable to set expectations about τ in terms of $S_1, \ldots, S_k$, the precision of estimates of effect size. It is reasonable to argue that studies should not be combined if the true effects are too different, for in that case they would be estimating dramatically different things. A natural criterion for judging the magnitude of between-study (between-effect size parameter) variation is the within-study variation estimated by the sampling standard error of the effect size estimates. There is at least some empirical evidence (from reviews in the physical and social sciences) that the estimated between-study variation of studies that have been combined in meta-analyses is slightly smaller than the typical sampling error variance: usually τ^2 is 25% to 100% the size of the average S_i^2 (Hedges, 1987, Schmidt, 1992).

A prior that has many desirable properties (suggested by DuMouchel) is

$$\pi(\tau) \propto S_{.}/(S_{.} + \tau)^2 \tag{11.34}$$

where S^2 is the harmonic mean of the sampling variances of the effect size estimates given by

$$S_{.}^2 = k/(S_1^{-2} + \cdots + S_k^{-2})$$

This prior has the advantage of having substantial mass at $\tau = 0$ while being highly dispersed (the expectations of τ and $1/\tau$ are both infinite). Indeed the first and 99th percentiles are $S_{.}/99$ and $99S_{.}$, so a very wide range of values of τ have non-negligible prior probability. Yet the distribution concentrates mass near $S_{.}$, since the first and third quartiles are about $S_{.}/3$ and $3S_{.}$.

When there is a substantial amount of data, the choice of prior will not greatly affect the results of analyses. However, when there are only a few studies, the choice of prior distribution may have a substantial effect on results. It is therefore especially important to experiment with alternative prior specifications when conducting meta-analyses of small data sets. We demonstrate the use of three prior distributions in the examples: the flat prior ($\pi(\tau) \propto 1$), the DuMouchel prior, and $\pi(\tau) \propto 1/\tau^2$.

Formulating informative prior distributions involves different considerations. Such distributions might come from the distribution of estimates from previous analyses of independent studies if they are both relevant and available. Informative priors might also be constructed on the basis of expert judgement. There is a considerable literature on the elicitation of prior distributions from experts, which may be of interest when the incorporation of expert judgement into meta-analyses is contemplated (Kadane *et al.*, 1980, Winkler, 1967).

11.6 Conclusions

The models given in this chapter can be applied in a wide variety of situations in which meta-analysis is appropriate, and they can be applied whether or not the sampling errors of effect size estimates can be taken as independent of one another. Bayesian analyses provide a way to include specific prior evidence (such as the results of previous studies or previous meta-analyses) or prior belief (such as expert opinion) into the combination of evidence across studies. Even when specific prior information is not available, Bayesian models permit the incorporation of the uncertainty about between-study variation into the analysis. This is critically important because the number of effect estimates is typically small and therefore estimates of between-studies variance components are likely to be poor (highly uncertain).

References

Box, G. E. P. and Tiao, G. C. 1973: *Bayesian inference in statistical analysis*. New York: John Wiley.

Brownson, R. C., Reif, J. S., Keefe, T. J., Ferguson, S. W. and Pritzl, J. A. 1987: Risk factors for adenocarcinoma of the lung. *American Journal of Epidemiology* **125**, 25–34.

Buffler, P. A., Pickle, L. W., Mason, T. J. and Contant, C. 1984: The causes of lung cancer in Texas. In Mizell, M. and Correa, P. (eds), *Lung cancer: causes and prevention*. New York: Verlag Chemie International, 83–99.

Butler, T. L. 1988: The relationship of passive smoking to various health outcomes among Seventh-Day Adventists in California. Unpublished doctoral dissertation, UCLA.

Carlin, J. B. 1992: Meta-analysis for 2 × 2 tables: A Bayesian approach. *Statistics in Medicine* **11**, 141–58.

Chalmers, I. 1988: *Oxford database of perinatal trials*. Oxford: Oxford University Press.

Correa, P., Fontham, E., Pickle, L. and Haensel, W. 1983: Passive smoking and lung cancer. *Lancet* 2, 595–7.

DerSimonian, R. and Laird, N. 1986: Meta-analysis in clinical trials. *Controlled Clinical Trials* 7, 177–88.

DuMouchel, W. H. 1990: Bayesian meta-analysis. In Berry, D. A. (ed.) *Statistical methodology in pharmaceutical sciences*. New York: Marcel Dekker, 509–29.

DuMouchel, W. H. and Harris, J. E. 1983: Bayes method for combining the results of cancer studies in humans and other species. *Journal of the American Statistical Association* **78**, 293–315.

Eddy, D. M., Hasselblad, V. and Shachter, R. 1992: *Meta-analysis by the confidence profile method: the statistical synthesis of evidence*. Boston: Academic Press.

Efron, B. and Morris, C. 1973: Combining possibly related estimation problems. *Journal of the Royal Statistical Society (B)* **35**, 379–421.

Fleiss, J. L. 1973: *Statistical methods for rates and proportions*. New York: John Wiley.

Fleiss, J. L. 1994: Measures of effect size for categorical data. In Cooper, H. and Hedges, L. V. (eds), *The handbook of research synthesis*. New York: Russell Sage Foundation, 245–60.

Fontham, E. T. H. *et al.* 1991: Lung cancer in nonsmoking women: a multicenter case–control study. *Cancer Epidemiology Biomarkers Prevention* **1**, 35–334.

Garfinkel, L. 1981: Time trends in lung cancer mortality among nonsmokers and a note on passive smoking. *Journal of the National Cancer Institute* **6**, 1061–6.

Garfinkel, L., Auerbach, O. and Joubert, L. 1985: Involuntary smoking and lung cancer: a case–control study. *Journal of the National Cancer Institute* **75**, 463–9.

Gelman, A., Carlin, J. B., Stern, H. S. and Rubin, D. B. 1995: *Bayesian data analysis*. London: Chapman & Hall.

Harville, D. A. 1977: Maximum likelihood approaches to variance components estimation and to related problems. *Journal of the American Statistical Association* **72**, 320–40.

Hedges, L. V. 1982: Estimation of effect size from a series of independent experiments. *Psychological Bulletin* **92**, 490–9.

Hedges, L. V. 1983: A random effects model for effect sizes. *Psychological Bulletin* **93**, 388–95.

Hedges, L. V. 1987: How hard is hard science, how soft is soft science? The empirical cumulativity of research. *American Psychologist* **42**, 443–55.

Hedges, L. V. and Olkin, I. 1983: Regression models in research synthesis. *American Statistician* **37**, 137–40.

Hedges, L. V. and Olkin, I. 1985: *Statistical methods for meta-analysis*. New York: Academic Press.

Humble, C. G., Samet, J. M. and Pathak, D. R. 1987: Marriage to a smoker and lung cancer risk. *American Journal of Public Health* **77**, 598–602.

Janerich, D. T. *et al.* 1990: Lung cancer and exposure to tobacco smoke in the household. *New England Journal of Medicine* **323**, 632–6.

Kabat, G. C. and Wynder, E. L. 1984: Lung cancer in nonsmokers. *Cancer* **53**, 1214–21.

Kadane, J. B., Dickey, J. M., Winkler, R. L., Smith, W. S. and Peters, S. C. 1980: Interactive elicitation of opinion for a normal linear model. *Journal of the American Statistical Association* **75**, 845–54.

Kass, R. E. and Wasserman, L. 1996: The selection of prior distributions by formal rules. *Journal of the American Statistical Association* **91**, 1343–70.

Laird, N. M. and Ware, J. H. 1982: Random effects models for longitudinal data. *Biometrics* **38**, 963–74.

Louis, T. A., Fineberg, H. V. and Mosteller, F. 1985: Findings for public health from meta-analysis. *Annual Review of Public Health* **6**, 1–20.

McCormick, K. A., Moore, S. R. and Siegel, R. A. (eds) 1994: *Clinical practice guideline development: methodological perspectives.* Washington, DC: US Agency for Health Care Policy and Research.

National Research Council 1992: *Combining information: statistical issues and opportunities for research.* Washington, DC: National Academy Press.

Raudenbush, S. W. 1994: Random effects models. In Cooper, H. and Hedges, L. V. (eds), *The handbook of research synthesis.* New York: Russell Sage Foundation, 301–21.

Rubin, D. B. 1981: Estimation in parallel randomized experiments. *Journal of Educational Statistics* **6**, 377–401.

Schmidt, F. L. 1992: What do data really mean? Research findings, meta-analysis, and cumulative findings in psychology. *American Psychologist* **47**, 1173–81.

Seltzer, M. 1993: Sensitivity analysis for fixed effects in the hierarchical model: a Gibbs sampling approach. *Journal of Educational Statistics* **18**, 207–35.

Seltzer, M. H., Wong, W. H. and Bryk, A. S. 1996: Bayesian analysis in applications of hierarchical models: issues and methods. *Journal of Educational and Behavioral Statistics* **21**, 131–67.

Shadish, W. R. and Haddock, C. K. 1994: Combining estimates of effect size. In Cooper, H. and Hedges, L. V. (eds), *The handbook of research synthesis.* New York: Russell Sage Foundation, 261–81.

Smith, A. F. M. 1973. Bayes estimates in one-way and two-way models. *Biometrika* **60**, 319–29.

Smith, T. C., Spiegelhalter, D. J. and Thomas, A. 1995: Bayesian approaches to random-effects meta-analysis: a comparative study. *Statistics in Medicine* **14**, 2685–99.

Winkler, R. L. 1967: The assessment of prior distributions in Bayesian analysis. *Journal of the American Statistical Association* **62**, 1105–20.

Wu, A. H., Henderson, B. E., Pike, M. D. and Yu, M. C. 1985: Smoking and other risk factors for lung cancer in women. *Journal of the National Cancer Institute* **74**, 747–51.

12 Functional neuroimaging and statistics

Ian Ford and Andrew P. Holmes

12.1 Introduction

This chapter provides a brief description of the role of statistics in the construction and analysis of neuroimages. Areas of application discussed include autoradiography, single-photon emission computed tomography (SPECT), positron emission tomography (PET), functional magnetic resonance imaging (fMRI) and electroencephalography (EEG).

12.1.1 Imaging modalities

Autoradiography is, in a sense, the simplest technique to describe. *In vivo* autoradiography is used in animal experiments. Here, an experimental animal is injected with a solution of radioactive material. This is taken up and transported by the blood to the brain. At the same time, the animal is subjected to some form of stimulus. Radioactively labelled materials are used which will be absorbed by the brain tissue in increasing amounts with increasing brain activity. Hence the brain becomes radioactive, with a spatial distribution which directly relates to local neuronal activity. The animal is then sacrificed and the brain fixed, frozen and then sliced. Slices of brain tissue are placed directly against photographic plates. The exposed plates therefore contain direct images of the levels of radioactivity in the brain. These images can then be scanned and analysed using quantitative densitometry. *In vitro* autoradiography is also used. Here, post-mortem human brains are obtained soon after death and frozen at $-80°C$. At a later stage, slices of tissue can be defrosted and dipped into buckets of radioactive material designed to adhere to brain sites for specific neurotransmitters. The construction of images then proceeds as for *in vivo* autoradiography. This technique can be used to study abnormality in receptor distributions for subjects who have died from neurodegenerative conditions such as Alzheimer's disease.

In both PET and SPECT, a radioactive tracer is administered to the subject being studied, either by injection or by inhalation. The tracer finds its way to the brain via the circulatory system. The radioisotope is incorporated into a molecule that is absorbed into brain tissue and resides there in concentrations that indicate levels of metabolic activity or the distribution of neuroreceptors. Different radiochemicals are required to map different measures of metabolic activity, such as glucose utilization or blood flow. PET and SPECT studies differ fundamentally in the type of isotope used. SPECT isotopes are gamma emitters that decay to release single photons from locations in the brain. PET isotopes emit positrons, which in turn cause the simultaneous release of pairs of photons at 180° to each other. The gamma emitters tend to have long half lives while positron emitters have very short half lives. These facts result in significant differences between the two modalities, both in the engineering of the imaging systems and in the applications that can be addressed. In both systems, banks of gamma detectors count the photons that are emitted from a patient's head. In some instruments, the detectors move during the scanning session, recording radioactive counts in each position. These data are then processed using reconstruction algorithms to produce images (maps) of radiation levels in the brain. Using a freely diffusible blood flow tracer, such as positron-emitting (^{15}O) water, quantitative estimates of regional cerebral blood flow (rCBF) can be repeatedly obtained on a single subject with relatively little radiation exposure. These images are indicative of brain activity, since an increase in local neuronal activity causes an increase in rCBF to supply the required glucose and oxygen. In the last decade this has led to a new field of human neuroscience, namely functional brain mapping.

More recently, developments in magnetic resonance imaging, which had previously been limited to studies of brain structure, have provided the opportunity to study brain function. BOLD (Blood Oxygenation Level Dependent) fMRI gives images indicative of the relative proportions of blood oxy and deoxyhaemoglobin, considered indicative of local neuronal function. Although the exact nature of the fMRI signal is still not fully understood, one explanation is that the increased rCBF supplies oxygen at a rate which outstrips demand, resulting in relatively oxyhaemoglobin-rich blood in the vicinity of an activation. However, the signal is sensitive to subject movement, artefactual effects from neighbouring major vessels, to proximate bone or air pockets in the skull, and to cardiac and respiratory cycles. Although these problems may make certain types of study difficult, fMRI has a number of major advantages over PET and SPECT. Firstly, the technique is based on electromagnetic radiation and does not involve the exposure of subjects to radioactive materials. Secondly, images can be obtained within a fraction of a second, rather than the minutes required to obtain images using the other approaches. This improved time resolution is important in providing information about temporal aspects of brain processes.

Further improvements in time resolution can be obtained by moving to another approach to brain imaging, namely EEG. In EEG electrical potentials on the surface of the brain are observed directly from a net of electrodes placed on the scalp. This approach provides excellent time resolution but has the disadvantage of providing poorer spatial resolution caused by problems in inferring the sources of the electrical activity within the brain.

12.1.2 Reconstruction

From all of these approaches, we obtain two-dimensional (2D) or three-dimensional (3D) maps of some measure of cerebral metabolic function. These maps normally consist of average levels of activity for square pixels (2D) or cuboidal voxels (3D) of tissue. For brevity, voxel-level data will be assumed from now on. By its nature, autoradiography is a direct imaging technique with levels of radioactivity being imaged from the impact of the Poisson emissions of radioactive particles from the brain tissue on the photographic plate. Hence autoradiography represents the gold standard against which other techniques based on radioactive emissions must be judged. A detailed discussion of tomographic image reconstruction is beyond the scope of this chapter. However, it is worthy of note that for PET and SPECT, the problem can be formulated as a Poisson regression model with a very large number of parameters (Herman, 1980, Vardi *et al.*, 1985, Green, 1990). In this model, the observations are the radiation counts accumulated by the detectors outside the patient's head and the parameters are the voxel-level intensities within the brain. Hence, at least in theory, standard statistical approaches can be taken for the estimation of the unknown parameters, although, in practice, non-statistical algorithms are often used for computational reasons (Snyder and Politte, 1983, Defrise *et al.,* 1989, 1990, Townsend *et al.*, 1991). Autoradiography or tomographic reconstruction of PET or SPECT images generates, in the first instance, a map of radiation levels across the brain. Often this is what is used for analysis purposes. However, if there is a requirement to measure metabolic activity in absolute units, then the relationship between the input function of radiation to the patient to the output measured by the detection process must be modelled. Some form of compartmental model is generally used to calibrate the radiation levels or to estimate parameters of interest.

12.1.3 Overview

In some cases, interest lies in studying an individual patient's scan for clinical reasons – for instance, to identify areas of unusually low metabolic activity associated with stroke or the presence of a tumour. Clinical applications are becoming more common, as the necessary equipment becomes cheaper and more widely available. However, the major use of these techniques has been in research. Initially, this work focused on cross-sectional studies of patient groups, defined by disease status, age or some other variable. These studies usually concentrated on the analysis of data in anatomically defined regions of the brain. In each subject, anatomical knowledge was used to identify specific regions of the brain, either directly from the functional image or with the aid of a structural image from an MRI or CT scan. Under the assumption that metabolic activity was uniform across these areas, a data value was created by averaging activity over all voxels in the region of interest (ROI). The ROI approach thus generates a multivariate data vector for each subject. ROI approaches are discussed in Section 12.2.

Functional mapping experiments seek to investigate the structure–function relationship of the healthy brain, by repeatedly imaging indicators of neuronal activity while the subject performs carefully designed tasks in a suitably designed experiment. The simplest activation experiments use a small number of conditions differing only by a single cognitive component. Condition-dependent changes in regional metabolic activity are small, necessitating replication of studies possibly within and across subjects and the development of statistical techniques to locate areas of the brain that have been stimulated by specific tasks. Without prior hypotheses regarding the anatomical localization of the cognitive component of interest, analysis must proceed at the voxel level. Voxel-by-voxel approaches are discussed in Section 12.3.

12.2   Statistical methods for ROI data in cross-sectional studies

12.2.1   The data

For a given subject j, in a treatment group or disease category i, the data will consist of a K vector of observations y_{ij}, $j = 1, \ldots, n_i$; $i = 1, \ldots, I$. These observations are on the same scale of measurement and hence can be thought of as repeated measures. It is worth noting that, unlike voxels, the K ROIs are not generally all of the same size or shape. Metabolic activity in the resting normal brain is largely left/right (LHS/RHS) symmetric. Specific stimuli, on the other hand, generate asymmetric responses and certain neurological illnesses appear to have associated asymmetries in brain function. For these reasons, K is often equal to $2K_0$, where K_0 is the number of anatomically distinct ROIs, and measurements are made on both sides of the brain. Occasionally, the data set includes a small number of centrally located ROIs.

K is usually large, particularly relative to $N = \sum n_i$. This reflects both the high per capita cost of these studies and logistical problems in recruiting and obtaining good-quality scans on normal controls and patients.

12.2.2   The normalization problem

In some PET and most SPECT studies, the elements of y_{ij} are reconstructed mean counts of radiation. There is non-trivial variability among subjects in the amount of radioactivity which is administered and in particular in the amount of radioactive material which penetrates and is trapped in brain tissue. This induces a scalar multiplicative source of variation in all regions in the same subject. This source of variability is largely spurious and may need to be adjusted for in some way. Even when kinetic models have been applied to provide measurements on an absolute scale, a 'subject effect' may still be present although possibly to a reduced degree. There are various sources of global variation, including between-subject variability in the general level of activation in the brain in any given context and even considerable variability within a subject over time (Camargo *et al.*, 1992, Yoshii *et al.*, 1988, Videen *et al.*, 1988, Martin *et al.*, 1991). The result is that usually one must analyse profiles of response across the brain rather than the actual levels. This can be done by first normalizing the data or by incorporating an implicit normalizing factor into the model used for analysis, as in a repeated measures ANOVA. The simplest approaches are based on normalizing the regional values by either dividing by or subtracting a measure of global activity. These approaches have the advantage of transparency and ease of interpretation. The user can readily interpret the normalized values as activity relative to a global subject level.

An alternative approach which will yield similar results to the ratio method is to take logarithms of the data first and then subtract the logarithmic means from the regional values. Statistical tests are then applied to the regional adjusted values. Friston *et al.* (1990) have suggested that analysis of covariance (ANCOVA) may provide more powerful tests of regional differences. This approach is based on modelling the relationship between the local regional value and the measure of global activity. An important factor in determining whether or not this will be beneficial is the magnitude of the correlation between the local and global values and whether this correlation is similar in the groups being compared. The higher the underlying correlation, the more powerful the corresponding test for a difference between groups is likely to be. It is possible that this correlation will vary across the brain and hence the power of the test to detect evidence of activation will vary. Since the ANCOVA is carried out separately for each region, normalized images, scaled to a common global mean using this approach, would not necessarily show the same patterns of activity as the original images. In particular the rank order of the ANCOVA-adjusted values would not necessarily be the same as for the original raw data. Of course, the correct approach to this problem depends on the actual underlying subject/source component of variation, be it additive, multiplicative or in the form of a more complex relationship. This is still a controversial subject.

Consider first the cross-sectional data context involving two groups. An appropriate ANCOVA would be based on the following model for the regional responses across groups and subjects for data in a given region k:

$$y_{ijk} = \mu_k + \alpha_{ik} + \beta_k \bar{y}_{ij.} + \epsilon_{ijk}$$

where y_{ijk} is the measure of blood flow in region k of subject j in group i, and $\bar{y}_{ij.}$ a measure of global blood flow. The parameters are μ_k, an overall mean, α_{ik}, the group effect, β_k, a regression coefficient, and ϵ_{ijk}, error terms which are independent across subjects. With the exception of the assumption of constant slope across the groups within each region, and the fact that the covariate is the mean of the response over regions, this model is not particularly problematic.

An alternative method, particularly in the study of patient populations, is to normalize with respect to activity in a brain region believed to be unaffected by the illness being studied.

It is difficult to obtain data to validate any particular method so, in practice, researchers tend to adopt a particular method and hope that strong signals in the data will show up despite flaws in the analytical approach applied. However, there is clearly great potential for confusion. McCrory and Ford (1991) illustrate some of the problems which can arise in a two-group SPECT study involving normal controls and sufferers from Alzheimer's disease. They consider transformations of the form:

(i) y_{ijk}

(ii) $y_{ijk}/\bar{y}_{ij.}$

(iii) y_{ijk}/y_{ij1}

(iv) y_{ijk}/y_{ij2}

Here y_{ij1} and y_{ij2} are levels of blood flow in the occipital and basal ganglia regions of the brain respectively, regions which are thought to be spared in Alzheimer's disease.

The transformed data were then compared between the groups applying two-sample t tests. It was seen that in (i) no significant differences were obtained because of the substantial between-subject variation. In (ii), tests for the regions where blood flow would be expected to be reduced did not reach statistical significance because global flow was also reduced. In fact, the regions showing significant differences were the basal ganglia and the occipital, exactly those which are probably unaffected by the disease. Apparent increases were seen in these regions in the Alzheimer subjects because of the reduction in global flow. In (iii) and (iv), tests for the regions which one would, a priori, have expected to be affected by the disease showed up as being significant, although the results after normalization to the basal ganglia were less well determined.

This example illustrates the point that many factors are at play in these apparently simple tests. The disease may be affecting either or both of the terms in the ratios. In addition, the variances and covariances of the two basic variables involved play a significant role in the outcome of these tests.

12.2.3   Correlation analyses

The brain can be thought of as a large and complex network of interconnected neurones. There are known connections between brain regions which are physically far apart. These connections should manifest themselves in PET and SPECT data as correlations between observations in different brain regions. Many diseases of the brain lead to neuronal death and it is natural, in studying the diseased, to investigate and compare patterns of correlation across the brain. Worsley *et al.* (1991) have proposed models for the interregional correlation structure in FDG PET scans on normal subjects. Their models focus primarily on the distance between brain regions and on additional simple features such as side of brain. As noted above, this is probably too naïve an approach to represent the overall pattern of correlation. Despite this, Worsley *et al.* had a moderate degree of success in fitting these models to their data. Tyler *et al.* (1988) and Worsley *et al.* (1991) also note, in the case of data with a symmetric LHS/RHS structure, that if one transforms to hemispheric SUMS and DIFFERENCES then the SUMS appear to be uncorrelated with the DIFFERENCES. This is useful, since it provides a data reduction mechanism to facilitate the study of correlations and other analyses based on separate analyses of the SUMS and DIFFERENCES.

Although this fact is interesting in resting normal subjects, it is important to carry out investigations in diseased groups. McCrory and Ford (1991) applied a similar analysis to SPECT scans in normal subjects and subjects with probable Alzheimer's disease. They obtained results similar to those of Tyler *et al.* (1988) for normal controls. There also appeared to be relatively little correlation among the regional DIFFERENCES. In the Alzheimer's disease group, the correlations between SUMS and DIFFERENCES and among DIFFERENCES were slightly higher but not to an extent that the authors thought outweighed the advantages of the data reduction achieved.

It should be clear that methodological and other factors, which lead to substantial random subject effects, can create difficulties in the interpretation of correlations calculated on raw data. A number of authors (Horwitz *et al.*, 1984, Metter *et al.*, 1984a, 1984b) have considered alternative approaches, either explicitly normalizing the data prior to calculating correlations or calculating partial correlations conditional on a measure such as subject global activity. However, different approaches to normalization can induce different apparent correlation structures and Ford (1986) has pointed out that, in certain circumstances, spurious correlations can be generated. Given the inadequacies of the available data, therefore, extreme caution should be exercised in the interpretation of any calculated correlations.

12.2.4   Factor analytic approaches

There have been a number of applications of factor analytic methods to PET ROI data. PET data sets often consist of a large number of ROIs for a – relatively speaking – small number of subjects. For instance, Horwitz *et al.* (1986) studied 59 regions in comparing two groups of 15 subjects. Rather than using a priori criteria to preselect a smaller number of regions for investigation, we postulate that the data have a fair degree of redundancy and that much of the linked activity and hence correlation structure in brain activity is explained by a small number of subnetworks. If these subnetworks can be identified, then more focused investigations of differences between disease groups or of correlations between PET data and clinical data can be carried out.

Needless to say, different authors have taken different approaches to this problem, making comparison of their results difficult. All, however, have applied some form of principal components factor analysis.

Once again the random subject effect is a problem. Given its presence, it is inevitable that the first principal component, calculated on the correlation matrix for the raw data, will be very similar to the average activity over the ROIs studied. Clark *et al.* (1985) carried out a principal components analysis on the 'correlation' matrix calculated by reversing the roles of subjects and ROIs. The product–moment correlation coefficient between the vectors of data on subject *i* and subject *j* was regarded as a distance measure between the two ROI profiles. The authors noted that this approach involved an automatic normalization factor for global activity.

Moeller *et al.* (1987) and Moeller and Strother (1991) described what they called the scaled subprofile model. In their approach, the data were first log transformed, the ROI values were then normalized to have zero mean for each subject and a principal components analysis was carried out using the between-ROI covariance matrix of the transformed data. The rest of the details are rather complex but the general approach is rather similar to the FANOVA technique (Yochmowitz, 1983). One feature of this approach is that, when analysing data from different groups, all subjects are included in the principal components analysis without any adjustment for the known group membership. This is understandable to the extent that the authors wished to go on to study group differences with respect to the factors selected. However, the principal components might be affected substantially by the relative sample sizes in the two groups.

Despite these misgivings, this approach has been applied with apparent success to a number of disease states.

Worsley *et al.* (1991) carried out separate principal components analyses on the regional SUMS and DIFFERENCES, taking advantage of the apparent independence of these two groups of variables. The DIFFERENCES are implicitly normalized for an additive subject effect. More recently, McLaughlin *et al.* (1992) carried out a SPECT study of blood flow. In this study 10 subjects were investigated in three conditions each (at rest and with two aural stimulation paradigms); 28 ROIs were identified and studied. The 30 scans (10 subjects by three conditions) were regarded as independent replications and a principal components factor analysis was carried out, followed by varimax rotation. The authors identified three subnetworks in their data (auditory/linguistic, attentional and visual imaging). No a priori normalization was applied.

12.3 Functional mapping – voxel-level approaches

Until recently, a detailed knowledge of the functional anatomy of the human brain was not available, the only information coming from lesion deficit studies (where function is inferred from the disabilities of subjects with focal brain injuries), or (comparatively) from invasive studies of primates. In the absence of a prior anatomical hypothesis, functional mapping studies have traditionally been analysed voxel by voxel. The approaches in common use are massively univariate. Typically, an activation study generates a 3D map (statistical parametric map) of (highly correlated) test statistics, each assessing the evidence for the presence of activation in a single voxel. The assessment of these statistic images presents a large multiple comparisons problem. Interest lies in identifying the locations of activation, not just in assessing whether or not there is any evidence at all of activation (omnibus test). Thus, this large multiple comparisons problem must be addressed with a technique providing strong control of familywise Type I error, so that the location as well as the presence of an activation can be reported.

12.3.1 Preprocessing

A prerequisite for the analysis of data pooled within or across subjects at the voxel level is that any given voxel represents the same anatomical region across images. Within a subject, images must be realigned to account for interscan movement. Between subjects, images must be spatially normalized to account for differences in individual anatomy, usually by warping the observed images (Friston *et al.*, 1995d) to 'match' a reference image in a standard space (Talairach and Tournoux, 1988). This can involve various image processing techniques, such as segmentation with prior knowledge, but a detailed description is beyond the scope of this chapter. The spatial normalization accounts for (large scale) intersubject anatomical variability, but is applied even to single-subject experiments to allow localization in the standard reference frame. In addition images are often smoothed with a spherical Gaussian kernel of FWHM ~4 mm (fMRI) to ~12 mm (PET). (FWHM, Full Width at Half Maximum, is a measure of resolution. A univariate Gaussian kernel has FWHM of $\sigma\sqrt{(8\ln 2)}$, where σ is the standard deviation of the Gaussian kernel.) Spatial smoothing is performed to improve signal to noise, reduce residual intersubject anatomical variability, and, for certain types of analysis, to condition the spatial autocovariance of the images to permit their consideration as lattice representations of continuous random fields, a topic we shall return to.

12.3.2   Experimental designs and data sets

The PET data set we shall consider involves the study of a single subject in a language experiment (Silbersweig *et al.*, 1994). The experiment was

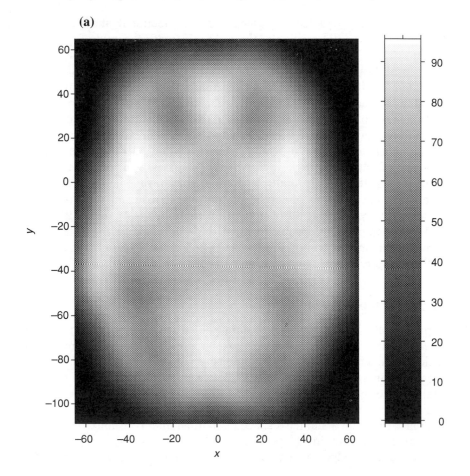

(b)

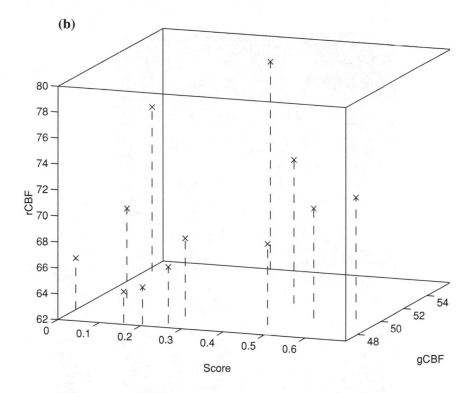

Fig. 12.1 PET data set. (a) Transverse slice of the first acquisition at the level of the intercommissural line ($z = 0$), after anatomical transformation to Talairach space, the current neuroanatomical reference space. The axes are graduated in millimetres, with x running from left to right, y from posterior to anterior. (b) Plot of rCBF vs. gCBF (global flow) vs. score across scans for the $2 \times 2 \times 4\,mm^3$ voxel centred at (30, −40, 8).

designed to investigate the potential of PET for investigating transitory events. The technique was subsequently used with hallucinating schizophrenics who were able to report reliably the onset of their hallucinations, permitting localization of the implicated brain region (Silbersweig *et al.*, 1995). During each of 12 scans, the subject was presented with short sentences of mixed content, at a fixed rate for each scan. The rates for each scan were chosen randomly from 12 rates ranging from occasional to almost continuous presentation. The subject indicated by a button press when he or she heard the stimuli, and for each scan a score was computed indicating the proportion of time spent under the stimulation condition. Voxels with rCBF positively correlated with the score across scans are assumed to be those activated by the stimulus. Figure 12.1 shows a slice of one scan and the data for a voxel in the primary auditory cortex.

The simplest fMRI experiments are simple activation experiments comparing an activation condition with a rest condition. Owing to drifts in baseline and low frequency aliasing of cardiac and respiratory effects,

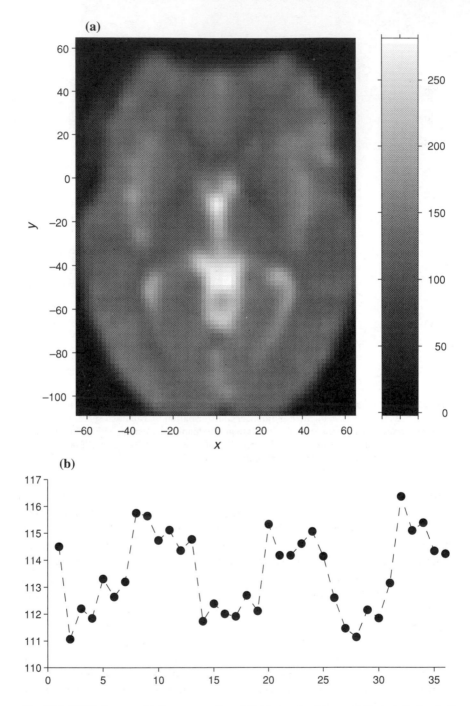

Fig. 12.2 fMRI data set. (a) Transverse slice of the first activation acquisition at the level of the intercommissural line ($z = 0$), after anatomical transformation to Talairach space and smoothing with a spherical Gaussian kernel of FWHM 5 mm. (b) Plot of signal vs. scan number for the $2 \times 2 \times 2\,mm^3$ voxel centred at $(50, -40, 8)$

the two conditions must be presented quickly, frequently and alternately, leading to designs where 20–40 s blocks of scans are acquired alternately under each condition. The following experiment is typical: 64 slice $3 \times 3 \times 3 \, \text{mm}^3$ BOLD/EPI acquisitions were made every 7 seconds; 16 blocks of six scans (42 s blocks) were used, the condition for successive blocks alternating between rest and auditory stimuli, starting with rest. During the activation condition, the subject was presented binaurally with bisyllabic words at a rate of 60 per minute. For various physical and psychological reasons the first few scans are atypical. Here we consider six blocks from the middle of the experiment, starting with a rest block (Fig. 12.2)

12.3.3 Formation of statistic image

Simple univariate models are built for the data at each voxel (across scans), and simple univariate statistics formed for the appropriate null hypothesis at that voxel. Let Y_j^k be the observed data at voxel k of observation j, where $k = 1, \ldots, K$ and $j = 1, \ldots, M$. A multivariate regression model is typically assumed, $Y = X\beta + \epsilon$.

Here Y is the data matrix, an $M \times K$ matrix with jkth element Y_j^k. Thus, the rows of Y ($\mathbf{Y}_j^\top$) are row vectors of length K consisting of the jth scan, and the columns of $Y = (\mathbf{Y}^1 \ldots \mathbf{Y}^k \ldots \mathbf{Y}^K)$ are column vectors of length M containing the data at voxel k across scans. X is the design matrix, an $M \times L$ matrix, where L is the number of model parameters. $\beta = (\beta^1 \ldots \beta^k \ldots \beta^K)$ is the matrix of parameters, an $L \times K$ matrix with kth column β^k, the parameters for the model at voxel k.

The $M \times K$ matrix ϵ contains the residual errors, with jkth element ϵ_j^k, and jth row ϵ_j. Standard multivariate analysis (assuming $\epsilon_j \sim N_K(0, \Sigma)$) is not feasible, since the number of observations is considerably less than their dimensionality, leading to singular estimates of the error covariance matrix Σ. An alternative approach is to impose a structure on Σ. For instance, we might assume the (standardized) error images to be strictly stationary, discrete Gaussian random fields, such that the correlation between the errors at two voxels is a function of their displacement (Friston *et al.*, 1995c). This leads to tests based on the theory of random fields, described below. A further possibility is to work with the first few principal components of the data. Friston *et al.* (1996) performed such multivariate analyses for problems where the presence but not the localization of an effect was of interest.

12.3.3.1 PET model

For our example PET experiment, let Y_j^k be the rCBF measurement at voxel k at observation $j = 1, \ldots, M$. Let $g_j = \bar{y}_j$ be the corresponding gCBF, and S_j the hallucination score. Using ANCOVA-style global normalization, a commonly used model is

$$Y_j^k = \mu^k + \rho^k S_j + \zeta^k(g_j - \overline{g}.) + \epsilon_j^k$$

or, as a multivariate regression (an *image regression*),

$$\mathbf{Y}_j = \boldsymbol{\mu} + \boldsymbol{\rho} S_j + \boldsymbol{\zeta}(g_j - \overline{g}.) + \boldsymbol{\epsilon}_j$$

This model would be extended to multi-subject parametric experiments by the inclusion of subject effects. Our omnibus null hypothesis is $H: \rho = \mathbf{0}$, the intersection of the voxel hypotheses $H^k: \rho^k = 0$. Computing the usual univariate t statistic for H^k at each voxel gives a t statistic image (Fig. 12.3). Under the null hypothesis, and assuming (at least) marginal normality of the residuals ($\epsilon_j^k \overset{iid}{\approx} N(0, \sigma^2)$), this statistic image has voxel values drawn from a Student's t distribution.

Because statistical models are foreign to most functional imagers, it has become common to illustrate complex models with an image of their design matrix (Fig. 12.3), even to such an extent that researchers will design experiments by drawing design matrices!

(a)

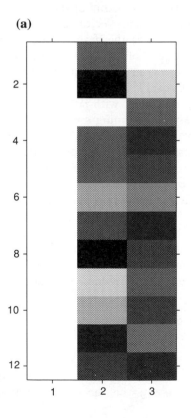

Fig. 12.3 Statistic images for PET data set (intercommissural plane). (a) An image representation of the design matrix. The columns are: ones, for the overall mean, the scan scores, and the centred gCBF. (b) Fitted score coefficient $\hat{\rho}$. (c) Residual variance estimates. (d) t statistic image. Mesh plots of the intercommissural plane of the volumetric images are used as they depict noise better than intensity images

(b)

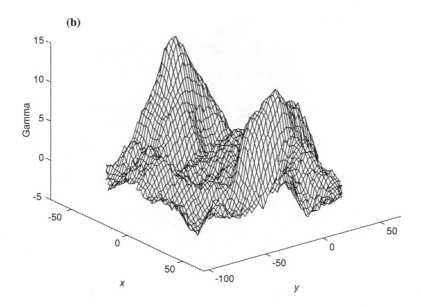

(c)

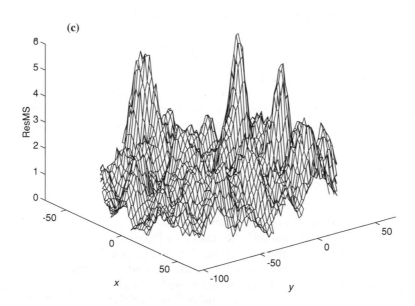

Fig. 12.3 (*continued*)

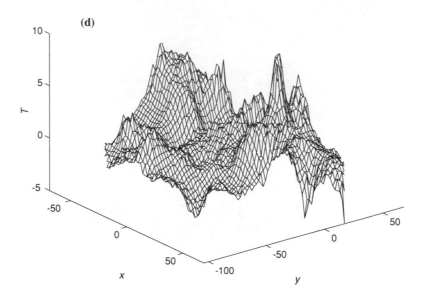

Fig. 12.3 (*continued*)

12.3.3.2   fMRI model

Again, a simple linear model is used to model the fMRI time series $\mathbf{Y}^k = (Y_1^k, \ldots, Y_j^k, \ldots, Y_J^k)$ of J observations at voxel k:

$$\mathbf{Y}^k = X\boldsymbol{\beta}^k + \boldsymbol{\epsilon}^k$$

In this time series setting, the columns of the design matrix can be thought of as discretized waveforms. However, a straightforward regression analysis is not possible for most fMRI time series, since for interscan intervals less than 6–8 s the measurements are correlated. This auto-correlation in the fMRI time series is a result of the haemodynamics of blood flow in the brain (BOLD fMRI gives images indicating brain activity by contrasting blood oxygenation levels, dependent on supply and demand). The observed fMRI time series may thus be considered as the actual neuronal activity time series smoothed out by the haemodynamic response. Temporally, the haemodynamic response to an impulse activation has approximately the form of a Poisson kernel, with a mean of 5–8 s, and varies around the brain. Many authors have simply ignored the temporal autocorrelation of the residuals, and continued with standard regression analyses, or have employed standard rank-based non-parametric methods, possibly obtaining false positives due to the incorrect assumptions. The problem is simply one of serially correlated regression, to which there are various solutions. Of those successfully applied to fMRI, one is to model the residual time series with a simple Box–Jenkins time series model, enabling the removal of the autocorrelation (Bullmore *et al.,* 1996). The approach we shall consider is due to Worsley and Friston, using results from the literature on serially correlated regression (Worsley and Friston, 1995, Friston *et al.*, 1995a).

Since the fMRI signal to a point response has the form of the haemodynamic response function, the signal is optimally recovered if the fMRI time series is smoothed by convolution with an approximation to the haemodynamic response function (matched filter theorem). Thus, Worsley and Friston proposed temporally smoothing the time series data at each voxel $\mathbf{Y}$ to give (dropping the voxel superscript k)

$$KY = KX\beta + K\epsilon$$

for K a Toeplitz matrix containing the discretized smoothing kernel in each row (a Gaussian kernel was chosen, with SD $\tau = \sqrt{8}\,\mathrm{s}$, giving $[K]_{ij} \propto \exp[-(i-j)^2/2\tau^2]$). The parameters β are the same, but are better estimated after convolution. Although the raw errors will be slightly correlated for most interscan intervals, this autocorrelation is swamped by the temporal smoothing. Thus, the components of the error vector ϵ are assumed independent, $\epsilon_j \overset{\text{iid}}{\sim} N(0, \sigma^2)$, such that the autocovariances of the smoothed errors $K\epsilon$ are completely specified by K and σ, reducing the problem to one of serially correlated regression with known auto-correlation function.

The least squares estimates of β are $\hat{\beta} = (X^{*\top}X^*)^{-1}X^{*\top}KY$, where $X^* = KX$. $\hat{\beta}$ is unbiased with $\mathrm{var}(\hat{\beta}) = \sigma^2(X^{*\top}X^*)^{-1}X^{*\top}VX^*(X^{*\top}X^*)^{-1}$, where $V = KK^\top$. This implies the following test statistic for a linear compound $\mathbf{c}^\top\beta$ at voxel k:

$$T = \frac{\mathbf{c}^\top\hat{\beta}}{\sqrt{\mathbf{c}^\top\hat{\sigma}(X^{*\top}X^*)^{-1}X^{*\top}VX^*(X^{*\top}X^*)^{-1}}}$$

with σ^2 estimated in the usual way by $\hat{\sigma}^2 = \mathbf{r}^\top\mathbf{r}/\mathrm{trace}(RV)$, where $\mathbf{r} = RKX$ is the vector of residuals for R, the residual forming matrix. By analogy with the χ^2 approximation for quadratic forms (Satterthwaite, 1946), the null distribution of T may be approximated by a t distribution with η degrees of freedom, where the effective degrees of freedom are given by

$$\eta = \frac{2E[\hat{\sigma}^2]^2}{\mathrm{var}(\hat{\sigma}^2)} = \frac{\mathrm{trace}(RV)^2}{\mathrm{trace}(RVRV)}$$

For our example language experiment of alternating epochs of baseline and activation conditions, a minimal design would have only two degrees of freedom, a mean for each condition, with conditions associated with

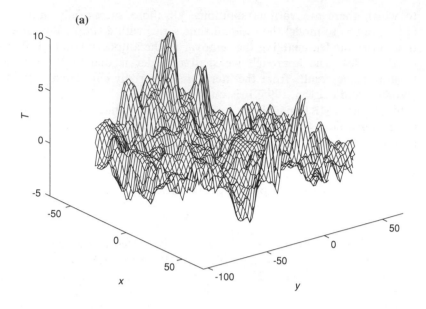

(a)

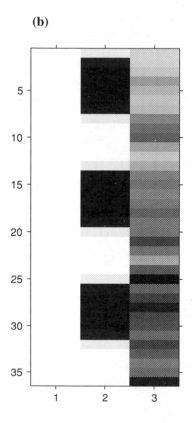

(b)

Fig. 12.4 Statistic images for fMRI data set.
(a) Mesh plot (intercommissural plane) of
'Gaussianized' t statistic image for $\beta_2 = 0$ at
each voxel. The effective degrees of freedom
of the t statistic are $\eta = 32.47$. (b) Design
matrix KX, shown as a grey-scale image with
black $= -1$, white $= +1$

scans reflecting the haemodynamic lag. One possible design matrix X for this has a column of ones, and a column containing a box-car waveform of blocks of zeros and ones, lagged 8 s from the actual experimental conditions to account for the haemodynamic delay. A lagged box-car can be thought of as a crude approximation of the haemodynamic response to a neuronal activation by the stimulus. However, its simplicity and success have ensured its use. For illustration, consider this approach, with the global measurement as a confounding covariate, leading to the design matrix (after convolution) shown in Fig. 12.4(b). The null hypothesis of no activation corresponds to zero amplitude of the box-car waveform, giving a t statistic image for the appropriate contrast of the fitted parameters as shown in Fig. 12.4(a)

12.3.4 Random field approaches

There remains the multiple comparisons problem of assessing these statistic images. The smoothness of the images leads to dependent tests at nearby voxels, making naïve corrections based on the Bonferroni or Šidák–Jogedo inequalities excessively conservative. The most fruitful parametric approaches have proceeded by assuming the statistic image is a strictly stationary discrete random field, regarding it as a good lattice representation of an underlying continuous random field with the same properties, and applying results from continuous random field theory. The simplest tests are single threshold tests, declaring significant evidence against the hypotheses at voxels with statistics above a given threshold u_α. Clearly the distribution of maximal voxel statistic is of interest here. Unfortunately the distribution of the maxima of a continuous random field has proved elusive, necessitating recourse to more esoteric topological measures.

Briefly, for a real-valued function $Z(x)$, defined over a compact subset $\Omega \subset \mathfrak{R}^D$, the excursion set above a threshold u is the subset of Ω for which Z exceeds u, $\{x : Z(x) > u, x \in \Omega\}$. These excursion sets can be characterized by the Euler characteristic χ_u, a topological measure which essentially measures the number of isolated parts of the excursion set less the number of 'holes', and is mathematically tractable.

For $Z(x)$, a real-valued stochastic process, as the threshold u increases the Euler characteristic tends (in probability) to the number of local maxima. For large u, near Z_{max}, $\Pr(Z_{max} > u) \approx \Pr(\chi_u > 0) \approx E[\chi_u]$ and the expected Euler characteristic approximates the P value for Z_{max}. For an observation $z(x)$, $x \in \Omega$ of the stochastic process, approximate adjusted P values for high $z(x)$ are given by $E[\chi_{z(x)}]$. Strong control over familywise Type I error follows from the fact that the expected Euler characteristic reduces with the size of Ω. This argument was introduced by Worsley *et al.* (1992) for strictly stationary, homogeneous Gaussian random fields, using the expected Euler characteristic derived by Adler (1981), a relatively simple function of the size of Ω, the threshold u, and the smoothness of the random field (Adler, 1981). Subsequently Worsley (1994) extended Adler's results, deriving the expected Euler characteristic for t, F and χ^2 fields.

Gaussian fields are easier to work with, and additional results are available. Thus t statistic images are often 'Gaussianized' by probability integral transform to have null marginal standard normal distributions. Unless the degrees of freedom are high, the resulting Gaussian statistic image is not a discrete Gaussian random field, and the ensuing test is more lenient than its counterpart for the raw t statistic image. An alternative, proposed by Worsley *et al.* (1992), is to assume homoscedasticity, and use a variance estimate pooled over all voxels when forming voxel statistics. The effective degrees of freedom of the resulting estimate are then sufficiently high that the t statistic can be considered Gaussian. Unfortunately most data sets exhibit considerable heteroscedasticity, and such variance pooling is inappropriate, possibly leading to invalid tests.

The application of these methods implies numerous assumptions, discussed by Holmes (1994).

12.3.4.1   Extensions

There are numerous extensions to the basic framework presented here. Recognizing that departures from the null hypothesis are distinguished not just by their height, Poline and Mazoyer (1993) proposed assessing their spatial extent. The statistic image is thresholded at a fairly low value u (usually at levels corresponding to (uncorrected) $P \in [0.001, 0.01]$) and the resulting clusters of suprathreshold voxels characterized by their size. The omnibus null hypothesis for clusters above a critical size s_α is rejected. Poline and Mazoyer estimated s_α by simulation. Later Friston *et al.* (1994) developed an approximate theoretical treatment, based on the theory of strictly stationary, continuous Gaussian random fields, assuming a Poisson model for the number of components of the excursion set (Adler, 1981). Clearly such an approach does not control experimentwise Type I error at the voxel level; the test has no localizing power within the identified clusters. (Assuming subset pivotality, strong control can be loosely claimed at the cluster level.) The loss of voxel-level strong control is offset by increased sensitivity. The arbitrariness of the threshold u is somewhat of a problem: intense focal activations are optimally detected with high u, or indeed the single threshold test, less intense spatially extended departures by a lower threshold.

Worsley *et al.* (1995a) extended results for the expected Euler characteristic to small, irregularly shaped subsets of $\Re^D$, enabling its use within extended regions of interest. Worsley *et al.* also extended and implemented an extension to 'scale space', enabling the search for activations over different smoothings of the original data, an approach originally suggested by Poline and Mazoyer (1994).

Worsley *et al.* (1995b) developed a theory leading to omnibus tests for statistic images, tests maintaining only weak control over experimentwise

Type I error. These were based on the sum of square voxel statistics, or the proportion of voxels with statistics exceeding a given threshold. Subsequently, multivariate methods were developed to address the same questions.

Poline *et al.* (1997) combined the single threshold and suprathreshold cluster tests, addressing the insensitivity of the latter to focal activations when a low primary threshold is used. They derived the asymptotic (high threshold) joint distribution of the size and peak intensity of a simply connected component of the excursion set of a strictly stationary, continuous Gaussian random field. The unconditional joint distribution was then obtained using a Poisson assumption for the number of components of the excursion set (Adler, 1981). The boundary of the rejection region was then chosen such that the marginal extrema probabilities for size and height were equal.

Recently Friston *et al.* (1995b) extended the suprathreshold cluster method to 'set-level inferences', obtaining a theoretical distribution for the number of suprathreshold clusters of size greater than a given size threshold. (The distribution reduces to those for Z_{max} and S_{max} for appropriate parameters.) This allows a P value to be computed for the set of suprathreshold clusters larger than a given size, again giving increased sensitivity at the expense of localization.

12.3.4.2 Results

As an example, consider the application of the single threshold test and the suprathreshold cluster size test to the example data sets. The PET and fMRI statistic images (Figs 12.3(d) and 12.4(a) respectively) were 'Gaussianized' by replacing each voxel t value with a standard normal variate with identical tail probability. These 'Gaussianized' statistic images are then considered as good lattice approximations of a strictly stationary, continuous Gaussian random field defined over the same volume, and with the same smoothness. The smoothness is estimated from the standardized residual images ϵ_j, with a correction factor applied to account for the 'Gaussianization' and the use of a variance estimate in standardizing the residuals. For the PET data set, the smoothness was equivalent to that of a white noise process smoothed with a Gaussian kernel of FWHM $16.4 \times 17.5 \times 13.5\,\text{mm}^3$. Dividing the volume of the brain by the smoothness given the number of *resolution elements*, or *resels*, indicative of the number of independent measurements in the statistic image. For the PET intracerebral volume of $66\,689$ $2 \times 2 \times 4\,\text{mm}^3$ voxels, this gives 273 resels. For this volume and smoothness, the expected Euler characteristic is 0.05 at threshold $u_\alpha = 4.328$, so the null hypothesis can be rejected at voxels with statistic exceeding this threshold (Fig. 12.5). Suprathreshold clusters of voxels were identified using a primary threshold of $\Phi^{-1}(1 - 0.001)$, identifying two significantly large clusters of voxels. Not surprisingly, given the auditory stimulus, the significant areas are the

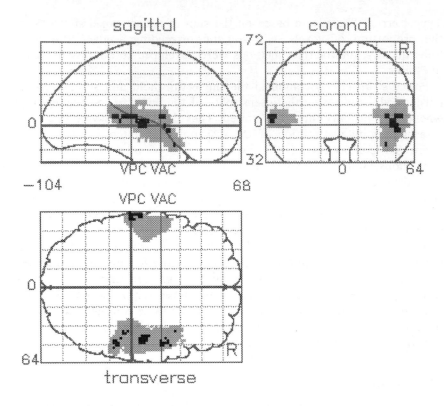

Fig. 12.5 Orthogonal 'glass brain' views of the significant voxels at $\alpha = 0.05$ (corrected) for the PET data set. The smoothness of the 'Gaussianized' t statistic image was estimated at $16.4 \times 17.5 \times 13.5 \, \text{mm}^3$, equivalent to 273 'resolution elements' (resels), for an intracerebral volume of 66 689 voxels. Voxels above the critical threshold u_α of 4.328 (3d.p.) are shown black. Suprathreshold clusters of voxels were identified using a primary threshold of $\Phi^{-1}(1 - 0.001)$, identifying two significantly large clusters of voxels, shown translucent grey

primary auditory cortices on either side of the brain. For the fMRI data set, similar but more widespread results are found (Fig. 12.6).

12.3.5   Non-parametric approaches

Holmes *et al.* (1996) introduced non-parametric multiple comparisons procedures for the assessment of functional mapping experiments, based on randomization/permutation test theory. By considering appropriate permutations of the labellings of the scans (labellings as 'rest' and 'active', or associated covariate such as scan score), and computing statistic images for each labelling, the permutation distribution for the entire statistic image can be obtained. From this null distribution of the statistic image, given the data and appropriate null hypothesis, the permutation distribution of any statistic summarizing the statistic image can be found.

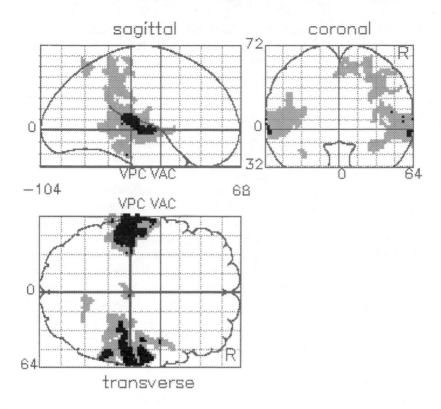

Fig. 12.6 'Glass brain' views of the significant voxels at $\alpha = 0.05$ for the fMRI data set. The smoothness of the 'Gaussianized' t statistic image was estimated at $8.8 \times 9.5 \times 7.7\,\text{mm}^3$, equivalently 2039 resels, for 162 993 intracerebral voxels. Suprathreshold clusters of voxels were identified using a primary threshold of $\Phi^{-1}(1 - 0.001)$

Summarizing each statistic image by its maximum statistic gives the permutation distribution for Z_{max}, the $100(1 - \alpha)$th percentile of which is the appropriate critical threshold for a single threshold test at level α. Summarizing each statistic image by the size of the largest cluster of voxels with values above a prespecified threshold gives the permutation distribution of S_{max}, and appropriate critical suprathreshold cluster sizes. Strong control over experimentwise Type I error is maintained (at the appropriate level) in both cases.

In addition to the usual attractions of non-parametric methods, namely minimal assumptions, guaranteed validity and exactness, flexibility and intuitiveness, the approach is especially attractive for small data sets such as the single-subject PET study presented here: t statistic images with low degrees of freedom exhibit a high (spatial) frequency noise, and the statistic image is rough. The properties of such statistic images are not well approximated by continuous random fields with the same distributions. The continuous fields have features smaller than the voxel dimensions, leading to critical thresholds for single threshold tests that are conservative for lattice representations of the continuous field. An extreme example is a 3D strictly stationary continuous random t field with three degrees of freedom, which almost certainly has a singularity (Worsley *et al.*, 1993).

12.3.5.1   'Pseudo' t statistic images

The noise in statistic images with low degrees of freedom results from the variability of the residual variance estimate, illustrated in Fig. 12.3. In PET it is reasonable to assume that the residual variability is approximately constant over small localities, suggesting that variance estimates could be locally pooled. A weighted local pooling of variance estimates is a smoothing of the estimated variance image (since the degrees of freedom are the same at every voxel). The smoothed variance image for the PET data is shown in Fig. 12.7(a), where weights from an isotropic 3D Gaussian kernel of FWHM 12 mm were used (the kernel was truncated at the edges of the intracerebral volume). Clearly variance estimates at proximate voxels are not independent. A theoretical distribution for such smoothed variance images has proved elusive, thus precluding further parametric analysis. The 'pseudo' t statistic image formed with this sample variance image is shown in Fig. 12.7(b); compare with Fig. 12.3. Effectively the noise is smoothed but not the signal!

The ability to consider statistic images constructed with smoothed variance estimates appears to make the non-parametric approach considerably more powerful than the parametric approaches discussed. Results for the PET data set are shown in Fig. 12.8. Here 1000 permutations (including the actual allocation) of the 12! possible

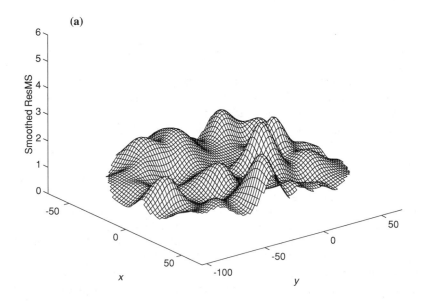

(a)

(b)

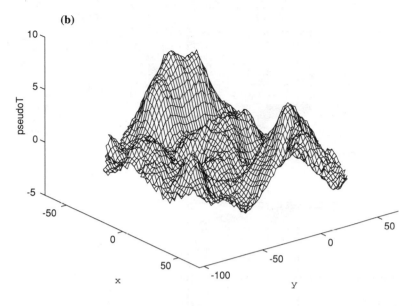

Fig. 12.7 Statistic images for PET data set. (a) Mesh plot (intercommissural plane) of estimated variance image smoothed with an isotropic Gaussian kernel of FWHM 12 mm, truncated at the edge of the intracerebral volume. (b) Mesh plot of 'pseudo' t statistic computed with smoothed variance estimate

permutations of scores to scans were considered, and the (approximate) permutation distribution of the maximum 'pseudo' t statistic computed. The resulting single threshold test identifies many more significant voxels than the parametric single threshold test using the expected Euler characteristic on the 'Gaussianized' t statistic.

Using raw t statistic images, the non-parametric approach on the whole agrees with the parametric approaches, a comforting observation. These methods permit great flexibility in the use of test statistics and are guaranteed to be robust.

12.3.6   Issues

12.3.6.1   Software

The vast quantities of data preclude the use of (most) professional statistical packages for routine analysis in functional neuroimaging. Most analyses have to be programmed from first principles, necessitating the implementation of even basic statistical algorithms most statisticians would take for granted. This has severely limited the statistical tools at the disposal of the researcher. Most units have customized software containing a few statistical tools which researchers use routinely.

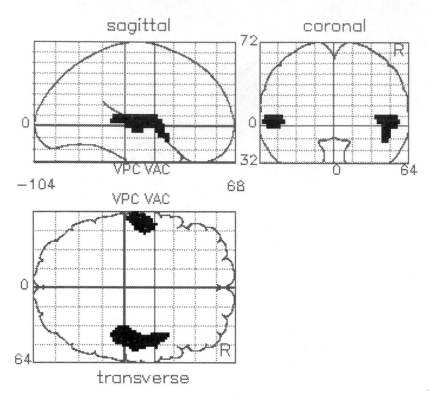

Fig. 12.8 'Glass brain' views of the significant voxels at $\alpha = 0.05$ from a non-parametric single threshold test using 'pseudo' t statistic images

Consequently, the most popular methods are those implemented in readily available software. The theory presented here is implemented in the popular SPM (Statistical Parametric Mapping) package developed by Dr Karl Friston and collaborators.

12.3.6.2 Modelling

Usually a model is chosen because it is implemented in the software rather than because it is appropriate. Model selection and checking procedures are rarely considered. Rarely is anything more complex than a fixed effects general linear model. Further, the small number of subjects makes the consideration of random subject effects prohibitively conservative for all but the strongest sensori-motor stimuli. Most inference is effected using fixed effects models, with results presented as 'case studies' for the subjects at hand. Single-subject analyses are common, particularly in fMRI. This has occasionally led to spurious claims in the literature, particularly in split-plot designs comparing activations between patient groups, where subject by condition interactions are routinely assumed negligible, although such effects are almost certainly present.

12.3.7   Alternative approaches to the analysis of activation studies

The model-based and non-parametric methods considered so far have been designed to try to control the multiple comparisons problems generated by the analysis of the data at the voxel level. Alternative approaches are possible to help to control the 'curse of dimensionality'. For simplicity, it is common to analyse voxels covering the entire brain. Often, there will be prior knowledge which will allow the exclusion of many voxels which include regions where activation is certain to occur or where one is certain that no activation can have occurred. Similarly, brain regions which are of no interest in the study being carried out could be excluded. In some contexts specific hypotheses can be formulated from previous studies. Here an ROI approach would be sensible, focusing on a small number of regions.

Finally, some investigators have used a two-stage approach. In the first stage of the experiment a pilot full voxel-based analysis is conducted to identify regions of the brain which might be activated. No adjustments are made for multiple comparisons as the aim of the pilot is to identify large ROIs which can be investigated in a confirmatory follow-up study.

12.4   Discussion

The field of neuroimaging has come a long way in a relatively short period of time. The earlier output from experiments based on PET was considered to be disappointing. However, the introduction of activation studies, with multiple studies being carried out in single subjects, along with improvements in electronics and in the available radiopharmaceuticals, have radically changed this situation. Nowadays, studies of brain function using PET and fMRI make headline news in the world's leading science journals. Developments in statistical methodology have made an important contribution, providing methods of analysis in which scientists in the field can have greater faith. The developing field of fMRI in particular presents a significant challenge, with large data sets collected in time and space. The underlying technology is still in the developmental stage with resulting difficulties in terms of the interpretation of fMRI images. Future experimentation will almost certainly involve a variety of technologies being applied together with PET, fMRI and EEG data being available on the same subjects. The simultaneous interpretation of these data, with their different time and spatial resolutions, will present a significant challenge. Similarly, the study of patient populations presents significant difficulty.

Many of the assumptions which permit the pooling of data across scans and normalization of images are unlikely to be valid in patient groups.

References

Adler, R. 1981: *The geometry of random fields*. New York: John Wiley.

Bullmore, E., Brammer, M., Williams, S. C. R., Rabe-Hesketh, S., Janot, N., David, A., Mellors, J., Howard, R. and Sham, P. 1996: Statistical methods of estimation and inference for functional MR image analysis. *Magnetic Resonance in Medicine* **35**, 261–77.

Camargo, E. E., Szabo, Z., Links, J. M., Sostre, S., Dannals, R. F. and Wagner, H. N. Jr. 1992: The influence of biological and technical factors on the variability of global and regional brain metabolism of 2-[18F]Fluoro-2-deoxy-D-glucose. *Journal of Cerebral Blood Flow and Metabolism* **12**, 281–90.

Clark, C., Carson, R., Kessler, R., Margolin, R., Buchsbaum, M., DeLisi, L., King, C. and Cohen, R. 1985: Alternative statistical models for the examination of clinical positron emission tomography fluorodeoxyglucose data. *Journal of Cerebral Blood Flow and Metabolism* **5**, 142–50.

Defrise, M., Townsend, D. W. and Clark, R. 1989: Three-dimensional image reconstruction from complete projections. *Physics in Medicine and Biology* **34**, 573–87.

Defrise, M., Townsend, D. W. and Geissbuhler, A. 1990: Implementation of three-dimensional image reconstruction for multi-ring tomographs. *Physics in Medicine and Biology* **35**, 1361–72.

Ford, I. 1986: Confounded correlations: statistical limitations in the analysis of interregional relationships of cerebral metabolic activity. *Journal of Cerebral Blood Flow and Metabolism* **6**, 385–8.

Friston, K. J., Ashburner, J., Poline, J.-B., Frith, C. D., Heather, J. D. and Frackowiak, R. S. J. 1995d: The spatial registration and normalisation of images. *Human Brain Mapping* **2**, 165–89.

Friston, K. J., Frith, C. D., Liddle, P. F., Dolan, R. J., Lammertsma, A. A. and Frackowiak, R. S. J. 1990: The relationship between global and local changes in PET scans. *Journal of Cerebral Blood Flow and Metabolism* **10**, 458–66.

Friston, K. J., Holmes, A. P., Poline, J.-B., Grasby, P. J., Williams, S. C. R., Frackowiak, R. S. J. and Turner, R. 1995a: Analysis of fMRI time series revisited. *NeuroImage* **2**, 45–53.

Friston, K. J., Holmes, A. P., Poline, J.-B., Price, C. J. and Frith, C. D. 1995b: Detecting activations in PET and fMRI: levels of inference and power. *NeuroImage* **4**, 223–35.

Friston, K. J., Holmes, A. P., Worsley, K. J., Poline, J.-B., Frith, C. D. and Frackowiak, R. S. J. 1995c: Statistical parametric maps in functional imaging: a general linear approach. *Human Brain Mapping* **2**, 189–210.

Friston, K. J., Poline, J.-B., Holmes, A. P., Frith, C. D. and Frackowiak, R. S. J. 1996: A multivariate analysis of PET activation studies. *Human Brain Mapping* **4**, 140–51.

Friston, K. J., Worsley, K. J., Frackowiak, R. S. J., Mazziotta, J. C. and Evans, A. C. 1994: Assessing the significance of focal activations using their spatial extent. *Human Brain Mapping* **1**, 214–20.

Green, P. J. 1990: Bayesian reconstructions from emission tomography data using a modified EM algorithm. *IEEE Transactions on Medical Imaging* **9**, 84–93.

Herman, G. T. 1980: *Image reconstruction from projections*. New York: Academic Press.

Holmes, A. P. 1994: *Statistical issues in functional neuroimaging*. PhD thesis, University of Glasgow (available at http://www.fil.ion.ucl.ac.uk/~andrew).

Holmes, A. P., Blair, R. C., Watson, J. D. G. and Ford, I. 1996: Non-parametric analysis of statistic images from functional mapping experiments. *Journal of Cerebral Blood Flow and Metabolism* **16**, 7–22.

Horwitz, B., Duara, R. and Rapoport, S. I. 1984: Intercorrelations of glucose metabolic rates between brain regions: application to healthy males in a state of reduced sensory input. *Journal of Cerebral Blood Flow and Metabolism* **4**, 484–99.

Horwitz, B., Duara, R. and Rapoport, S. I. 1986: Age differences in inter-correlations between regional cerebral metabolic rates for glucose. *Annals of Neurology* **19**, 60–7.

Martin, A. J., Friston, K. J., Colebatch, J. G. and Frackowiak, R. S. J. 1991: Decreases in regional cerebral blood flow with normal aging. *Journal of Cerebral Blood Flow and Metabolism* **11**, 684–9.

McCrory, S. J. and Ford, I. 1991: Multivariate analysis of SPECT images with illustrations in Alzheimer's disease. *Statistics in Medicine* **10**, 1711–8.

McLaughlin, T., Steinberg, B., Christensen, B., Law, I., Parving, A. and Friberg, L. 1992: Potential language and attentional networks revealed through factor analysis of rCBF data measured with SPECT. *Journal of Cerebral Blood Flow and Metabolism* **12**, 535–45.

Metter, E. J., Riege, W. H., Kameyama, M., Kuhl, D. E. and Phelps, M. E. 1984a: Cerebral metabolic relationships for selected brain regions in Alzheimer's, Huntingdon's, and Parkinson's diseases. *Journal of Cerebral Blood Flow and Metabolism* **4**, 500–6.

Metter, E. J., Riege, W. H., Kuhl, D. E. and Phelps, M. E. 1984b: Cerebral metabolic relationships for selected brain regions in healthy adults. *Journal of Cerebral Blood Flow and Metabolism* **4**, 1 7.

Moeller, J. R. and Strother, S. C. 1991: A regional covariance approach to the analysis of functional patterns in positron emission tomographic data. *Journal of Cerebral Blood Flow and Metabolism* **11**, A121–35.

Moeller, J. R., Strother, S. C., Sidtis, J. J. and Rottenberg, D. A. 1987: Scaled subprofile model: a statistical approach to the analysis of functional patterns in positron emission tomographic data. *Journal of Cerebral Blood Flow and Metabolism* **7**, 649–58.

Poline, J.-B. and Mazoyer, B. M. 1993: Analysis of individual positron emission tomography activation maps by detection of high signal-to-noise ratio pixel clusters. *Journal of Cerebral Blood Flow and Metabolism* **13**, 425–37.

Poline, J.-B. and Mazoyer, B. M. 1994: Enhanced detection in brain activation maps using a multifiltering approach. *Journal of Cerebral Blood Flow and Metabolism* **14**, 639–42.

Poline, J.-B., Worsley, K. J., Evans, A. C. and Friston, K. J. 1997: Combining spatial extent and peak intensity to test for activations in functional imaging. *Human Brain Mapping* **5**, 83–96.

Satterthwaite, F. E. 1946: An approximate distribution of estimates of variance components. *Biometrics* **2**, 110–14.

Silbersweig, D. A., Stern, E., Schnorr, L., Frith, C. D., Ashburner, J., Cahill, C., Frackowiak, R. S. J. and Jones, T. 1994: Imaging transient, randomly-occurring neuropsychological events in single subjects with positron emission tomography: an event-related countrate correlational analysis. *Journal of Cerebral Blood Flow and Metabolism* **14**, 771–82.

Silbersweig, D. A. *et al.* 1995: A functional neuroanatomy of hallucinations in schizophrenia. *Letters to Nature* **378**, 176–9.

Snyder, D. L. and Politte, D. G. 1983: Image reconstruction from list-mode data in an emission tomography system having time-of-flight measurements. *IEEE Transactions on Nuclear Science* **20**, 1843–9.

Talairach, J. and Tournoux, P. 1988: *Co-planar stereotactic atlas of the human brain*. Stuttgart: Theime.

Townsend, D. W., Geissbuhler, A., Defrise, M., Hoffman, E. J., Spinks, T. J., Bailey, D. L., Gilardi, M.-C. and Jones, T. 1991: Fully three-dimensional reconstruction for a PET camera with retractable septa. *IEEE Transactions on Medical Imaging* **10**, 505–12.

Tyler, J. L., Strother, S. C., Zatorre, R. J., Alivisatos, B., Worsley, K. J. and Diksic, M. 1988: Stability of regional cerebral glucose metabolism in the normal brain measured by positron emission tomography. *Journal of Nuclear Medicine* **29**, 631–42.

Vardi, Y., Shepp, L. A. and Kaufman, L. 1985: A statistical model for positron emission tomography. *Journal of the American Statistical Association* **80**, 8–20.

Videen, T. O., Perlmutter, J. S., Mintun, M. A. and Raichle, M. E. 1988: Regional correction of positron emission tomography data for the effects of cerebral atrophy. *Journal of Cerebral Blood Flow and Metabolism* **8**, 662–70.

Worsley, K. J. 1994: Local maxima and the expected Euler characteristic of excursion sets of χ^2, F, and t fields. *Advances in Applied Probability* **26**, 13–42.

Worsley, K. J., Evans, A. C., Marrett, S. and Neelin, P. 1992: A three-dimensional statistical analysis for CBF activation studies in human brain. *Journal of Cerebral Blood Flow and Metabolism* **12**, 900–18.

Worsley, K. J., Evans, A. C., Marrett, S. and Neelin, P. 1993: Detecting and estimating the regions of activation in CBF activation studies in human brain. In Uemura, K. *et al.* (eds), *Quantification of brain function: tracer kinetics and image analysis in brain PET*. Amsterdam: Elsevier, 535–44.

Worsley, K. J., Evans, A. C., Strother, S. C. and Tyler, J. L. 1991: A linear spatial correlation model, with applications to positron emission tomography. *Journal of the American Statistical Association* **86**, 55–67.

Worsley, K. J. and Friston, K. J. 1995: Analysis of fMRI time-series revisited—again. *NeuroImage* **2**, 173–81.

Worsley, K. J., Marrett, S., Neelin, P. and Evans, A. C. 1995a: A unified statistical approach for determining significant signals in location and scale space images of cerebral activation. *NeuroImage* **2**, S71.

Worsley, K. J., Poline, J.-B., Vandal, A. C. and Friston, K. J. 1995b: Tests for distributed, nonfocal brain activations. *NeuroImage* **2**, 183–94.

Yochmowitz, M. G. 1983: Factor analysis of variance model (FANOVA). In Kotz, S. and Johnson, N. (eds), *Encyclopedia of statistical sciences, volume 3*. New York: John Wiley.

Yoshii, F. *et al.* 1988: Sensitivity of cerebral glucose metabolism to age, gender, brain volume, brain atrophy, and cerebrovascular risk factors. *Journal of Cerebral Blood Flow and Metabolism* **8**, 654–61.

13 Localizing brain activation in a single subject using functional magnetic resonance imaging

S. Rabe-Hesketh, M. J. Brammer and
E. T. Bullmore

13.1 Introduction

Functional magnetic resonance imaging (fMRI) is a non-invasive technique for measuring changes in cerebral blood oxygenation related to brain activity. In about 5 minutes, a sequence of three-dimensional images is acquired from which the temporal and spatial characteristics of neuronal activity can be deduced. The most important objective is usually to determine which brain regions are associated with a given mental task. The localization of brain function has important clinical applications, for example for the planning of brain surgery (Gandhe *et al.*, 1994). It is also very exciting for researchers in psychiatry and psychology attempting to map brain function in normal subjects and to detect abnormalities in patient groups. In this chapter, we will describe the difficulties associated with detecting and localizing activation in the brain of a single subject (other aspects of fMR image analysis are reviewed in Rabe-Hesketh *et al.*, 1997).

Firstly, we briefly describe the principles underlying fMRI. We will attempt to give only a superficial explanation of the physics of fMRI (see Foster and Hutchison (1985) and Cohen and Weisskopf (1991) for more detailed introductions). The subject's head is inside a strong magnetic field which causes the hydrogen nuclei inside the brain to spin. The frequency of the spin (i.e. the number of cycles per second) is proportional to the magnetic field strength. A short pulse of radiowaves of the same frequency is transmitted towards the brain. Since the radiowaves and the nuclei are in resonance, the nuclei absorb the energy from the radiowaves and move into a higher energy 'excited' state. After the pulse, the nuclei 'relax' back into their lower energy state, and emit a radiowave which is measured as the fMRI signal. The strength of the radiowave emitted by each volume element (voxel) varies spatially owing to differences in the density of the nuclei and in the amount of relaxation that has occurred at the time the signal is measured. Although most of the hydrogen nuclei are in tissue water, the exact relaxation rate depends on the type of tissue containing the water, such as grey matter or cerebrospinal fluid. Also, hydrogen nuclei in deoxygenated blood relax slightly faster than those in oxygen-rich blood. It is this latter effect, called BOLD (Blood Oxygen Level Dependent) contrast (Ogawa *et al.*, 1990) that is utilized in the fMRI method described in this chapter.

The connection between neural activation and the BOLD effect is believed to be as follows. Cortical activity typically causes increased glucose consumption and regional cerebral blood flow without commensurate increase in oxygen consumption (Fox and Raichle, 1986). The net effect of activation is therefore (somewhat paradoxically) a local increase in concentration of oxyhaemoglobin, causing an increase in the signal. This increase occurs gradually and is only detectable after a 'haemodynamic delay' which lasts about 4–6 seconds, but is locally variable.

There are several important issues that need to be considered when attempting to localize activation imaged through BOLD contrast as described above. These issues include data quality and preprocessing (Section 13.2), experimental design (Section 13.3), modelling and detecting activation (Sections 13.4 and 13.5 respectively) and finally localizing the activated regions anatomically (Section 13.6). We will describe our own methodology in each of these areas, illustrating it, wherever possible, on an fMRI data set. At the same time we will review some of the approaches taken by other researchers.

13.2   Image quality and preprocessing

Signal change due to neural activation in the human brain (i.e. BOLD contrast) is very subtle, amounting to about 3–7% of the baseline signal (Turner *et al.*, 1993) when a magnetic field strength of 1.5 tesla is used. This contrast is very small compared with signal contrast between tissue types and we can therefore only detect activation by looking for changes occurring at each location as we follow it over time. In order for changes in activation to occur, the subject needs to perform several different mental tasks or experience different sensations during the acquisition of a sequence of images (see next section). Adding to the problem of a low BOLD contrast, the signal is corrupted by high levels of noise comprising 'physiological noise', related to breathing and cardiac cycles, as well as measurement error associated with the instrument ('thermal noise' etc.).

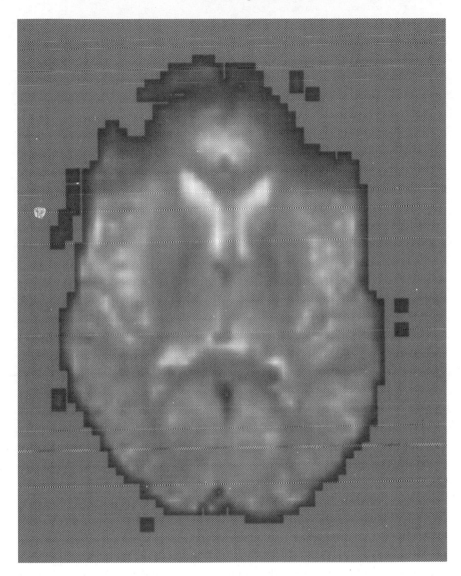

Fig. 13.1 One slice of a functional image at one time point

Owing to instrumental instability, or 'temporal drift', there is a slowly varying, roughly linear trend superimposed onto the signal of interest.

Functional MR images have a high spatial and temporal resolution. For example, the data used to illustrate various points in this chapter consist of 100 MR images acquired at 3 s intervals for each of 10 slices which are 5 mm thick and separated by an interslice gap of 0.5 mm. Each slice in the data set consists of a matrix of 64×128 voxels whose in-plane dimensions are $3 \times 3 \text{ mm}^2$. Other technical details of data acquisition are described in Brammer *et al.* (1997a). Figures 13.1 and 13.2 show a single

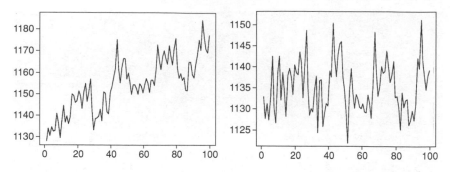

Fig. 13.2 Auditory time series at a voxel before (left) and after (right) movement correction

image slice at a single time point and a time series at a single voxel respectively.

The spatial and temporal resolutions are not quite as good as implied by the voxel dimensions ($3 \times 3 \times 5\,mm^3$) and time intervals (3 s) because of the presence of spatial and temporal autocorrelations. These auto-correlations are due to the effects of breathing and cardiac cycles as well as motion artifacts and haemodynamics, all of which are gradual in space and time. Spatial autocorrelations are further increased by the point spread function inherent in the instrument and during the construction of the 3D image through filtered Fourier transformation.

Signal-to-noise ratio in fMRI may be improved at the expense of spatial or temporal resolution by locally averaging the image, for example by convolving the images with a Gaussian kernel. Poline and Mazoyer (1994) and Worsley (1998) point out that the signal is optimally enhanced only if the filter is appropriate for the size (and shape) of the activated region (matched filter theorem). Since there is no reason to assume that all activated regions in the brain are of the same size (and shape), these authors suggest multi-filtering or multi-scale approaches in which a sequence of filters of different widths is applied.

A fundamental difficulty with fMRI is subject movement (Hajnal *et al.*, 1994). Even slight movement during the acquisition of the image sequence can lead to apparent temporal changes in the signal which are unrelated to changes in cerebral blood flow. Subject movement may be corrected for by finding, for each image in the sequence, that rigid transformation (rotation and translation) which minimizes some measure of discrepancy between corresponding voxel values. After applying a rigid transformation to each image, the voxel grids are no longer aligned with each other and approximate values need to be computed for some common grid using, for example, tricubic splines (see Hill *et al.* (1994) for a discussion of movement correction). For the data described here, we have used the sum of absolute differences between each image and the mean image as the measure of discrepancy and tricubic splines for interpolation.

Even if the realignment has been successful, there remains a movement-related effect determined by the nuclei's previous location within the magnet. These effects may be removed by regressing the time series on a second-order polynomial function of the instantaneous and lagged movement parameters (Friston *et al.*, 1996). As can be seen in Fig. 13.2, this method often removes the linear trend from the time series.

Another problem with fMRI is spatial distortion caused by magnetic field inhomogeneity, for example due to differences in susceptibility between air and bone in the sinuses (Mansfield *et al.*, 1994). These distortions may make it difficult to localize regions in the functional image anatomically and several authors have therefore attempted to correct them; see for example Jezzard and Balaban (1995). An alternative approach is described in Section 13.6.

13.3 Experimental design

Because of the low signal-to-noise ratio, subjects usually perform two very different tasks A and B while a large number of images (between 50 and 100) are being acquired. The sequence of experimental tasks can be thought of as an 'input' function so that the signal is simply the response (in terms of BOLD contrast) to this input function.

In order to be able to estimate the signal of interest, the input function needs to be sufficiently different from that part of the trend in the time series which is due to the gradual instrumental drifts. For this reason, the two tasks are usually alternated periodically, each condition lasting somewhere between 10 and 40 s. In this type of single subject (N of 1) trial, it is generally recommended that 'treatment' sequences be determined randomly (see, for example, Senn, 1993). One way of doing this in fMRI would be to determine randomly the order of A and B in each pair of conditions. However, this is very rarely done in practice. While it would be preferable to carry out randomization in order to justify significance testing and especially randomization testing, use of a deterministic sequence is probably much less problematical in fMRI than in clinical N of 1 trials where blindness is an issue. (In fMRI the subject is neither blind to the conditions nor can knowledge of the condition bias his or her response, so the problem of subjects being able to guess the sequence of conditions does not apply.)

The first fMRI studies concentrated on the visual system (Kwong *et al.*, 1992). Here the periodically alternated tasks were A: looking at a flashing screen, and B: looking at a dark screen. These studies correctly identified the primary visual cortex as being activated by visual stimulation and therefore served to verify fMRI.

The data described here were acquired using two active tasks, seeing and hearing with different periodicities for the two tasks. We will analyse only the auditory task which worked as follows. During the active condition, the subject heard, via pneumatically driven headphones (to block out the banging noises made by the scanner), a recorded voice reading aloud from a book; during the control condition, the subject received no auditory–verbal stimulation. Both conditions lasted 39 s, corresponding to 13 images.

We would like to note that most fMRI studies carried out at the Institute of Psychiatry involve higher-level, cognitive processing tasks such as linguistic or working memory exercises instead of simple sensory or motor tasks. The two tasks must be designed in such a way that they differ significantly only in the one function which is being investigated. This is difficult to do and involves the assumption that no other brain activity is associated with either task, for example boredom with the control task or frustration with the active task. It may also be difficult if not impossible to know to what extent the subject was actually performing the task or was distracted by other thoughts. Finally, the BOLD contrast associated with these higher-level functions tends to be weaker than for functions such as hearing and seeing. Despite these difficulties, interesting results are emerging and researchers are planning ever more complicated studies, for example studies where the input function is not directly determined by the experiment such as in sporadically occurring hallucinations.

13.4   Modelling the experimental effect

Analysis of fMRI is usually done in two steps. Instead of applying some full spatio-temporal model to the entire data set, the experimental effect is first estimated separately from the time series at each voxel and then the image of estimated effect sizes is analysed. This section reviews approaches to the first (time series modelling) step of the analysis.

13.4.1   Models

The simplest model for the time series at a voxel which is activated by the experimental task is

$$Y(y) = \beta b(y) + \epsilon_t \qquad t = 1,,\ldots,n \qquad (13.1)$$

where $Y(t)$ is the intensity value observed at time point t, $b(t)$ is the box-car function which has value 1 during condition A and value -1 during condition B, and ϵ_t is the residual term. Any linear trend in the time series may be removed before fitting the model or may be accommodated by adding the terms $\alpha_0 + \alpha_1 t$ to (13.1). The regression coefficient β represents the amplitude or magnitude of the response and its estimate is proportional to the mean difference between the images during conditions A and B or the covariance between the input function and the time series. Both the mean difference and covariance or correlation have been used by many researchers as estimates of the experimental effect; see for example Kwong *et al.* (1992) and Bandettini *et al.* (1993).

The main problem with this model is that it is inadequate to cope with haemodynamically mediated delay between the input function and the observed fMRI time series. Such delay has been found to be present and to be highly variable between voxels (see, for example, Bullmore *et al.*, 1996b). For this reason, Bandettini *et al.* (1993) allowed the box-car function to be delayed with respect to the observed signal by d time points, giving the model

$$Y(t) = \beta b(t - d) + \epsilon_t \tag{13.2}$$

Since we would not expect the signal to have exactly the same shape as the input function, a more general model is given by

$$Y(t) = \beta f(t; \theta) + \epsilon_t \tag{13.3}$$

where f is a general smooth periodic function parameterized by θ. One approach to defining this function is to make the following assumptions (Friston *et al.*, 1994a, Lange and Zeger, 1997). If we could cause a brief moment or 'spike' of neuronal activity, this would be accompanied by a delayed, gradual rise and fall in blood flow, which is described by the *response function* $g(t; \theta)$ for some shape and delay parameters θ. (This idea of a response function is similar to the concept of a point spread function in optics which causes a point source to be imaged as a 'blob'.) Continuous neuronal activation can be thought of as a sequence of spikes of activation. The amount of blood flow observed at time t is simply the sum of the amounts of blood flow $g(s; \theta)$ remaining at time t that were caused by spikes of activation at earlier time points t s. The total haemodynamic effect at time t is therefore given by the convolution

$$f(t; \theta) = \sum_{0 \leq t - s \leq n} h(t - s)g(s; \theta) \tag{13.4}$$

where $h(t - s)$ is simply an indicator variable which is equal to one if activation was present at time $t - s$ and to zero otherwise. Note that for fMRI we assume that neuronal activation is present during condition A and absent during condition B so that

$$h(t) = [b(t) + 1]/2 \tag{13.5}$$

Friston *et al.* (1994a) suggest the Poisson distribution for the response function

$$g(s; \lambda) = \frac{\lambda^s e^{-\lambda}}{(s)!} \tag{13.6}$$

where the parameter λ determines the delay of the peak of blood flow relative to the spike of neuronal activation, as well as the shape of the response function (i.e. its dispersion and asymmetry). The authors assume

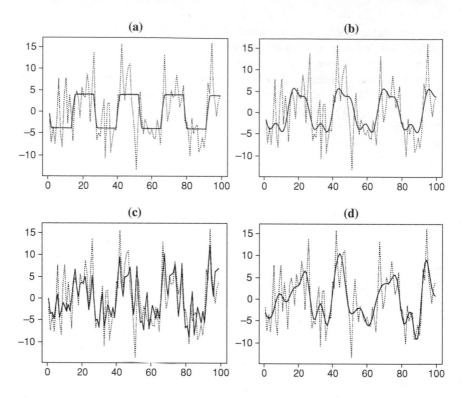

Fig. 13.3 Models fitted to the time series in Fig. 13.2: (a) box-car convolved with a Poisson; (b) sinusoidal regression model; (c) non-parametric periodic model allowing the amplitude to change; (d) Daubechies 8 wavelet using dyadic resolution levels 4 and 5

that λ is constant throughout the image. We have estimated λ together with the amplitude to obtain a least squares fit to the movement-corrected time series of Fig. 13.2. The estimated curve is shown in Fig. 13.3(a). Note that this is not very smooth because of the small delay ($\lambda = 0.43$, corresponding to a delay of 0.43 s) relative to the box-car function which starts with condition B (i.e. $b(1) = -1$).

Lange and Zeger (1997) use the more flexible two-parameter gamma family $\Gamma(\lambda, u)$ for g

$$g(s; \lambda, u) = \frac{1}{\Gamma(u)} \lambda^u s^{u-1} e^{-\lambda s} \qquad u, \lambda \geq 0 \qquad (13.7)$$

and allow both the shape and scale parameters (λ and u respectively) to depend on the voxel location. Estimation of the shape and delay parameters in (13.3) is complicated because the model is not linear in these parameters (see Lange and Zeger (1997) for details on their method of parameter estimation in the Fourier domain).

Bullmore *et al.* (1996a) and Friston *et al.* (1995) suggest linear models involving sinusoidal terms which also allow flexibility in the shape and delay of the signal. The former is given by the first few terms of a Fourier series:

$$Y(t) = \gamma_1 \sin(\omega_0 t) + \delta_1 \cos(\omega_0 t) + \gamma_2 \sin(2\omega_0 t) + \delta_2 \cos(2\omega_0 t)$$
$$+ \gamma_3 \sin(3\omega_0 t) + \delta_3 \cos(3\omega_0 t) + \epsilon_t \tag{13.8}$$

Here ω_0 is the angular frequency (in radians per time point) of the box-car function. If there are n_c repetitions of conditions A and B, then $\omega_0 = 2n_c\pi/n$. The frequencies ω_0, $2\omega_0$ and $3\omega_0$ are the fundamental frequency and the first and second harmonics respectively. Note that the power at the fundamental frequency, $\gamma_1^2 + \delta_1^2$, plays a similar part to β^2 in (13.2) and (13.3) since

$$\gamma_1 \sin(\omega_0 t) + \delta_1 \cos(\omega_0 t) = \sqrt{\gamma_1^2 + \delta_1^2} \sin(\omega_0 t - \Phi) \tag{13.9}$$

where $\Phi = -\tan^{-1}(\delta_1/\gamma_1)$ corresponds to the delay parameters d and λ in (13.2) and (13.3) respectively. Under the null hypothesis, the standard error of the estimated power at the fundamental frequencies is approximately $\sqrt{\{2[SE(\hat{\gamma}_1)^4 + SE(\hat{\delta}_1)^4]\}}$. The standardized measure of experimental effect is therefore given by

$$P = \frac{\hat{\gamma}_1^2 + \hat{\delta}_1^2}{\sqrt{2[SE(\hat{\gamma}_1)^4 + SE(\hat{\delta}_1)^4]}} \tag{13.10}$$

The fit of this model (six parameters) to the time series is given in Fig. 13.3(b). Here, the delay relative to the negative sine wave (corresponding to BABA etc.) was only 0.36 s.

There are also several methods of detecting activation which do not employ any explicit models for the experimental effect. For example, an early approach was simply to compare the distribution of intensities during conditions A and B using a Kolmogorov–Smirnov test. Fuzzy clustering (Scarth *et al.*, 1996) and principal components analysis (Synchra *et al.*, 1994) have also been used to identify groups of voxels with similarly shaped waveforms without the necessity to make any assumptions about the activation patterns.

Klose *et al.* (1996) suggest a method which assumes that the signal is periodic in shape but may have a time-varying amplitude. For each pair of conditions A and B, the corresponding part of the time series is normalized by dividing by the mean difference in intensity during the two conditions; the mean normalized time course for pairs of conditions is then calculated. Multiplying this average time course by the pair-specific differences gives the estimated signal. The estimated signal for our time series (involving 26 parameters for the shape of a full cycle plus another four for the amplitudes of the cycles) is shown in Fig. 13.3(c). Although this function is probably overparameterized, allowing the amplitude to change with time is an interesting idea which would be useful when there are learning effects during the scan.

Brammer *et al.* (1997b) model the signal using wavelets. This approach allows the smoothness and the approximate periodicity of the estimated signal to be determined by an appropriate choice of resolution levels of the dyadic decomposition (see Unser, 1996). In Fig. 13.3(d), for example, we have fitted a Daubechies 8 wavelet to the time series using resolution levels 4 and 5 (counted from fine to coarse) where the periodic response from the auditory stimulation should be concentrated. The fit is not strictly periodic but seems reasonably good at distinguishing between signal and noise. Wavelets may also be useful for non-periodic designs such as hallucination studies.

13.4.2   Modelling temporal autocorrelations

Many of the models described above are simple linear models and the effect size of interest is a regression coefficient. If standard errors are required for the estimated effect sizes, then it is important to model the temporal autocorrelations adequately in the time series. Simply ignoring autocorrelations and carrying out a standard regression analysis would yield standard error estimates that tend to be too low.

Bullmore *et al.* (1996a) model the autocorrelations of the random part of the time series by a first-order autoregressive process,

$$\epsilon_t = \zeta \epsilon_{t-1} + v_t \tag{13.11}$$

where v_t are independently normally distributed. The regression co-efficients δ_i and γ_i and the autoregression parameter ζ can be estimated simultaneously by maximum likelihood. Since the estimation needs to be repeated over 300 000 times in a typical fMRI data set (and even more often if randomization testing is used, see Section 13.5.1.1), Bullmore *et al.* use the computationally more expedient method of 'pseudo-generalized least squares' (Cochrane and Orcutt, 1949, Hibbs, 1974) which yields very similar results in practice. The method works as follows. The regression is first estimated by ordinary linear least squares. The estimated residuals c_t are then used to estimate the autoregression parameter ζ and the model is transformed as

$$\begin{aligned} Y(t)^* &= Y(t) - \zeta Y(t-1) \\ X(t)^* &= X(t) - \zeta X(t-1) \end{aligned} \qquad t = 2, \dots, n \tag{13.12}$$

where $X(t)$ is the tth row of the design matrix (whose columns are $\sin(k\omega_0 t)$, $\cos(k\omega_0 t)$, $k = 1, 2, 3$). The final regression parameters as well as their standard errors are estimated by linear least squares for the transformed model. In a number of fMRI time series used by the authors to develop this model, the residuals from the transformed model were no longer significantly correlated by the Box–Pierce test (Box and Pierce, 1970), suggesting that a first-order autoregressive process is adequate to model the autocorrelations.

Worsley and Friston (1995) assume that the observed time series can be generated by convolving uncorrelated data (unobserved) with a Gaussian kernel and that the regression model is appropriate for these uncorrelated data. The regression coefficients may then be estimated by first convolving the design matrix with the Gaussian kernel and then applying the usual least squares procedure. Both the covariance matrix of the estimated parameters and the effective residual degrees of freedom are functions of the Gaussian kernel (see also Watson, 1955). Instead of estimating the width of the Gaussian kernel from the time series, Worsley and Friston smooth the time series with a Gaussian kernel and assume that this same kernel adequately accounts for the autocorrelation structure.

13.5   Detecting activation

When the experimental effect at each voxel has been estimated, a necessary next step in many investigations is to identify regions of activation in the image. The question therefore is which of the estimated effects are real. The simplest approach is to apply a threshold to the effect estimated at each voxel. More sophisticated approaches also take local neighbourhood information into account by considering clusters of activation. These two approaches are described in Sections 13.5.1 and 13.5.2 respectively.

13.5.1   Hypothesis testing

An obvious problem with performing hypothesis tests at each voxel is the high risk of obtaining a large number of false positives. In order to keep the number of false positives reasonably small, authors usually try to make the voxelwise Type I error α as small as possible without losing too much power to detect activation. The apparently activated regions are then displayed as coloured blobs in a grey-scale image of the brain. Colour coding activated regions according to the size of the observed effect (or according to the significance levels) may help assess which of the blobs are more likely to be true positives. Further considerations are the size of clusters of blobs, large clusters providing more evidence for activation than small ones, as well as any prior expectation about where activation is likely to occur. Finally, a region would have to be consistently identified in a number of studies before it is generally accepted as being associated with a specific function.

However, some researchers are not happy with this informal approach to the problem of false positives and try to obtain strong control over the imagewise Type I error, thus inevitably increasing the risk of not detecting weak activation. The Bonferroni correction is conservative to the extent that voxels are correlated (since the tests are not independent, which means that there are effectively fewer independent comparisons than there are voxels). Worsley and Friston (1995) therefore suggest modelling the standardized measures of experimental effect estimated at each voxel as a lattice representation of a continuous, stationary Gaussian random field. Gaussian random field theory can then be used to derive the approximate probability that at least one voxel in the image exceeds a given threshold. Details of this approach are given in Chapter 12.

Holmes *et al.* (1996) point out that the statistic image can only be approximated by a continuous field if it is sufficiently smooth and if sufficient degrees of freedom were available for estimating the variance required for standardizing the test statistic. If these two conditions are not met, the continuous field would have features which are smaller than the voxel size. This is the main reason why groups using Gaussian field theory smooth the images by convolving them with a Gaussian filter, thus risking the elimination of small activated regions. Holmes *et al.* also remark that departures from the assumed distribution will have the greatest effect in the tails which are of primary importance in deriving the threshold.

13.5.1.1   Non-parametric methods

In order to avoid making ambitious assumptions about the distribution of the test statistic, Bullmore *et al.* (1996a) introduced randomization testing to fMRI (see Edgington (1980) and Manly (1991) for introductions to randomization testing). The idea behind the method is simply that under the null hypothesis of no activation, the temporal ordering of the data is irrelevant; any observed value would have been equally likely to have arisen in any position in the series (the data are *exchangeable*). (Strictly speaking the null hypothesis of this test is therefore complete randomness, whereas we would expect unactivated voxels to show some temporal autocorrelations. It seems unlikely, however, that any trends induced by the autocorrelations at unactivated voxels would happen to have the same periodicity as the experiment. Further, Bullmore *et al.* (1996a) compare the permutation distribution of the test statistic with the distribution of the test statistic derived from a 'null' image acquired without a periodic experimental stimulus and find a very close agreement between these distributions.)

By repeatedly permuting the data and re-estimating the test statistic, one obtains an approximate empirical null distribution. The threshold value of the test statistic corresponding to a two-tailed significance level α is just the $100(1 - \alpha/2)$ percentile of this permutation distribution. This method was applied to our example image and the result is shown in Fig. 13.4 (left).

Holmes *et al.* (1996) show how randomization testing can also be adapted to control the imagewise Type I error. Instead of testing each voxel against the empirical sampling distribution of voxel values, the largest test statistic in the image is tested against the distribution of the largest test statistic obtained from a large number of permutations of the

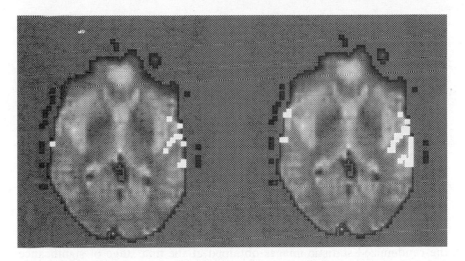

Fig. 13.4 Average functional image with activation superimposed. The activation was determined by applying a threshold of $\alpha = 1/2000$ to (i) P values from time series (left) and (ii) the product of P values from time series and from cluster size (right)

image sequence. It is therefore not necessary to introduce Gaussian field theory in order to control the imagewise Type I error.

13.5.2   Incorporating spatial context

It is probably safe to assume that activation is unlikely to occur at a single isolated voxel and that a number of contiguous voxels exceeding a threshold provide more evidence for underlying true activation than a single voxel (since such clusters are less likely to come about by chance).

Friston *et al.* (1994b) derive an expression for the probability of at least one activated *cluster* containing S voxels or more under the Gaussian field assumptions. Here, a cluster is defined as a set of contiguous voxels (i.e. each voxel is a nearest neighbour of another voxel in the set), all exceeding the threshold T. Poline and Mazoyer (1993) and Forman *et al.* (1995) simulate images, assuming they are realizations of a Gaussian field, to derive approximate P values for cluster sizes at various thresholds. A drawback of these cluster size methods is that the choice of threshold (and hence cluster size) determines to what type of underlying activation the method is sensitive. For example, a high threshold picks up strong activation concentrated in a small area but misses diffuse activation, spread out into a larger area and vice versa. Poline *et al.* (1997) have therefore developed a method which combines significance testing based on peak height and spatial extent and is sensitive to both types of activation.

Bullmore *et al.* (1996a) combine peak height and spatial extent in the following two-stage significance test. In the first stage, they perform distribution-free hypothesis testing as described in Section 13.5.1.1, but by permuting entire images instead of permuting each time series independently. This results in a collection of temporally randomized but spatially connected statistic images which are thresholded using the same threshold as for the observed image (to achieve a voxelwise significance of $\alpha = 0.05$). Each voxel in the observed image is also assigned a P value P_t (for 'temporal') using the percentiles of the randomization distribution.

The false positive voxels in the observed image would be expected to be randomly scattered (apart from some clustering that may result from the correlation between spatially adjacent time series), whereas true activated voxels are more likely to be found within a cluster of other activated voxels. In the second stage of the significance test, the authors therefore use the number of voxels constituting each eight-connected cluster (m_c) as the test statistic. Assuming that all the activated voxels in the randomized statistic images obtained at the first stage of significance testing are false positives, the authors obtain an empirical null distribution of m_c by counting the number of voxels constituting each eight-connected cluster in the randomized images. The percentiles of this distribution provide the P value P_s (for 'spatial') for m_c.

Finally, the two stages of significance testing are combined in a heuristic way by thresholding the product of P values $P_t P_s$ at each voxel. Figure 13.4 shows an fMRI slice averaged over time with the activated voxels superimposed in white. Unlike the image on the left, that on the right uses spatial information as outlined above.

13.6   Localizing activation anatomically

When the regions of activation within an fMR image have been identified, the remaining problem is to map these activated regions to anatomical locations. The problem with fMRI is the relatively poor anatomical contrast making it difficult to recognize anatomical features in the image itself. One approach is therefore to acquire a structural image with superior anatomical contrast and to overlap or register the two images. Brammer *et al.* (1997a) use an approach similar to the realignment used for movement correction. Firstly, the structural image is rescaled to have the same voxel dimensions as the time-averaged functional image. Then it is histogram matched to the average functional image and finally rotated and translated to minimize the sum of absolute differences between voxels. The blobs on the functional image are then transferred to the corresponding locations in the structural image as shown in Fig. 13.5.

For brain experts, this may be sufficient to identify anatomical structures by referring to a brain atlas if necessary. The most popular atlas is that by Talairach and Tournoux (1995), who defined a rectangular coordinate system for the brain of a middle-aged female.

A more formal approach to identifying anatomical structures is to

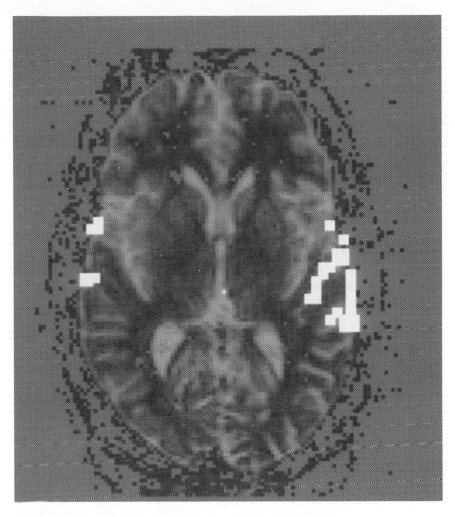

Fig. 13.5 Structural (EPI) image with activated regions superimposed

register the structural image to the Talairach atlas. This is usually done by manually locating the AC–PC line (superior aspect of the anterior commissure to inferior aspect of the posterior commissure) in the image and aligning it with the corresponding coordinate axis of the Talairach atlas. The three coordinate axes are then rescaled to match the image to the atlas as closely as possible. A problem with this approach is the amount of user input required to determine the AC–PC line and the questionable accuracy associated with it (Nadeau and Crosson, 1995). To avoid these problems every time a functional image is analysed, Brammer *et al.* have carefully registered images of 12 subjects to the Talairach atlas, using the AC–PC line as well as several reference points, and averaged these registered images to derive a template image. All future images may

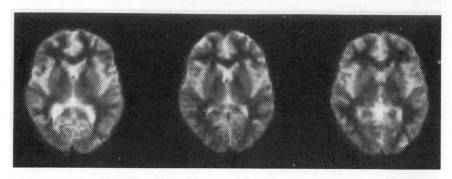

Fig. 13.6 Images from three subjects registered in standard space

then simply be registered with the Talairach template by using essentially the same method as in movement correction and functional to structural image registration. This final step, also called registration into 'standard space', allows an automatic allocation of Talairach coordinates to the activated regions. This step is also essential for group comparisons.

A problem with this allocation of coordinates as a method of identifying anatomical structures is the substantial variation between the shapes or proportions of brain structures between individuals. Some form of 'elastic' matching or warping is probably required to ensure that corresponding anatomical structures overlap between the image and atlas (see Little and Hawkes (1997) for a review of such methods). To illustrate the variation in shape between individuals, Fig. 13.6 shows one image slice from three different subjects registered into standard space.

13.7   Concluding remarks

We have described and illustrated the methods of analysis which are routinely applied to functional images acquired at the Institute of Psychiatry. At the same time we have reviewed some of the large number of alternative methods advocated by other groups. Functional MRI is still a relatively new technique, its first application to humans being as recent as 1992 (Kwong *et al.*, 1992), and no standard approach to the analysis of such images has yet evolved. This is partly because of difficulties encountered when attempting to apply and compare alternative approaches objectively. Applying alternative approaches is difficult because of the amount of time and effort required to implement them. Even if solutions from several approaches were available for the same data set, a further problem would be how to compare these solutions when the true locations of activation in the particular brain that was imaged (i.e. the 'ground truth') are not known.

However, we believe that whatever method is implemented, there are several important issues that should be addressed. These include allowing for spatially varying haemodynamic delay and taking account of temporal autocorrelations in time series analyses. Further we believe that it is dangerous to place too much emphasis on control over Type I error at the expense of increasing Type II error. Finally, we feel that randomization testing is an elegant way of avoiding possibly unrealistic assumptions regarding the distribution of the test statistic.

Acknowledgements

ETB is supported by the Wellcome Trust. This chapter would not have been possible without the support of our colleagues at the Institute of Psychiatry, in particular Ian Wright, Steve Williams and Andy Simmons.

References

Bandettini, P. A., Jesmanowicz, A., Wong, E. C. and Hyde, J. S. 1993: Processing strategies for time-course data sets in functional MRI of the brain. *Magnetic Resonance in Medicine* **30**, 161–73.

Box, G. E. P. and Pierce, D. A. 1970: Distribution of residual autocorrelations in autoregressive integrated moving average time series models. *Journal of the American Statistical Association* **65**, 1509–26.

Brammer, M. J., Bullmore, E. T., Simmons, A., Williams, S. C. R., Grasby, P. M., Howard, R. J., Woodruff, P. W. R. and Rabe-Hesketh, S. 1997a: Generic brain activation mapping in fMRI – a nonparametric approach. *Magnetic Resonance Imaging* **15**, 736–70.

Brammer, M. J., Wright, I. C., Woodruff, P. W. R., Williams, S. C. R., Simmons, A. and Bullmore, E. T. 1997b: Wavelet analysis of periodic and non-periodic experimental designs in functional magnetic resonance imaging of the brain. *NeuroImage* **5**, S479.

Bullmore, E. T., Brammer, M. J., Williams, S. C. R., Rabe-Hesketh, S., Janot, N., David, A. S., Mellers, J. D. C., Howard, R. and Sham, P. 1996a: Statistical methods of estimation and inference for functional MR image analysis. *Magnetic Resonance in Medicine* **35**, 261–77.

Bullmore, E. T., Rabe-Hesketh, S., Morris, R. G., Williams, S. C. R., Gregory, L., Gray, J. A. and Brammer, M. J. 1996b: Functional magnetic resonance imaging of a large scale neurocognitive framework. *NeuroImage* **4**, 16–33.

Cochrane, D. and Orcutt, G. H. 1949: Application of least squares regression to relationships containing autocorrelated error terms. *Journal of American Statistical Association* **44**, 32.

Cohen, M. S. and Weisskopf, R. M. 1991: Ultra-fast imaging. *Magnetic Resonance Imaging* **9**, 1–37.

Edgington, E. S. 1980: *Randomisation tests*. New York: Marcel Dekker.

Forman, S. D., Cohen, J. D., Fitzgerald, M., Eddy, W. F., Mintun, M. A. and Noll, D. C. 1995: Improved assessment of significant activation in functional magnetic resonance imaging (fMRI): use of a cluster-size threshold. *Magnetic Resonance in Medicine* **33**, 636–47.

Foster, M. A. and Hutchison, J. M. S. 1985: NMR imaging – method and applications. *Journal of Biomedical Engineering* **7**, 171–82.

Fox, P. T. and Raichle, M. E. 1986: Focal physiological uncoupling of cerebral blood flow and oxidative metabolism during somatosensory stimulation in human subjects. *Proceedings of the National Academy of Science* **83**, 1140–4.

Friston, K. J., Frith, C. D., Turner, R. and Frackowiak, R. S. J. 1995: Characterising evoked haemodynamics with fMRI. *NeuroImage* **2**, 157–65.

Friston, K. J., Jezzard, P. and Turner, R. 1994a: The analysis of functional MRI time series. *Human Brain Mapping* **1**, 153–71.

Friston, K. J., Williams, S. C. R., Howard, R., Frackowiak, R. S. J. and Turner, R. 1996: Movement-related effects in fMRI time series. *Magnetic Resonance in Medicine* **35**, 346–55.

Friston, K. J., Worsley, K. J., Frackowiak, R. S. J., Mazziotta, J. C. and Evans, A. C. 1994b: Assessing the significance of focal activations using their spatial extent. *Human Brain Mapping* **1**, 210–20.

Gandhe, A. J., Hill, D. L. G., Studholme, C., Hawkes, D. J., Ruff, C. F., Strong, A. J., Cox, T. C. S. and Gleeson, M. J. 1994: Combined and 3D rendered multimodal data for planning skull base surgery: a prospective evaluation. *Neurosurgery* **35**, 463–71.

Hajnal, J. V., Myers, R., Oatridge, A., Schwieso, J. E., Young, I. R. and Bydder, G. M. 1994: Artifacts due to stimulus correlated motion in functional imaging of the brain. *Magnetic Resonance in Medicine* **31**, 283–91.

Hibbs, D. A. 1974: Problems of statistical estimation and causal inference in time series regression models. In Costner, H. L. (ed.), *Sociological methodology 1973–1974*. San Francisco: Jossey-Bass, 252–308.

Hill, D. L. G., Hawkes, D. J., Studholme, C., Summers, P. E. and Taylor, M. G. 1994: Accurate registration and transformation of temporal image sequences. *Proceedings of the 2nd Conference of the Society of Magnetic Resonance*, vol. 411, 820.

Holmes, A. P., Blair, R. C., Watson, J. D. G. and Ford, I. 1996: Nonparametric analysis of statistic images from functional mapping experiments. *Journal of Cerebral Blood Flow and Metabolism* **16**, 7–22.

Jezzard, P. and Balaban, R. S. 1995: Correction for geometric distortion in echo planar images from B_0 field variations. *Magnetic Resonance in Medicine* **34**, 65–73.

Klose, U., Wildgruber, D., Britsch, P. and Grodd, W. 1996: Evaluation of fMRI data using pixel specific target functions. *NeuroImage* **4**, S71.

Kwong, K. K. *et al.* 1992: Dynamic magnetic resonance imaging of human brain activity during primary sensory stimulation. *Proceedings of the National Academy of Science* **89**, 5675–9.

Lange, N. and Zeger, S. L. 1997: Non-linear Fourier time series analysis for human brain mapping by functional magnetic resonance imaging. *Applied Statistics* **46**, 1–29.

Little, J. and Hawkes, D. 1997: Registration of multiple medical images acquired from a single subject: why, how and what next? *Statistical Methods in Medical Research* **6**, 239–65.

Manly, B. J. F. 1991: *Randomisation and Monte Carlo methods in biology*. London: Chapman & Hall.

Mansfield, P., Coxon, R. and Glover, P. 1994: Echo planar imaging of the brain at 3.0T. *Journal of Computer Assisted Tomography* **18**, 339–43.

Nadeau, S. E. and Crosson, B. 1995: A guide to the functional imaging of cognitive processes. *Brain* **8**, 143–62.

Ogawa, S., Lee, T. M., Kay, A. R. and Tank, D. W. 1990: Brain magnetic resonance imaging with contrast dependent on blood oxygenation. *Proceedings of the National Academy of Science* **87**, 9868–72.

Poline, J.-B. and Mazoyer, B. M. 1993: Analysis of individual positron emission tomography activation maps by detection of high signal-to-noise pixel clusters. *Journal of Cerebral Blood Flow and Metabolism* **13**, 425–37.

Poline, J.-B. and Mazoyer, B. M. 1994: Analysis of individual brain activation maps using hierarchical description and multiscale detection. *IEEE Transactions on Medical Imaging* **13**, 702–10.

Poline, J.-B., Mazoyer, B. M., Evans, A. C. and Friston, K. J. 1997: Combining spatial extent and peak intensity to test for activations in functional imaging. *NeuroImage* **5**, 83–6.

Rabe-Hesketh, S., Bullmore, E. T. and Brammer, M. J. 1997: The analysis of functional magnetic resonance images. *Statistical Methods in Medical Research* **6**, 215–37.

Scarth, G., Wenneberg, A., Somoriai, R., Hindmarsh, T. and McIntyre, M. 1996: The utility of fuzzy clustering in identifying diverse activations in fMRI. *NeuroImage* **4**, S89.

Senn, S. 1993: *Cross-over trials in clinical research*. Chichester: John Wiley.

Synchra, J. J., Bandettini, P. A., Bhattacharya, N. and Lin, Q. 1994: Synthetic images by subspace transforms I. Principal components images and related filters. *Magnetic Resonance Imaging* **21**, 193–201.

Talairach, J. and Tournoux, P. 1995: *Coplanar stereotactic atlas of the human brain*. New York: Thieme.

Turner, R., Jezzard, P., Wen, H., Kwong, K. K., Bihan, D. Le. Zeffiro, T. and Balaban, R. S. 1993: Functional mapping of the human visual cortex at 4 and 1.5 Tesla using deoxygenation contrast EPI. *Magnetic Resonance in Medicine* **26**, 277–9.

Unser, M. 1996: A practical guide to the implementation of the wavelet transform. In Adroubi, A. and Unser, M. (eds), *Wavelets in medicine and biology*. Boca Raton, FL: CRC Press, 37–73.

Watson, G. S. 1955: Serial correlation in regression analysis: I. *Biometrika* **42**, 327–41.

Worsley, K. J. 1998: Testing for a signal with unknown location and scale in a χ^2 random field, with an application to fMRI. *Annals of Statistics* (in press).

Worsley, K. J., Evans, A. C., Marrett, S. and Neelin, P. 1992: A three-dimensional statistical analysis for CBF activation studies in human brain. *Journal of Cerebral Blood Flow and Metabolism* **12**, 900–18.

Worsley, K. J. and Friston, K. J. 1995: Analysis of fMRI time series revisited— again. *NeuroImage* **2**, 173–81.

Author index

Aalen, O.O. 62, 63, 68, 69
Abrams, K.R. 36, 49, 53, 54
Adler, R. 295, 296, 297
Agodoa, L.Y. 16
Agresti, A.A. 166, 180
Ahlbom, A. 92
Aitkin, M. 192, 230
Akritas, M.G. 166
Albert, P.S. 177, 192, 194
Alivisatos, B. 283
Altman, D.G. 19, 156
Altman, N.S. 166
Amara, I.A. 145
Andersen, P.K. 20, 54, 77, 78, 84
Anderson, D.A. 192
Anderson, G.L. 179
Anderson, J. 112
Anderson, J.A. 112
Anderson, R.D. 193
Angus, J.W. 150
Arbuthnot, J. 3
Archer, V. 88
Arnold, S.F. 166
Ashburner, J. 285, 286
Ashby, D. 36, 49, 165
Auerbach, O. 259, 271
Azzalini, A. 181

Bacchetti, P. 113
Bahadur, R.R. 180
Bailey, D.L. 279
Baker, R.J. 136
Balaban, R.S. 310, 313
Balagtas, C.C. 180
Balla, D. 128
Bandettini, P.A. 315, 317
Barinaga, M. 61
Barnes, F. 92
Barrett-Connor, E. 67

Bayley, N. 128
Becchetti, P. 108, 112
Beck, G.J. 177
Becker, M.P. 180
Benard, A. 163
Berger, J.O. 47
Bernardinelli, L. 230
Bernardo, J.M. 37
Berzuini, C. 55
Best, N.G. 38, 39, 195, 230, 244
Bhapkar, V.P. 165
Bhattacharya, N. 317
Bihan, D.Le. 310
Birch, M.W. 161
Bishop, Y.M.M. 181
Bjertness, E. 68, 69
Blair, R.C. 298, 320
Bloch, D.A. 103, 165
Blumen, I. 61
Bonney, G.E. 189
Borch-Johnsen, K. 77
Borgan, O. 20, 76, 77, 78, 80, 82, 84, 85, 86, 87, 89, 91, 95, 96, 98
Bowman, J. 92
Box, G.E.P. 187, 254, 272, 318
Brammer, M.J. 293, 309, 311, 315, 316, 318, 320, 321, 322
Brayne, C.E.G. 244
Breiman, L. 101
Breslow, N.E. 14, 75, 127, 136
Britsch, P. 317
Brook, R.H. 229
Brown, G.W. 157, 159
Brownson, R.C. 259, 271
Bryk, A.S. 127, 130, 230, 254
Buchsbaum, M. 284

Buffler, P.A. 259, 271
Bullmore, E.T. 293, 309, 311, 315, 316, 318, 320, 321, 322
Butler, T.L. 259, 271
Bydder, G.M. 312

Cahill, C. 286
Camargo, E.E. 281
Campbell, M.J. 156
Carey, J.R. 61
Carey, V. 183, 187
Carlin, B.P. 39, 119, 233
Carlin, J.B. 254, 272
Carr, G.J. 156
Carr-Hill, R.A. 141
Carroll, R.J. 215
Carson, R. 284
Casella, G. 231
Chalmers, I. 251
Chan, W.S. 141
Chen, S. 108
Cheng, T.-C. 92
Chhikara, R.S. 71
Chinchilli, V.M. 9, 145
Christensen, B. 285
Christiansen, C.L. 230, 233
Cicchetti, D. 128
Clark, C. 284
Clark, L.A. 101, 111
Clark, R. 279
Clayton, D.G. 38, 39, 54, 68, 89, 127, 136, 230
Clifford, P. 213
Cochran, W.G. 161
Cochrane, D. 318
Cohen, J.D. 321
Cohen, M.S. 309
Cohen, R. 284
Colebatch, J.G. 281
Collett, D. 19, 54

Committee on the
   Biological Effects of
   Ionizing Radiation 88
Conaway, M.R. 193, 196
Congdon, R. 127
Conover, W.J. 166
Contant, C. 259, 271
Copas, J.B. 226
Cornell, J. 16
Correa, P. 259, 271
Cowie, C.C. 16
Cowles, M.K. 39, 233
Cox, D.R. 8, 19, 20, 75,
   102, 181, 182, 189
Cox, T.C.S. 309
Coxon, R. 313
Crosson, B. 323
Crouchley, R. 68
Crowder, M.J. 9, 145, 156,
   159, 177
Crowley, J. 108, 110, 112
Cuzick, J. 68

Daley, J. 229
Daniels, M. 7
Dannals, R.F. 281
David, A. 293
David, A.S. 316, 318, 320,
   321
Davidian, M. 9, 145
Davis, C.S. 159, 165
Davis, J.W. 67
Davis, R. 112
Davis, S.D. 187
Dawber, T.R. 175
Dawson, J.D. 156
de Bruijn, N.G. 38
Deckert, T. 77
Deddens, J.A. 88
Defrise, M. 279
de Leeuw, J. 230
DeLisi, L. 284
DerSimonian, R. 252, 255
DeStavola, B.L. 19, 55
Detels, R. 119
Dickey, J.M. 273
Diggle, P.J. 9, 141, 145,
   156, 166, 177, 183, 204,
   209, 210, 211, 213, 214
Diksic, M. 283
Di Serio, C. 60, 65, 67
Dixon, W.J.E. 25
Dockery, D.W. 175, 177
Dolan, R.J. 281
Draper, D. 229

Drum, M. 197
Duara, R. 283, 284
DuBois, R.W. 229
DuMouchel, W.H. 254
Durbin, J. 163

Eaves, L. 68
Eddy, D.M. 257
Eddy, W.F. 321
Edgington, E.S. 320
Efron, B. 230, 254
Eggers, P.W. 16
Ekholm, A. 180
Elder, J.F. 123
Elliott, C.D. 128
Epstein, A.M. 229
Errington, R.D. 36, 49
Evans, A.C. 283, 285, 295,
   296, 297, 300, 321

Fahey, J.L. 119
Fahrmeier, L. 177, 194
Feller, W. 62
Ferguson, S.W. 259, 271
Ferris, B.G. 175, 177
Feychting, M. 92
Fieger, A. 186
Fienberg, S.E. 181
Fineberg, H.V. 251
Fisher, W.D. 104
Fitzgerald, M. 321
Fitzmaurice, G.M. 177,
   179, 180, 181, 182, 187,
   213
Fleiss, J.L. 16, 253
Fleming, T.R. 102, 106,
   123
Folks, J.L. 71
Fontham, E.T.H. 259,
   271
Ford, I. 282, 283, 284, 298,
   320
Forman, S.D. 321
Foster, M.A. 309
Fox, P.T. 310
Fox, W. 7
Frackowiak, R.S.J. 281,
   285, 286, 289, 293, 296,
   313, 316, 321
Freedman, L.S. 36
French, M.A.H. 119
Friberg, L. 285
Friedman, J.H. 101, 104
Friedman, M. 163
Frison, L. 156

Friston, K.J. 281, 285, 289,
   293, 296, 297, 313, 315,
   316, 319, 321
Frith, C.D. 281, 285, 286,
   289, 297, 316

Gandhe, A.J. 309
Ganiats, T.G. 67
Garfinkel, L. 259, 271
Gatsonis, C.A. 229
Gehan, E.A. 107
Geissbuhler, A. 279
Gelfand, A.E. 38, 53, 119,
   194, 231
Gelman, A. 39, 254, 272
Geman, D. 194
Geman, S. 194, 233
Gemand, D. 233
George, E.I. 231
Geweke, J. 43
Ghosh, M. 156
Gibbons, R.D. 195
Gilardi, M.-C. 279
Gilks, W.R. 38, 39, 54, 195,
   230, 231, 233
Gill, R.D. 20, 78, 84
Gillings, D.B. 145
Gilmour, A.R. 193
Giltinan, D.M. 9, 145
Ginsberg, R.B. 61
Giorgi, J.V. 119
Gleeson, M.J. 309
Glickman, M.E. 229, 230
Glonek, G.F.V. 180, 183
Glover, P. 313
Goldstein, H. 127, 130, 136,
   195, 229, 230
Goldstein, L. 76, 82, 84, 85,
   87, 88, 89, 96, 98
Gordon, L. 112
Grambsch, P.M. 102, 123
Grandinetti, A. 67
Grasby, P.J. 293
Grasby, P.M. 311, 322
Gray, J.A. 315
Green, A. 77
Green, P.J. 241, 279
Greenhouse, J. 49
Gregory, L. 315
Grieve, A.P. 214
Grizzle, J.E. 156
Grodd, W. 317
Gupta, P. 119

Haddock, C.K. 253

Haensel, W. 259, 271
Haenszel, W. 13
Hafner, K.B. 156
Hajnal, J.V. 312
Hand, D.J. 9, 145, 156, 159, 177
Hardman, G. 141
Harrington, D. 106
Harrington, D.P. 180, 183
Harris, J.E. 254
Hart, J.D. 166
Harville, D.A. 254
Hasselblad, V. 257
Hastings, W.K. 232
Hauck, W.W. 194
Hawkes, D.J. 309, 312, 324
Hayes, R.B. 2
Heagerty, P.J. 184
Heath, A.F. 213
Heather, J.D. 285
Heckman, J.J. 61, 211
Hedeker, D. 195
Hedges, L.V. 252, 253, 255, 272
Henderson, B.E. 259, 271
Herman, G.T. 279
Hettmansperger, T.R. 157
Heumann, C. 186
Hewitt, J. 68
Heyman, E.R. 159, 160
Hibbs, D.A. 318
Hill, D.L.G. 309, 312
Hills, S.E. 38, 39
Hindmarsh, T. 317
Hodges, J.L. 163
Hoffman, F.J. 279
Holland, P.W. 181
Holmes, A.P. 289, 293, 296, 297, 298, 320
Hornung, R. 88
Horwitz, B. 283, 284
Hougaard, P. 61, 62, 68, 77
Howard, R.J. 293, 311, 313, 316, 318, 320, 321, 322
Huang, X. 108
Huber, P.J. 182
Humble, C.G. 259, 271
Husebye, E. 68, 69
Hutchison, J.M.S. 309
Hyde, J.S. 315

Iachine, I. 66, 68
Iman, R.L. 166

James, I.R. 119

Janerich, T.D. 259, 271
Janot, N. 293, 316, 318, 320, 321
Jencks, S.F. 229
Jesmanowicz, A. 315
Jewell, N.P. 108, 112, 194
Jezzard, P. 310, 313, 315
John, E. 92
Johnson, W.E. 163, 164, 165, 167
Jones, R.H. 9, 145
Jones, T. 279, 286
Jorgensen, B. 71
Joubert, L. 259, 271

Kabat, G.C. 259, 271
Kadane, J.B. 38, 231, 273
Kalbfleisch, J.D. 37, 164, 179, 194
Kaldor, J. 230
Kameyama, M. 283
Karim, M.R. 187, 194
Kass, R.E. 38, 46, 47, 271
Kastner, C. 186
Kaufman, L. 279
Kay, A.R. 310
Keefe, T.J. 259, 271
Keiding, N. 20, 77, 78
Keller, J.B. 112
Kenward, M.G. 9, 145, 211, 213, 214
Kepner, J.L. 166
Kessler, R. 284
King, C. 284
King, E.B. 114
Kingsley, J.A. 119
Kirby, A.J. 38
Klose, U. 317
Knudson, A.G. 62
Koch, G.G. 145, 156, 159, 160, 163, 166
Kogan, M. 61
Korn, E.L. 189, 192
Kreft, I.G. 230
Kreiner, S. 77
Kruskal, W.H. 157
Kshirsagar, A.M. 9, 145, 166
Kuhl, D.E. 283
Kuo, L. 39
Kwong, K.K. 310, 313, 315, 324

Lachin, J.M. 163, 164, 165, 167

Laird, N.M. 177, 179, 180, 181, 182, 183, 192, 196, 209, 252, 254, 255
Lammertsma, A.A. 281
Landis, J.R. 159, 160
Lang, J. 180
Lange, N. 119, 239, 315, 316
Langer, R.D. 67
Langholz, B. 76, 77, 80, 82, 84, 85, 86, 87, 88, 89, 91, 95, 96, 98
Lausen, B. 102, 110
Law, I. 285
LeBlanc, M. 108, 110, 112
Lee, T.M. 310
Leeper, E. 91
Lehmann, E.L. 163
Lenhart, G. 229
Lesaffre, E. 180
Leung, S.S. 141
Leyland, A. 230
Li, H.G. 226
Liang, K.Y. 9, 141, 145, 156, 166, 177, 180, 182, 183, 184, 189, 192, 194, 204, 210
Liddle, P.F. 281
Liedo, P. 61
Lin, Q. 317
Lindsey, J.K. 9, 145
Linet, M. 92
Links, J.M. 281
Lipsitz, S.R. 180, 183, 187, 189
Littell, R.C. 230
Little, J. 324
Little, M.P. 62
Little, R.J.A. 132, 196, 210, 213, 214
Lock, S. ix
London, S. 92
Longford, N. 230
Longford, N.T. 229, 230
Louis, T.A. 130, 251
Love, S.B. 19
Lowrie, E.G. 16
Lubin, J. 88
Lundin, F. 88

McCabe, G.P. 150, 151, 153
MacCarthy, P. 61
McCormick, K.A. 251
McCrory, S.J. 282, 283
McCullagh, P. 180, 193, 197

McDonald, J.W. 180
McIntyre, M. 317
Mack, W. 88
McLaughlin, T. 285
McMillan, A. 88
McNeil, A.J. 38
McNemar, Q. 161
Madansky, A. 160, 161
Maddala, G.S. 135
Mallal, S. 119
Manly, B.J.F. 320
Mansfield, P. 313
Mantel, N. 13
Manton, K.G. 61, 63, 66
Marek, P. 107
Margolin, R. 284
Marrett, S. 295, 296, 300
Martin, A.J. 281
Martin, S. 141
Mason, T.J. 259, 271
Mason, W.M. 193
Matthews, J.N.S. 156
Mazoyer, B.M. 296, 312, 321
Mazziotta, J.C. 296, 321
Medina, R.A. 16
Meinhardt, T. 88
Mellers, J.D.C. 316, 318, 320, 321
Mellors, J.W. 119, 293
Metropolis, N. 232
Metter, E.J. 283
Meyer, J. 68
Michiels, B. 214
Mildvan, A.S. 61
Miller, M.E. 159
Miller, R.G. 102
Milliken, G.A. 230
Mintun, M.A. 281, 321
Moeller, J.R. 284
Molenberghs, G. 180, 184, 214
Monterrosa, A. 16
Montomoli, C. 230
Mood, A.M. 157, 159
Moolgavkar, S.H. 62
Moore, D.S. 150, 151, 153
Moore, S.R. 251
Morens, D.M. 67
Morris, C. 230, 254
Morris, C.N. 230, 233
Morris, R.G. 315
Moses, L.E. 165
Moss, A.R. 113
Mosteller, F. 251

Muenz, L.R. 189
Muirhead, C.R. 62
Mullen, E. 128
Müller, H.G. 166
Munoz, A. 113
Myers, R. 312

Nadeau, S.E. 323
National Research Council 252
Naylor, J.C. 38, 231
Neelin, P. 295, 296, 300
Nelder, J.A. 136, 180
Neuhaus, J.M. 192, 194
New York State Department of Health 229
NHS Executive 229
Nightingale, F. 6
Noll, D.C. 321
Normand, S.-L.T. 229, 230
Nuttal, D. 230

Oakes, D. 68, 76, 84
Oatridge, A. 312
O'Brien, P.C. 165
Ochi, Y. 193
Ogawa, S. 310
O'Hagan, A. 34, 47
Olkin, I. 252, 253
Olshen, R.A. 101, 112
Orcutt, G.H. 318
Orozco, D. 61
O'Sullivan, F. 112

Page, E.B. 163
Palesch, Y.Y. 165
Pan, H. 230
Parmar, M.K.B. 36
Parving, A. 285
Pathak, D.R. 259, 271
Peacock, S. 141
Pearson, E.S. 4
Pendergast, J. 166
Pepe, M.S. 179
Pericchi, L.R. 47
Perlmutter, J.S. 281
Peters, J. 92
Peters, S.C. 273
Petersen, T. 32
Peto, J. 107
Peto, R. 107
Petrakis, N.L. 114
Phelps, M.E. 283
Pickle, L.W. 259, 271

Pickles, A. 68
Pierce, D.A. 318
Pike, M.D. 259, 271
Plewis, I. 127
Pocock, S.J. 7, 21, 156, 165
Pogoda, J. 88
Poline, J.B. 285, 289, 293, 296, 297, 312, 321
Politte, D.G. 279
Potthoff, R. 166
Pregibon, D. 101, 111
Prentice, R.L. 75, 107, 164, 179, 180, 181, 184, 193
Price, C.J. 297
Pritzl, J.A. 259, 271
Pugh, J.A. 16
Puri, M.L. 157, 167

Qaqish, B. 180, 183, 184
Quetelet, A. 5

Rabe-Hesketh, S. 293, 309, 311, 315, 316, 318, 320, 321, 322
Racine-Poon, A. 38
Rae, A.L. 193
Raftery, A.E. 46, 47
Raichle, M.E. 281, 310
Rapoport, S.I. 283, 284
Rasbash, J. 127, 133, 195, 230
Raudenbush, S.W. 127, 130, 141, 230, 255
Raz, J. 166
Read, C.B. 6
Reed, D. 67
Reif, J.S. 259, 271
Rice, N. 230
Richardson, S. 38, 230, 231, 241
Richardson, W.S. 2
Riege, W.H. 283
Rinaldo, C.R. 119
Ripley, B.D. 39
Ritter, L.L. 184
Roberts, G.O. 39
Robertson, W.H. 210, 213
Robinson, D.H. 166
Rogers, W.H. 229
Rolph, J.E. 229, 230
Rosenberg, W. 2
Rosenbluth, A.W. 232
Ross, G.W. 67
Rotnitzky, A.G. 179, 182
Rottenberg, D.A. 284

Roy, S.N. 166
Royall, R.M. 182
Royston, P. 156
Rubin, D.B. 132, 210, 254, 272
Rubinstein, L.V. 189
Ruff, C.F. 309
Rutter, M. 68
Ryan, L. 239
Ryan, T.J. 230

Sackett, D.L. 2
Samet, J.M. 259, 271
Sansó, B. 53
Sarton, G. 5
SAS Institute Inc. 32, 33, 187
Satterthwaite, F.E. 293
Savitz, D. 92
Scarth, G. 317
Schmidt, F.L. 272
Schneider, E.C. 229
Schnorr, L. 286
Schumacher, M. 102, 110
Schwertman, N.C. 157, 159
Schwieso, J.E. 312
Scottish Office 229
Segal, M.R. 101, 103, 106, 108, 112, 119
Self, S.G. 189
Seltzer, M. 254
Sen, P.K. 156, 157, 163, 166, 167
Senn, S. 2, 313
Senthilselvan, A. 112
Shachter, R. 257
Shadish, W.R. 253
Sham, P. 293, 316, 318, 320, 321
Shaper, A.G. 165
Shapiro, S.S. 167
Sharples, L.D. 38
Shaw, J.E.H. 38, 231
Sheldon, T.A. 141
Shepp, L.A. 279
Shoesmith, E. 4
Sidtis, J.J. 284
Siegel, R.A. 251
Siegmund, D. 102
Silberg, J. 68
Silbersweig, D.A. 286, 287
Simmons, A. 311, 318, 322
Simonoff, E. 68
Simpson, G.M. 150
Singer, B. 61

Skene, A.M. 231
Smith, A.F.M. 37, 38, 39, 194, 231, 254
Smith, D.M. 210, 213
Smith, P. 141
Smith, P.W.F. 180
Smith, T.C. 254
Smith, W.B. 9, 145, 166
Smith, W.S. 273
Snyder, D.L. 279
Sobel, E. 92
Somoriai, R. 317
Sonju, T. 68, 69
Soong, S.-J. 108
Sostre, S. 281
Sparrow, S. 128
Speizer, F.E. 175, 177, 189
Spengler, J.D. 175
Spiegelhalter, D.J. 36, 38, 39, 54, 195, 229, 230, 231, 244, 254
Spinks, T.J. 279
Spiro, A. 130, 175, 177
Stallard, E. 61, 63, 66
Stangl, D.K. 55
Statistical Sciences Inc. 32, 38, 39, 187
Steenland, K. 88
Steinberg, B. 285
Stepniewska, K.A. 19
Stern, E. 286
Stern, H.S. 254, 272
Sternio, J.L.F. 130
Stigler, S.M. 4, 38
Stiller, C.A. 62
Stiratelli, R. 192
Stokes, M.E. 145
Stone, C.J. 101
Stram, D.O. 175, 189
Strehler, B.L. 61
Strong, A.J. 309
Strother, S.C. 283, 284, 285
Stroup, W.W. 230
Studholme, C. 309, 312
Summers, P.E. 312
Sutherland, I. 7
Synchra, J.J. 317
Szabo, Z. 281

Talairach, J. 285, 322
Tank, D.W. 310
Tarone, R.E. 106, 107
Taylor, J.M.G. 119
Taylor, M.G. 312
Teller, M.N. 232

Tellet, A.H. 232
Thall, P.F. 153, 165
Therneau, T.M. 102, 123
Thisted, R.A. 38
Thomas, A. 39, 54, 195, 230, 244, 254
Thomas, D.C. 75, 78, 88, 92
Thomas, N. 229, 230
Thompson, G.L. 166
Thompson, R. 136
Thorogood, J. 233
Tiao, G.C. 254, 272
Tidwell, P.W. 187
Tierney, L. 38, 231
Todd, J.A. 119
Tournoux, P. 285, 322
Townsend, D.W. 279
Tsai, W.-Y. 108, 112
Tsiatis, A.A. 36
Tukey, J.W. 128
Turner, R. 293, 310, 313, 315, 316
Tutz, G. 177, 194
Tvrdik, J. 92
Tyler, J.L. 283, 285

UKTSSA 233
Unser, M. 318

Vail, S.C. 153
Van Houlwelingen, H.C. 233
Vandal, A.C. 296
van der Leeden, R. 230
van Elteren, P. 163
Vardi, Y. 279
Vaupel, J.W. 61, 63
Verbyla, A.P. 213
Videen, T.O. 281
Vines, K. 39
Vonesh, E.F. 9, 145

Wachtel, H. 92
Wagner, H.N. Jr. 281
Wagoner, J. 88
Walker, J. 229
Walker, S.H. 163
Wallis, W.A. 157
Wang, M.-C. 108, 112
Ware, J.H. 106, 107, 130, 175, 177, 189, 192, 209, 254
Wasserman, L. 271
Watson, G.S. 319
Watson, J.D.G. 298, 320

Wedderburn, R.W.M. 136, 183
Wehrly, T.E. 166
Wei, L.J. 163, 164, 165, 167, 189
Weisberg, H.I. 130
Weisskopf, R.M. 309
Wen, H. 310
Wenneberg, A. 317
Wertheimer, N. 91
White, H. 182
White, L.R. 67
White, R.M. 119
White, S.J. ix
Whittaker, J. 39
Whittaker, J.C. 215
Whittemore, A.S. 88, 112, 189, 192
Wild, P. 39
Wildgruber, D. 317

Wilk, M.B. 166
Williams, S.C.R. 293, 311, 313, 315, 316, 318, 320, 321, 322
Winkler, R.L. 273
Wolfinger, R.D. 230
Wolfram, S. 71
Wong, E.C. 315
Wong, G.Y. 193
Wong, W.H. 254
Woodhouse, G. 127, 133, 195, 230
Woodruff, P.W.R. 311, 318, 322
Worsley, K.J. 283, 285, 289, 293, 295, 296, 297, 300, 312, 319, 321
Wrensch, M.R. 114
Wu, A.H. 259, 271
Wu, M.C. 215

Wynder, E.L. 259, 271

Yang, M. 141, 230
Yashin, A.I. 61, 66, 68
Ying, Z. 108
Yochmowitz, M.G. 284
Yoshii, F. 281
Young, I.R. 312
Yu, M.C. 259, 271

Zahl, P.-H. 63, 66
Zajicek, G. 62
Zatorre, R.J. 283
Zeffiro, T. 310
Zeger, S.L. 9, 141, 145, 156, 166, 177, 180, 182, 183, 184, 187, 189, 192, 194, 204, 210, 315, 316
Zerbe, G.O. 163, 166
Zhao, L.P. 180, 181, 184

Subject index

Absolute risk 89
Accelerated failure time
  models 14, 29–34
Acceleration factor 31
Acceptance–rejection
  criterion 39
Activation studies 303
AIDS 107, 113
Allowable splits 103–5
Alzheimer's disease 282, 283
Analysis of covariance
  (ANCOVA) 281, 282, 290
Analysis of variance
  (ANOVA) 176
Arbuthnot, John 3–4
Asymptotic approximation
  methods 38
Asymptotic null distribution
  159
Asymptotic variance
  formulae 95
Autism, language ability in
  128–30
Auto-correlation plots 43
Autoradiography 279
Available case missing value
  restrictions 214
Average man 4–5

Bayes estimates 262
Bayes factors 46–8
Bayes information criterion
  (BIC) 47
Bayesian analysis 231
Bayesian inference 271
Bayesian meta-analysis
  251–75
Bayesian methods 10
Bayesian models 34
Bayley developmental
  quotient (DQ) 128, 132
Bessel function 71, 72

Bias 229
BOLD 310
  fMRI 278
BOLD/EPI acquisitions 289
Bonferroni inequality 295
Box–Jenkins time series
  model 293
Boxplots 150
Brain activation 309–27
Breast cancer, cohort study
  114–18
Breslow estimator 78
BUGS software 39, 195,
  244–6
Burn-in 237, 246

CART 101–6, 109–11, 114
Case neighbourhood data
  sets 94
Ceiling effects 127, 135–6
  choice of measuring
    instrument 138–9
  parent report of receptive
    language 136–8
Censored data 60–1
  mixed models for 135–6
Censored observations 127
Censored patients 13
Censoring 78
Cerebral blood oxygenation
  and brain activity 309
Childhood leukaemia 97
Classification and Regression
  Trees. See CART
Clinical prior 16
Clinical trial, epileptic
  patients 151
CODA 39
Cognitive development 127
Cohort data 77–8
Cohort sampling
  design 75

techniques 75
Cohort studies 107
  breast cancer 114–18
  HIV 118–23
Colorado Plateau 87–91
Competing risks 65–6
Complete case analysis 208
Complete case missing
  variable restrictions 214
Complexity parameter 109
Composite link function
  (CLF) 136
Computed X-ray
  tomography (CT) 11
Conditional associations
  180
Conditional Bayes estimates
  262
Conditional distribution
  263, 266, 268
Conditional expectation 176
Conditional log odds ratios
  181
Conditional mean 261
Conditional metrics 180
Conditional probabilities
  180
Conditional regression
  models 188–96
Confidence intervals 90, 261
Confounding factors 86
Contingency table 159, 160
Convergence criteria 39
Correlation analyses 283–4
Cost–complexity algorithm
  109–10
Cost–complexity pruning
  109
Counter matching 80–1
  design 87
  neighbourhood-stratified
    91–8

Counting processes
　notation 20
　theory 85
Covariance matrix 158, 161,
　168
Covariate information
　16–17
Cox, Sir David 7
Cox partial likelihood 75,
　78
Cox regression model 22–3,
　75–7, 85
Cox–Snell residuals 27
Cross-over phenomena
　63–4, 67
Cross-sectional studies
　233–5
　ROI data 280–5
Cumulative baseline hazard
　90
Cumulative distribution
　function (cdf) 157
Cumulative hazard rates,
　estimation 84–6
Cumulative radon exposure
　86
Cut-points 104

Delayed-type
　hypersensitivity (DTH)
　skin tests 119–23
Delta-betas 29
Dental fillings, duration of
　69–71
Deviance residuals 27–8
Differential ability scales
　(DAS) 128, 138–9
Directed acyclical graphs
　(DAGs) 39
Distribution-free methods
　for incomplete repeated
　measurements from two
　samples 163–5
Divine providence 3–4
Drop-out 203–8, 210–13,
　215–17, 222, 226
　models 216, 224, 225

EEG 303
Effect size, exchangeable
　254–65
Effect size estimates 259,
　271, 272
Effect size measurement
　253–4

EGRET 84
Electromagnetic fields
　(EMFs) 91–2
Emission tomography 11
Empirical Bayes estimates
　69
Empirical variogram
　ordinates 210
End-stage renal disease
　(ESRD) 14
　background 15
　Bayesian parametric
　　models 49
　Cox proportional hazards
　　regression model 22–3
　descriptive methods 17–19
　deviance residuals 27–8
　martingale residuals 27–8
　model application 39–43
　plot of log-log $S(t)$ versus
　　log(t) for overall survival
　　26
　prior information 15–16
　semi-parametric
　　proportional hazards
　　regression models 24
　study 15–55
　study design 16–17
EPICURE 84
Epidemiology 60
Epileptic patients 167–8
　clinical trial 151
　seizure counts 151
EPILOG 84
Equivalence prior 16
Euler characteristic 295, 296
Evidence-based medicine
　(EBM) 2
Experimental designs and
　data sets 286–9
Exponential relative risk
　function 84
Extensions 296–7
Extrapyramidal side effects
　148

F distribution 55
Factor analysis 284–5
False protectivity 60, 65–7
FANOVA technique 284
Fisher information matrix
　182
Fisher, Sir Ronald Aylmer
　3, 6–7
Fixed effects

analysis 259
　approach to performance
　　assessment 229
　models 235, 251–3
Floor effects 127, 135–6
　choice of measuring
　　instrument 138–9
fMRI 11, 286, 287, 292–5,
　297–9, 302, 303, 309–27
　BOLD 278
　detecting activation 319–22
　experimental design
　　313–14
　hypothesis testing 319–21
　image quality and
　　preprocessing 310–13
　incorporating spatial
　　context 321–2
　localizing activation
　　anatomically 322–4
　modelling experimental
　　effect 314–19
　modelling temporal
　　autocorrelations 318–19
　signal-to-noise ratio 312
　spatial distortion 313
　subject movement 312
　Fourier transformation 312
Frailty
　distribution 62, 70, 71
　effect on relative risk
　　63–7
　models 59–74
　phenomenon 60, 66
　theory 61
　use of term 60
Functional magnetic
　resonance imaging. *See*
　fMRI
Functional mapping 285
Functional neuroimaging
　277–307
　software 301–2

Galen 1
Gamma distribution 62, 71
GAUSS program system 70
Gauss–Hermite quadrature
　195
Gaussian kernel 319
Gaussian random fields
　295–7
Gehan statistic 107
General association statistic
　160

General sampling designs 81–3
Generalized estimating equations (GEE) 176, 183–4, 187–8
Generalized inverse Gaussian distributions 71
Generalized likelihood ratio statistic 222
Generalized linear model (GLM) 136
GENMOD procedure 187
Gibbs sampling 38, 39, 142, 232–3, 237, 244
Glomerular filtration rate (GFR) 15
Gosset, W.S. ('Student') 6
Growth curve models 127, 130–3, 176
 parent report of expressive language 133–5

Haemodialysis 15
Harvey, William 1
Hazard estimates 45
Hazard function 31
Hazard ratio 16, 67
Heterogeneity 61
Hierarchical models 229, 251, 254, 256
HIV 107, 113–14
 cohort study 118–23
Hotelling's T^2s statistic 158, 165–6
Hyperprior 240
Hypothesis test 22

Image formation 289
Image reconstruction 279
Image regression 290
Imaging 10–11
Imaging modalities 277–9
Importance density 54
Improper prior distribution 47
Incomplete repeated measurements from two samples, distribution-free methods for 163–5
Independent-increments process 38
Individual hazard rate 61
Influential observations 29
Informative prior 263–5, 265–7

Institutional performance comparison 229–49
Intensity process 20
Intrinsic Bayes factors (IBFs) 47
Iteration 246
Iterative generalized least squares (IGLS) 141

Kaplan–Meier survival curves 17–19, 70–1, 112, 113, 118
Kaplan–Meier survival estimate 107
Kelvin, Lord 2
Kernel function 164, 168
Kidney transplant data 233
Kruskal–Wallis test 156

Labour
 pain relief during 153–6
 pain scores in 168–9
Language ability in autism 128–30
Language development 127–43
Laplace transform 61–2, 69, 71
Last observation carried forward 207–8
Least absolute deviations (LAD) 105–6
Least squares (LS) 105–6
 estimates 293
Left truncation 77, 107–8
Likelihood 68–9
Likelihood analysis 71
Likelihood-based inference 212
Likelihood equations 182
Likelihood-ratio goodness-of-fit statistics 186
Log-hazard ratio 16
Log-likelihood 70
Log-normal baseline intensity 51
Log-normal distribution 31, 49
Log-rank statistic splitting 110
Log-rank test 19
Logistic regression model 183
Longitudinal data 127–43
 analysis 9–10

layout and notation 146–7
 regression models for 175–201
Longitudinal studies
 missing values in 203–28
 notation 177
 with non-normal responses 145–73
Lung cancer, uranium miners 87–91

Magnetic resonance imaging (MRI) 11
Mann–Whitney–Wilcoxon test 156, 167
MANOVA 141
Mantel–Haenszel correlation statistic 162, 167
Mantel–Haenszel mean score statistic 161, 167
Mantel–Haenszel randomization model 159
Mantel–Haenszel randomization model statistics 162
Mantel–Haenszel statistics 159, 160
MAREG 186
Marginal expectation 176, 186
Marginal metrics 180
Marginal probabilities 180
Marginal regression models 178–81
Markov chain model 189, 190, 192
Markov chain Monte Carlo (MCMC) 47, 53, 54
 advantages 230
 computation 244–6
 introduction 231–3
 method 38, 195, 229–49
 reversible jump 240–1
Markov chains 232
Martingale residuals 27–8
Martingales 85
Masking 102
Matched case-control studies 84
Matching 86–7
Mathematica 71
Maximized log likelihoods 222

Maximum likelihood estimates 22, 182, 223, 224, 252
Medical statistics, recent advances 8–11
Meta-analysis 251–75
competing classes of models for 251–3
Missing values
in longitudinal studies 203–28
modelling 210–16
Missingness, definitions 210–11
Mixed models
application 127
for censored data 135–6
Mixed parameter models 181–2
MIXOR 195
MMKD result 214, 215, 222
Model checking 25–9, 32
Model comparisons 21–2, 32, 46–8, 53
Modelling strategies 21–2
Monte Carlo integration 231–2, 257
Mullen scales 128, 138
Multi-level models 229
Multiple hypergeometric randomization model distribution 160
Multiple unit model 68
Multiplicative intensity model 20
Multi-sample problem
with complete data 151, 167–8
with incomplete data 153–6, 168
Multi-sample repeated measures design 148
Multi-state models 25
Multivariate generalizations of univariate distribution-free methods 157–9
Multivariate growth curve models 139–41
Multivariate multi-sample median test 157
Multivariate multi-sample rank sum test 157
Multivariate regression 290

Multivariate survival data 67–71

'Neighbourhood walk' methods 97
Neighbourhood-stratified counter matching 91–8
Nested case–control sampling 78–80, 84
Neuroimages, construction and analysis 277–307
Nightingale, Florence 3, 5–6
Nodes 102, 103
summaries 111–12
Non-normal repeated measures 156–66
Non-normal responses, longitudinal studies with 145–73
Non-parametric approaches 298–301
Non-parametric distribution on two mass points 240
Non-parametric methods 320
Non-temporal models 34–7
Normal mixture model 240
Normal–normal conjugate model 34, 36
Normalization problem 281–3
Null distribution 165
Null hypothesis 157, 160
Numerical integration (quadrature) methods 38

Odds ratio 186–7
Ohio children's wheeze data 177, 184, 185, 187, 191–2, 194–5
One-sample problem 166–7
One-sample repeated measures design 148
Oswald function 221

Pain relief during labour 153–6
Pain scores in labour 168–9
PANSS score 226
Parametric models 48–9
Parametric regression model 53
Partial likelihood 20, 83–4, 87

Pattern mixture models 213–14
Pearson, Karl 4
Performance assessment, fixed effects approach to 229
Peritoneal dialysis 15
Pervasive developmental disorder (PDD) 128–30
PET 11, 278, 279, 283, 284, 286, 287, 289–90, 297, 300, 301, 303
Poisson distribution 21
Pooling 86–7
Population strata 86, 87
Positive and negative symptom rating scale (PANSS) 204–5
Posterior density 257, 258, 262, 268
Posterior distribution 256–9, 261, 262, 264, 265, 267–70
Posterior mean conditional 256
Posterior standard deviation 261–2
Power calculations 95–7
Predictive distribution 55
Preprocessing 285–6
Prior distribution 263, 265, 271–3
Probability density function 31, 193
Probability distribution 80, 85
PROC LIFEREG 33
Proper prior distribution 47
Proportional frailty model 61–3
Proportional hazards 31
Proportional hazards models 75–100
Proportional hazards regression model 14
Pseudo t statistic images 300–1

Quetelet, Adolphe 3, 4–5
Quetelet's index 118

Radon excess relative risk 89
Radon exposure 88

Random effects 244
distribution 237
meta-analysis 16
models 192–4, 214–15, 229, 235–7, 251–3
Random field approaches 295–8
Random intercept models 229
Randomization tests 159–63, 318
Rank measures of association 156–7
Rank statistics 106, 110
Ranks 237
Recursive partitioning methods 101
Reference prior 16
Region of interest (ROI) 280, 284
cross-sectional studies 280–5
Regional cerebral blood flow (rCBF) 278
Regression coefficients 86, 89
estimation 83–4
Regression models 27
for longitudinal data 175–201
survival data 13–58
Relative risk 64–6, 86, 89, 96
effect of frailty 63–7
function 77
Renal replacement treatment (RRT) 14, 15
Repeated event model 68
Repeated measures ANOVA 281
Repeated measures design 146–7
Repeated measures setting 157
Residuals 25–9
Resolution elements (resels) 297
Right censoring 78
survival data 106–7
Risk set sampling designs 75–100
Robust standard errors 186

Sampling of controls 78–83
Sampling variances 272

SAS PHREG 84
SAS PROC MIXED 230
Scalar random effect 217
Scale parameter 31
Schizophrenia trial data 148–50, 203–7, 217–26
Schwarz criterion 47
Seizure counts 151
Selection models 211–13
Semi-parametric models 37–8
Semi-parametric proportional hazards model 19–29
Semi-parametric proportional hazards regression model 23–5, 29
Semi-parametric regression model 41, 45
Serum albumin 15
Several-sample median test 159
Shape parameter 31
Shapiro–Wilk test of normality 167
Shared frailty model 68
Shrinkage 229
Sidák–Jogedo inequality 295
Simpson–Angus (SA) ratings for schizophrenic patients 149–50
Simulation methods 38
Single-subject analyses 302
Six Cities Study of Air Pollution and Health 177
Small sample problems 229
Smoking 88
Smoothing 112
Software
functional neuroimaging 301–2
tree-structured survival analysis 112–13
Spearman rank correlation coefficient 156
SPECT 11, 278, 279, 282, 283
Spikeplots 128, 137
Split–complexity 110
Split functions 103, 105–8
Split points 104
Splits 102, 103–5
Splus 101, 112, 210, 221
SPM (Statistical Parametric Mapping) package 302

Standard error intervals 261
Standard errors 112
Standard normal cumulative distribution function 258
Standard normal probability density function 257
Statistical Methods in Medical Research 8
Statistics in Medicine 8
Stratified log-rank test 19
Stratified models 25
Stratified proportional hazards model 86
Stratum-specific cumulative baseline hazard rates 87
Stratum-specific cumulative hazards 95
Student's *t* distribution 240, 290
Suprathreshold cluster method 297
Survival analysis 8–9, 59
tree-structured 101–25
Survival data
regression models 13–58
right-censored 106–7
Survival rates, from previous epoch as predictor 242–4
Survival tree pruning via split complexity 110
Survival tree size via graphical methods 111

Tarone–Ware (TW) statistic 106–7
TEACCH 128
Temporal autocorrelation 318
Time-dependent covariates 24, 108
Tomographic reconstruction 279
Transitional models 188–91
Tree size determination 109
Tree-structured regression methodology 103–12
Tree-structured survival analysis 101–25
examples 113–14
software 112–13

Truncation 78
Type I error 285, 297, 319, 320, 321

Unbalanced designs 208–10
Uninformative prior 256, 267
United States
  Environmental Protection
  Agency (USEPA) 259–60, 270, 271
Univariate distribution-free
  methods 156
University of Iowa Mental
  Health Clinical Research
  Center 148
Uranium miners, lung
  cancer 87–91

Variance–covariance matrix
  164–5
Variance matrix 218

Variogram 209–10, 219, 223
Variograms 217
Very high current
  configuration (VHCC)
  92–7
Vineland measure of
  expressive language 133
Vineland parent report
  measure 136
Vineland receptive measure
  130
  with and without censoring
  137
Voxel-level approaches 285

Wei–Johnson statistic 164, 165, 169
Wei–Lachin omnibus chi-
  square statistic 168, 169
Wei–Lachin vector of test
  statistics 167, 168

Weibull accelerated failure
  time model 49
Weibull baseline intensity
  50, 51
Weibull distribution 31, 49
Weibull hazard function 31
Weighted conditional
  logistic regression
  likelihood 84
Weighted mean effect size
  256
Weighted sum of squares
  256
Weighting matrix 183, 188
Western Australian HIV
  (WAHIV) database 119
Wilcoxon signed rank test
  166

XLISP-STAT 38

YS*s process 213–14